Beyond Madness

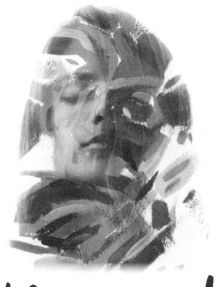

Beyond Madness

THE PAIN AND POSSIBILITIES OF SERIOUS MENTAL ILLNESS

Rachel A. Pruchno, PhD

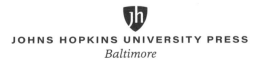

JOHNS HOPKINS UNIVERSITY PRESS
Baltimore

Note to the Reader: This book is not meant to substitute for medical care, and treatment should not be based solely on its contents. Instead, treatment must be developed in a dialogue between the individual and his or her physician. This book has been written to help with that dialogue.

Johns Hopkins University Press
2715 North Charles Street
Baltimore, Maryland 21218-4363
www.press.jhu.edu

Library of Congress Cataloging-in-Publication Data

Names: Pruchno, Rachel, author.
Title: Beyond madness : the pain and possibilities of
serious mental illness / Rachel A. Pruchno.
Description: Baltimore : Johns Hopkins University Press, 2022. |
Includes bibliographical references and index.
Identifiers: LCCN 2020045431 | ISBN 9781421441429 (hardcover) |
ISBN 9781421444598 | ISBN 9781421441443 (ebook)
Subjects: LCSH: Mental illness. | Mental illness—United States. |
Mental illness—United States—Treatment. | Patients—
Decision making. | Performance.
Classification: LCC RC454 .P688 2021 | DDC 616.8900973—dc23
LC record available at https://lccn.loc.gov/2020045431

A catalog record for this book is available from the British Library.

Special discounts are available for bulk purchases of this book.
For more information, please contact Special Sales at
specialsales@jh.edu.

*For my husband, whose love and support enabled me
to survive my journey and write this book*

CONTENTS

Beyond Madness

Prologue

JOE WAS A 17-year-old high school basketball star.

Sharon was a 51-year-old social worker.

Michelle was a 31-year-old housewife with four young children.

And Sophie, my daughter, was 16 when a doctor diagnosed a serious mental illness.

"I've met with Sophie several times since she's been in the hospital this week," the attending psychiatrist said over the phone. "There's no doubt about it. Your daughter has bipolar disorder." The doctor kept talking, but I didn't hear anything else she said. Finally, the doctor said, "Goodbye."

I placed the receiver back in its cradle. Steadying myself, I thought about how, for nearly a decade, Sophie's illness had crept into my life and overtaken it. Little by little, normal had disappeared. Still, I wondered about this new diagnosis. Psychiatrists, psychologists, and social workers had treated Sophie for years. Why hadn't anyone ever said anything about bipolar disorder? And why hadn't I, as a psychologist, recognized and understood what was happening to my daughter?

As a young child, Sophie had been smart, fearless, and headstrong. It had been almost impossible for my husband, Josh, and me to teach her right from wrong. But we weren't the only ones to have problems with our beautiful daughter. When Sophie ripped the pages out of a library book and tossed them in the air, her pre-K principal, a seasoned administrator, had given Sophie plastic gloves and bags and told her to empty all the trash cans in the school. Sophie had walked from room to room collecting the garbage with a huge smile on her face. By the end of the day, a dozen children had begged the principal for a turn to empty the rubbish.

Ever since Sophie could talk, she'd dazzled anyone who listened with her imagination. She'd convinced her kindergarten teacher that I'd been pregnant and delivered a child that year, although that had not happened. By the age of 8, Sophie would lie without flinching. She grew adept at playing her teacher and me against one another, telling me she had no homework while telling the teacher she'd done the work but had forgotten to bring it to school. Caught in a fib, Sophie would say she didn't care about the time-outs, extra homework, or other consequences the teachers and I imposed in hopes of disciplining her. I had wondered whether this indifference was evidence of a spirited personality or proof of a disturbed one. I'd tried to convince myself it was the former, but my suspicions that it was the latter grew. Should I have recognized these as the first signs of bipolar disorder?

By the time she was 9, Sophie had become more rebellious, refusing even the simplest requests. She ignored basic house rules. She began arguing when she woke up and didn't stop until she was asleep. Josh and I chose our battles and negotiated. We ignored her. We gave her extra attention. We put her in time-out. We offered rewards for good behavior. We pointed out the natural consequences of bad behavior. We reprimanded her using every strategy the parenting books we read suggested. Nothing worked.

I wondered now whether Sophie's bipolar disorder should have been evident to me by the clutter in her bedroom. I'd often find heaps of random things—her toothbrush, crayons, and jewelry—tangled and scattered on the floor. Her school papers were equally disorganized. I'd tried every way I could think of to help Sophie organize her work. Together, Sophie and I had put her papers in a large accordion file. We'd punched holes in the papers and put them in a binder. We'd put the papers in color-coded folders matching her notebooks. But no matter what we tried, Sophie's schoolwork ended up scrunched at the bottom of her backpack or buried on the floor of her locker. Her elementary school teachers had said she would outgrow the disorganization. They were wrong.

Although her fifth-grade teacher insisted that Sophie was by far the smartest kid in class, Sophie completed less than half the homework that year and nearly failed. When Sophie complained that she couldn't pay attention in class, I took her to the pediatrician, who diagnosed attention deficit hyperactivity disorder (ADHD) and started her on medication. Almost immediately, Sophie said it helped. Indeed, it seemed to. She completed her homework. Her grades improved, and she took responsibility for organizing her schoolwork. Even her classmates noticed how much calmer Sophie had become. I was convinced we'd identified the problem and solved it.

But we hadn't. In middle school, Sophie made up stories for me about play practice or visits with girlfriends so she could sneak around with boys. She'd gnaw on her fingernails until they bled. She'd twirl her hair around her finger or pull it out strand by strand until there'd be a bald spot the size of a quarter on the back of her head. She'd bounce her knees up and down at the dinner table and fiddle nonstop with her necklaces.

I knew Sophie's behavior wasn't normal. I'd taken her to the pediatrician and had gotten her medication. But the strange behavior continued. The pediatrician suggested I take Sophie to a psychiatrist. When I did, a second medicine was added. Then, when I told the psychiatrist that Sophie was cutting herself with razor blades and burning her arm with a cigarette lighter, she added a third. It didn't help either.

The summer before her sophomore year of high school, we hired a well-respected educational consultant to evaluate Sophie. After three days of testing and a bill of $5,000, the consultant concluded that Sophie lied to compensate for her poor organizational skills. "Being disorganized is a big part of ADHD," she'd said. "The school has to accommodate her disability." The consultant charged us another $2,000 to develop a 504 Plan—a plan ensuring that the school must make accommodations and protect the civil rights of a person with a disability. Section 504 of the Federal Rehabilitation Act of 1973 mandated that schools cannot discriminate against students diagnosed with a disability. Given Sophie's disability, the consultant recommended that she be provided with a second set of textbooks to be kept at home, extra time to complete tests, well-organized teachers who gave highly structured assignments, and weekly communication between her teachers and me. Even with these supports, Sophie didn't do her work.

Many of Sophie's behaviors—the lying, homework avoidance, and laziness—were characteristic of normal kids, although I don't remember lying to my parents when I was a kid and I always did my homework. Her self-cutting and conversations with strangers on the internet may not have been normal, but they certainly were not uncommon. But when my 15-and-a-half-year-old daughter tied bedsheets together and shimmied out of her second-floor bedroom window in the middle of the night to have sex in a motel room with a man she'd met on the internet, I was sure this was not normal. Still, none of the professionals with whom Sophie met on a regular basis had diagnosed bipolar disorder or any other serious mental illness. Why not?

One afternoon, after one of Sophie's regular appointments, her psychiatrist pulled me aside and said, "I think Sophie's very troubled." She gave me a prescription for a fourth medicine and said, "Make sure Sophie takes her medicine every day" and "She needs a therapist she can talk to." Had the psychiatrist suspected Sophie had bipolar disorder?

Over the next year, Sophie met weekly with her therapist. She swallowed her medications every morning. She attended a summer program for kids with ADHD recommended by her guidance counselor. She also had a knockdown, hair-pulling fight with a girl in the school cafeteria. Her clothes often reeked of marijuana. She got pregnant and had an abortion. The psychiatrist tried new medications. The therapist tried to help Sophie understand that her behaviors were not moving her toward her goal of gaining independence. Still, no one had ever mentioned bipolar disorder.

On April 15, 2009, Josh and I filed our income taxes. That evening we discovered Sophie making plans to run away with a pervert she'd met on the internet.

"Sophie, he's a crazy person. You're putting yourself in danger," I'd wailed after reading exchanges between them on the computer surveillance software we'd installed at her therapist's suggestion.

Sophie's eyes glazed. "But Mom, I love him. I have to be with him."

"Sophie, you said he's violent and has killed people," Josh said. "Do you understand he's likely to kill you?"

"Yes," she sighed.

"Do you want to die?" Josh asked.

"No, of course not," Sophie said.

"So, you don't want to die, but you want to go to him knowing it's likely he'll kill you," Josh said, scratching his head.

"Yes. Dad, I have to be with him, I've never loved anyone like I love him. He loves me too." Sophie sobbed and bolted out of the room.

Terrified, I followed her into her bedroom. She sat on her bed staring into space. In a calm voice, she said, "Mom, I feel like I'm going to hurt myself."

We rushed her to the crisis center's emergency room. After Sophie had spent a week in the hospital, the doctor called me and said, "Your daughter has bipolar disorder."

Reading the American Psychiatric Association's *DSM-IV*—the manual used at that time by clinicians to diagnose mental illness—I saw how well the bipolar diagnosis fit Sophie's behaviors. She'd had trouble concentrating in school. She'd vividly described racing thoughts. Sometimes she'd be giddy, blabbering nonstop. Other times she'd cry without reason. After nights when she complained she couldn't sleep, I'd find her bedroom filled with the remnants of an unfinished art project or homemade beauty treatment, the room a mess of glittery beads or cucumber glop.

The hospital doctor changed Sophie's medications again. I worried whether the medicines would work. Would Sophie be able to concentrate in school? I also worried whether the medication would dull the artistic flair that enabled Sophie to write exquisite poetry and sketch drawings that her art teacher said should be hanging in a museum. I worried whether Sophie would be able to go to college, get married, and have a normal life.

Yet part of me felt relief getting this diagnosis. Sophie's bizarre behaviors were signs of an illness. She didn't hate me. I wasn't a bad mother. We can fix this, I thought.

But I understood the seriousness of bipolar disorder all too well.

I was 12 years old when my mother was diagnosed with manic depression, the illness now labeled bipolar disorder.

Before Josh and I adopted Sophie, we'd had many discussions about the babies we would and would not consider adopting. We didn't feel we could adequately parent a baby with cerebral palsy, Down syndrome, spina bifida, cystic fibrosis, or fetal alcohol syndrome. Recognizing that the genetics underlying mental illnesses are complex and the accuracy of diagnosed and reported conditions questionable, we hadn't ruled out a baby whose parents or grandparents had suffered from mental illness. Turning my back on a baby that, given my mother's genes, I could have birthed myself had felt wrong to me anyway. Even more, a part of me had convinced myself that, if my child did have a mental illness, I would be able to fight—and conquer—the demons that had stolen my mother from me. As a child, there was little I could do to help my mother, but now, as an adult, let alone a psychologist, I was sure I could fix the problem.

Or could I?

I was about to find out.

CHAPTER 1

Preliminary Points

I LEARNED A lot about mental health in graduate school, but very little about mental illness. Over more than fifty years, my family taught me about that.

My first glimpse of mental illness came in 1966 when I was 12. That October, my 43-year-old mother—the beautiful woman with a master's degree in economics who had put her career on hold to raise my two younger brothers and me—started crumbling. It began with hand-wringing and insecurity over what to cook for dinner. She paced. She cried. She lost so much weight that her clothes drooped on her slender frame. Her once-pink cheeks turned ashen. Some days, she'd lay in bed curled in a fetal position. Other days, her endless cries of "I'm a terrible mother" echoed through the house. My mother's illness frightened me, making me cry myself to sleep almost every night. My father, brothers, and I told her she was wrong, but my mom didn't seem to understand what we were saying. During the summer that followed, mom became a whirlwind. She'd wake at four o'clock in the morning and have the house clean and dinner made by the time I had woken. She'd read books about foreign economies as she sat on our backyard patio. She insisted that my brothers and I not bother her. She must have gained ten pounds that summer.

In the Human Development and Family Studies graduate program I attended at Penn State from 1978 to 1982, I learned that mental health is a state of happiness, satisfaction, and interest in life. I was taught how to measure mental health with scientific rigor and to assess how individual characteristics (such as age, sex, and race), experiences (such as unemployment, death of a loved one, and divorce), and support from family, friends, and community influence a person's mental health. I was trained to develop and evaluate interventions designed to promote mental health, and I learned that incidents early in life can have lasting effects.

My family and my education taught me that, other than sharing an adjective, mental illness and mental health have little in common. Yet throughout my professional career as a research psychologist, I have seen the terms "mental illness" and "mental health" used interchangeably. Sometimes mental health has been described as the absence of mental illness. Even the names of some of our federal agencies create bewilderment about the distinction between mental illness and mental health. We have the Substance Abuse and Mental Health Services Administration (SAMHSA), but no Substance Abuse and Mental Illness Services Administration. We have a National Institute of Mental Health (NIMH), but not a National Institute of Mental Illness. Further confounding things are the missions of these agencies. NIMH's charge is "to transform understanding and treatment of mental illness," while SAMHSA's objective is "to reduce the impact of substance abuse and mental illness on America's communities."

This is not merely an issue of jargon. Nor is it due to society's desire to focus on the positive. It is, instead, a reflection of the unresolved tension between the goals of promoting mental health on one hand and caring for people with mental illnesses on the other. To be sure, health and illness, whether physical or mental, are often used to label end points along a continuum. But it is more appropriate to think about mental health and mental illness as being two separate entities. It is normal for mental health to vary from excellent to poor over the course of a person's life. Mental illness, on the other hand, is a sickness that typically is enduring. Some mental illnesses are relatively mild in severity, while others have the ability to destroy or completely debilitate people.

Philosophers, scholars, and physicians have struggled to define and diagnose mental illnesses. Lacking concrete evidence for mental illnesses, some have attributed the odd behaviors exhibited by people with these illnesses to invisible energy coursing through magnetic channels in our bodies. Others have blamed demonic possession, disrupted blood circulation, or sensory overload. Still others have claimed that mental illnesses are not real, while some have even blamed parents for their children's strange behaviors. When Sigmund Freud suggested that almost everyone struggles with a neurotic conflict, the line between mental illness and mental health nearly vanished. Psychoanalytic theory and its treatment, psychoanalysis, introduced a new type of patient, one who could function effectively in society but who wanted to function even better—"the worried well."

The current edition of the American Psychiatric Association's *Diagnostic and Statistical Manual of Mental Disorders* (DSM-5) chronicles more than three hundred maladies. While useful for determining what insurance companies will pay for and which children are eligible for special services in school, the manual has cast many normal human responses and feelings as mental illnesses, expanding the definition of mental illnesses so that an astonishing one in four US adults and one in five children can be labeled with a diagnosable mental illness every year.

These proportions are even greater from a lifetime perspective. When something becomes ordinary, as it does when it characterizes so many people, we begin to wonder whether it really is a problem. After all, if 47.6 million Americans live with mental illness, how bad can it be?

While all mental illnesses have the potential to impair a person's ability to function, the reality is that most mental illnesses do not stop people from going to school, working, or raising families. People with obsessive-compulsive disorders, anxiety disorders, trauma- and stress-related disorders, eating disorders, and personality disorders such as borderline personality disorder often experience high levels of distress and impairment. Yet most people with these conditions are able to lead purposeful lives. They take medications, go to therapy, and develop coping strategies.

In contrast, the disorders discussed in this book are "serious mental illnesses." Unless these illnesses are treated continuously and vigilantly, they have the potential to impair a person's emotions, thinking, social relationships, and ability to take care of basic needs. During the 1980s, these illnesses were called "chronic mental illnesses"; in the early 1990s, they were referred to as "severe and persistent mental illnesses"; and by 1995, with the advent of managed care, the label became "serious mental illnesses."

An explosion of research since 2000 using functional magnetic resonance imaging (a measure of brain activity) has confirmed that schizophrenia, bipolar disorder, and depressive disorders are brain disorders with biological roots. Moreover, there is good evidence that brain abnormalities often are visible even before behaviors lead to diagnosis. I focus primarily on these disorders because they have the greatest likelihood of keeping people from being able to function successfully and the greatest potential to destroy families and harm communities.

As if coping with delusions, hallucinations, wild mood swings, and crushing depression were not enough, people with serious mental illnesses face a challenge not experienced by people with other chronic illnesses such as diabetes, cancer, and heart disease: stigma. People with serious mental illness do not bear the physical markings originally associated with the term "stigma," and most do not look different from people without serious mental illness, but public attitudes about mental illnesses have left many individuals disgraced or discredited by illnesses that are feared and seen as shameful. Even as science has revealed that serious mental illnesses are biological illnesses, public attitudes about people who suffer these illnesses have become increasingly negative. A series of studies found that in 2010 people were more likely to report an unwillingness to have someone with schizophrenia as a friend, in-law, neighbor, or coworker than they were in 1950. Today, more than half of all Americans believe that people with serious mental illness are dangerous. Beliefs that these illnesses are contagious and can be transmitted through close contact prevail, despite scientific evidence to the contrary and despite decades of efforts to educate the public otherwise.

Not surprisingly, many people hide their serious mental illnesses and their odd behaviors. Nine years after my mother's death, in the first professional paper I published, my colleagues and I suggested that, because the lives of family members are linked, change in one person's life causes change in the lives of other family members. We discussed how a woman giving birth transformed her mother into a grandmother and how marriage in one generation creates in-laws in another. I didn't dare tell my coauthors how my mother's mental illness had changed me. I didn't tell them that my mother's illness made me worry that someday I too might suffer from crippling depression and unrestrained mania. Why? Because stigma about mental illnesses reaches far beyond its victims. I didn't want my colleagues to think poorly of me or my mother. And so, for more than forty years, I didn't tell anyone other than my husband about my mother's illness.

* * *

This book is about the modern experience of serious mental illness. It shows what life is like for many of the 11.2 million adults and 1.9 million children living with serious mental illness and for their families, the 20 million people who have a front-row seat to the ravages of serious mental illness.

Preparing to write this book, I realized that for readers to understand serious mental illnesses, they must see what these illnesses do to real people—not to wealthy rock stars, but to everyday people to whom they would more easily relate. I knew I would tell my own stories—as the daughter of a mother and mother of a daughter with serious mental illness—but I soon realized that I needed to enlist the help of people diagnosed with schizophrenia, depression, and bipolar disorder in order to show the many facets of serious mental illnesses. I looked carefully, hoping to find the right mix of people to help me tell this important story—people with serious mental illnesses who were not afraid to talk about their illness, who would spend hours telling me their stories, and who were willing to bear with my poking and prodding them as I ensured that I understood and accurately could tell their stories.

In chapter 2, you'll meet the heroes of this book—Joe, Sharon, and Michelle—and see the first hints of their mental illnesses unfold, just as they were experienced. You'll learn how genetics and environment combine to create these illnesses, which can surface at any time during a person's life. You'll understand the importance of increasing awareness and knowledge about illnesses such as schizophrenia, depression, and bipolar disorder and why efforts to decrease stigma are important. You'll see the powerful effect of a model program designed to educate high school students about mental illness.

Chapter 3 reveals one of the paradoxes of serious mental illness. Early treatment is critical. However, long waits in emergency rooms, shortages of psychiatric hospital beds and doctors, and brief hospital stays keep very ill people from getting the care they need. You'll read about Virginia senator Creigh Deeds and see what happened when a psychiatric bed could not be found in all of Virginia for his son. You'll learn about the role asylums once played and how what started out as a good idea turned sour. You'll see firsthand what happens when crisis care is not provided, and, through Joe's experiences, you'll learn how President John F. Kennedy's efforts to free people with mental illness from institutions made it more difficult, not easier, to get care. Through Michelle's story, you'll see what crisis care looked like by the late 1980s. As Sharon's story unfolds, you'll see how serious mental illnesses can become criminalized, and as my daughter's story continues, you'll witness the struggles my family had getting crisis care for her. Turning to the science and some model programs, I show that there really are better ways to help people in crisis.

As chapter 4 unfolds, you will learn what happens after people are diagnosed with schizophrenia, bipolar disorder, or depression. You will see the challenges people with serious mental illness and their families face as they begin to live with a very serious illness. As I share the experiences I had once my daughter was diagnosed with bipolar disorder, you will understand the initial challenges faced by people with serious mental illnesses and their families: finding health care providers, identifying treatment regimens that can quell the symptoms of mental illness, and deciding what to tell other people about the situation. For each challenge, I offer strategies that I hope you will find helpful.

In the United States, approximately half of all people with serious mental illness do not get treatment. Chapter 5 will explain that some of these people want treatment while others do not. Among people who want but do not get treatment, some cannot afford treatment, others cannot find treatment, and still others forgo treatment because they do not want anyone to find out they are sick. There also are many reasons why people do not want treatment. Some people do not believe they are sick. Others believe that the medications dull their creativity, while others find the physical side effects of the medications unacceptable. Still others believe that alcohol and street drugs are better ways to quell their symptoms. Strategies for helping people cope with obstacles to care are described, although the main premise of the chapter is that, to be effective, approaches must be responsive to the concerns of the person with mental illness. Ubiquitous, one-size-fits-all tactics will fail.

Tragedies surrounding serious mental illness are the focus of chapter 6. Most tragedies result from the myth that before a person with a serious mental illness can be helped, they must hit "rock bottom." This myth stems from laws established to protect the rights of people to make decisions about health care on their own, without interference from government or other people. Yet many people with a serious mental illness do not understand that they are sick and do not have the ability to make health care decisions on their own. Requiring people to hit rock bottom has resulted in countless drug abuses, suicides, homicides, incarcerations, and cases of homelessness. I suggest that an alternative model—shared or supported decision-making—is a much better alternative. This model, frequently used when older people become demented and are unable to make decisions on their own, enables people with brain illnesses to participate in decision-making along with family members or friends whom they trust.

Living with serious mental illness is hard work. Chapter 7 shows how Joe and Michelle have succeeded and now help others by volunteering in peer programs. We see how Sharon's experience with mental illness made her a better social worker. The importance of community support for people with serious mental illness is highlighted, and model programs are described. In this chapter, we see that having a serious mental illness is filled with challenges, but it is not a death sentence.

There are many reasons why we should pay more attention to serious mental illness than we do. Certainly, an illness affecting 13.1 million Americans is a powerful reason. Another good reason to pay attention to serious mental illness is that it is expensive. In 2012, the annual economic costs associated with serious mental illness in the United States were $467 billion, making serious mental illness the third-costliest medical condition, trailing only heart conditions and traumatic injury. But paying attention to serious mental illness is also important because it has the potential to devastate people. Paying attention is the right thing to do.

The term "madness" used in the book's title refers both to being "out of one's mind" and to being "foolish or extremely stupid." I use the word "madness" because it captures the ability of serious mental illness to rob its victims of the ability to think and feel, making them seem "out of their minds." More importantly, I use the term because it reflects society's irrational response to people with serious mental illness. Community resources are inadequate, many psychiatrists and psychologists choose to treat the "worried well" while avoiding treating people with serious mental illnesses, and psychiatric hospital beds are scarce. As such, many very sick people having nowhere else to go end up living on the streets, locked up in jails, or dead.

There is much we don't know about the causes and treatments of serious mental illness, but scientific advances in medicine, psychology, criminal justice, and social work have identified ways to make life better for these people. Tragically, these advances have not trickled into the lives of everyday people. As a result, millions of very sick people and their families continue to suffer needlessly. For this book, I've used my skills as a research psychologist to read hundreds of scientific articles and summarize what is known about serious mental illness. I've gone back to original sources documented in the notes section at the back of the book. I've talked with experts and visited places that are doing a good job taking care of people with serious mental illness. Then, driven by the passion of a mother forced to watch the daughter she loves be defeated by bipolar disorder, I've identified what families and communities can do right now to make life better for people with serious mental illness.

And so, with this book my hope is that, by taking a step back and assessing our situation, we will learn that there are better approaches right in front of our eyes just waiting to be embraced.

CHAPTER 2

Breaking Brains

JOE KNEW THAT Satan had invaded his grandmother's body. Now Satan was waiting for an opportunity to kill Joe.

But 17-year-old Joe also believed he was God. If Joe struck first, he could kill Satan, enabling his spirit followers to capture and imprison Satan's soul. Without their leader, the forces of evil would collapse and good would triumph.

Joe hid behind the American history textbook he pretended to study. He stared at Satan. Grandma swayed back and forth in her rocking chair and turned the pages of her *Reader's Digest*. Her glasses slid down her nose. A shawl covered her shoulders, warming her from the Catskills' cold February night.

Joe wondered when Satan would strike. While most of the country still reeled from the assassination of President Kennedy just three months ago and the nuclear standoff in Cuba between the Soviet Union and the United States about a year earlier, Joe had more important things on his mind. His blue eyes, offering a sparkling contrast to the dark hair that he wore parted on the side and slicked back, gave no hint of his inner turmoil.

Joe stretched his long legs, draping them over the edge of the living room couch. His six-foot height and muscular 165 pounds made him a formidable forward, one of the quickest athletes on the Roscoe Central High School basketball team. Just recently, Joe had made several key plays, sending the game into overtime three times, and then led his team to victory over its archrivals, the boys from Livingston Manor. Stripey, Joe's black-and-white dog, let out a sigh as she nestled into her bed. The creaking of Grandma's rocker filled the room.

Although Grandpa had died of a heart attack the previous year, Joe still felt his presence. Grandpa's rocking chair sat undisturbed in the corner. The handsome walnut desk Grandpa had built held the three-foot model of the USS *Wilkes* (DD-67) he had crafted to commemorate his service on the ship during World War I. On the desk were portraits of Grandpa's four children—Mary Georgianna, Antoinette, John Mauritius, and Frederick William. Frederick William was Joe's Uncle Fred. The youngest of Grandpa's children, Uncle Fred was just seventeen and a half years older than Joe. Joe loved the picture of his mother Mary Georgianna—everyone called her "Georgie"—it was the best photo of her he'd ever seen.

Since Grandpa's death, Grandma had slept in the guest room. She'd said there were too many sad memories in the bedroom she had shared with her beloved husband of forty-two years.

Joe had loved listening to Grandpa tell stories. One of Joe's favorite stories was of Grandpa driving in the country on a hot day with Grandma's cousin Merrill. Their car had overheated, so Grandpa made several trips down a steep bank to a brook to get water for the radiator. Each time Grandpa poured water into the radiator, Merrill howled, "Praise the Lord. He did it." At the end of the story Grandpa would shake his head and wryly say, "Maybe I should get some praise too?" Although Joe knew all the stories by heart, he missed hearing Grandpa tell them.

Joe had lived with his maternal grandparents since 1949, when he was 2 years old. Grandpa had been the disciplinarian, Grandma the softy. They had been a good team. Both loved Joe dearly, though they rarely hugged or kissed him. That just wasn't their way.

When Joe was very young, Grandma would read to him each night after dinner. He'd cuddle in her lap while she rocked them both in her rocking chair. Sometimes he'd be lulled to sleep. When Joe was older, Grandma had read *A Tale of Two Cities* to him. It was one of her favorite books and became one of his favorites too as they read and discussed it, chapter by chapter. Grandma had taught Joe the names of all the constellations in the sky and let him stay up late, even on school nights, when the northern lights were visible. Hoping Joe would become a good Christian, Grandma made sure Joe attended Sunday School every week at the local Presbyterian Church.

As a teenager, Joe cheerfully helped his grandmother maintain the house. In the winters, he disposed of the ashes from the woodstove and coal furnace. He shoveled the snow, no small job given the annual snowfalls of close to one hundred inches that were common in Roscoe. In the summer, he mowed the lawn, usually without being reminded.

Joe snuck another peak at Satan. The smell of the pork chops Grandma had fried for their 5:30 dinner lingered. Grandma was a great cook, and pork chops were Joe's favorite. As Joe, Grandma, and Uncle Fred bowed their heads that evening before eating, they uttered their usual prayer: "God, we thank you for this food, for rest and play and all things good, for wind and rain and sun above, but best of all for those we love. Amen." After the blessing, Uncle Fred asked, "Who won the game this afternoon?" Joe grunted, "We did," offering no details. Uncle Fred and Grandma chatted as they ate, but Joe heard little of their conversation. He was busy attending to the battle of good and evil raging inside his head.

Even then, Joe was unaware that Satan would enter Grandma's body later that night.

Had there been warning signs of things to come? As a young boy, Joe had played happily with the neighborhood children in the woods behind his grandparents' home and in Willowemoc Creek across the road. When other kids weren't around, Joe enjoyed fishing, skipping rocks, and playing games he'd make up. In third grade, when Joe's teacher caught him daydreaming, she'd gently remind him to pay attention to the lesson. In seventh grade, Joe's grades began to slip. He was easily distracted and withdrawn. His grandparents worried. They'd seen this behavior before. Their daughter Georgie, Joe's mother, had first been hospitalized in Middletown State Mental Hospital when she was in high school and then again when Joe was 10. The first time she was diagnosed with schizophrenia, the second time with manic depression.

Eager to help Joe, Grandma and Grandpa got a referral from the school to a psychologist, Dr. William Lyle. State funds had paid for the first several therapy sessions. After that, Grandma had given Dr. Lyle $1 for each session. It was all the family could afford, but Dr. Lyle was a generous man and he liked Joe.

As a young teenager, Joe had grumbled each week as Uncle Fred had driven him the fifteen miles to Dr. Lyle's office in Liberty. Taught from an early age to keep his feelings to himself, 13-year-old Joe was embarrassed by Dr. Lyle's questions about what he was thinking and how he was feeling. Recently, Joe imagined that the black, middle-aged Dr. Lyle was Martin Luther King Jr. Even though Joe believed that his illusions were real, Joe never told anyone about this fantasy or any of the others.

From the time Joe was little, he'd had imaginary conversations with God. His grandmother's Christian tradition, reinforced by his Sunday School education, taught Joe the importance of praying and silently communicating with God. Each evening, as Joe lay awake in bed thinking about his day, he tried to envision what it would be like to be God. Joe imagined God answering him, explaining in detail what His life was like.

In the past few weeks, Joe had become convinced that God was talking to him. God's voice was a low baritone, much like Grandpa's voice had been, and listening to God made Joe feel warm inside. God told Joe that many worlds had slowly developed intelligent life and complex civilizations, but they had failed because people had quarreled and fought. Time after time, God had developed vast cosmoses that people had destroyed.

During the past few days, Joe had come to believe he was God. He had made himself human out of loneliness. Joe had supernatural powers. He traveled in cutting-edge spaceships. Of course, there was no time to sleep, and it was impossible to focus on homework or mundane conversations with his teachers or coach.

Lying on the couch, Joe had figured out that Satan had disguised himself as Grandma and was planning to kill him because he is God.

As the dining room clock struck eleven o'clock, Grandma rose from her chair, laid her *Reader's Digest* on the rocker, and said goodnight to Joe.

Joe watched Satan, disguised as Grandma, walk up the stairs. He waited a few minutes, went outside to tie Stripey to her doghouse for the night, and walked into the kitchen. Joe knew this was the time to act. Within an hour, Uncle Fred would be back from his nightly trip to the Rockland House Bar.

Rifles hung in the gun rack in the dining room. Joe knew where the ammunition was, but he didn't dare touch the rifles. Only Uncle Fred was allowed to use those. Joe opened the door to the closet where Uncle Fred kept his shotguns. He stared at the double-barreled 12-gauge and the single-shot 16-gauge. Carefully Joe picked up the single-shot 16-gauge. Like most country boys, Joe had been well trained in gun safety. He'd completed rifle club, hunter safety, and firearm safety classes by the time he was 15 and often used the gun to hunt rabbits, grouse, and deer. Joe always got his prey. Joe took three 16-gauge shells from Uncle Fred's hunting vest. He put one shell in the gun and the other two in his pocket.

Joe crept upstairs. He shivered as the chilly air hit him—with the exception of the bathroom, the upstairs of the house was unheated. The door to Grandma's bedroom was open. She was kneeling in prayer beside her bed. Her hands were clasped, her head was bowed, and her eyes were closed—just the way she'd taught Joe to pray. She wore the pink nightgown Joe had given her last Christmas, her freshly brushed silver hair falling to her waist.

Satan praying? Clearly Satan had heard God's approach and was trying to deceive Joe. Joe slipped past the bedroom. He stood by his bedroom door, trying desperately to gather his thoughts. He held the shotgun in his right hand, his left hand near the trigger. Joe's heart pounded. How should he respond to Satan's treachery?

Suddenly Joe reversed course, barging into Grandma's bedroom. She had just climbed into bed. She looked up and stared at Joe. Joe pointed the gun at Satan's chest and pulled back the hammer with his thumb, cocking the shotgun. Grandma reached her hands toward Joe and pleaded, "Joe. Don't. You've never been mean to me."

Schizophrenia

Illnesses on the schizophrenia spectrum include schizophrenia, other psychotic disorders, and schizotypal disorder. They are defined by abnormalities in one or more of the following: delusions, hallucinations, disorganized thinking, abnormal motor behavior, and negative symptoms, so named because they are an absence as much as a presence (inexpressive faces, blank looks, monotone and monotonic speech, lack of interest in the world, inability to feel pleasure).

Schizophrenia is not as common as other mental illnesses, affecting 7 or 8 individuals out of 1,000 during their lifetime. It is, however, one of the most disabling mental illnesses. Schizophrenic delusions—beliefs that are fervently embraced despite solid evidence to the contrary, such as Joe's belief that he was God—usually start between the ages of 16 and 30, with men typically experiencing symptoms a little earlier than women. The delusions Joe experienced are known as "positive" symptoms of schizophrenia, so named because they are thoughts or behaviors that the person did not have before they became ill. Other positive symptoms include hallucinations, thought disorders, and movement disorders.

Hallucinations are altered sensory experiences faced by nearly two-thirds of people with schizophrenia. Interestingly, Joe never experienced hallucinations. Hallucinations can occur in any of the five senses (vision, hearing, smell, taste, or touch), with auditory hallucinations being most common. Auditory hallucinations can be either internal, seeming to come from within one's own mind, or external, in which case they can seem to be as real as another person speaking. The voices are usually male, unpleasant, and abusive, ordering people to do harm. Sometimes, however, the voices are friendly, warning people of danger. For some people, the voices talk to each other inside the person's head. Other times, people with schizophrenia talk to the voices they hear, making it appear to outsiders as if they are talking to themselves. Hallucinations can involve seeing people or objects that are not there, smelling odors that no one else detects, and feeling things like invisible fingers touching their bodies when no one is near. Not surprisingly, the sensory overload from hallucinations makes it difficult for people to concentrate or socialize.

The narrator in Edgar Allan Poe's "The Tell-Tale Heart" experienced auditory hallucinations. He says, "The disease has sharpened my senses—not destroyed—not dulled them. Above all was the sense of hearing acute. I heard all things in the heaven and in the earth. I heard many things in hell." What the narrator was hearing ("There came to my ears a low, dull, quick sound, such as a watch makes when enveloped in cotton. I knew that sound well too. It was the beating of the old man's heart.") was not heard by people around him. As the narrator felt the noise growing louder and louder, the visiting policemen chatted pleasantly and smiled, hearing nothing.

Thought disorders are unusual or dysfunctional ways of thinking. Sometimes people with schizophrenia have trouble organizing thoughts or connecting them logically. They may talk in "word salads," making it difficult for others to understand them. Some people with schizophrenia experience "thought blocking"—they stop speaking abruptly in the middle of a thought. When asked why they stopped talking, they explain that the thought was taken out of their head. Sometimes people with schizophrenia make up meaningless words, what psychiatrists call "neologisms." People with movement disorders may be agitated, repeating the same motion over and over. People with schizophrenia can also seem flat or trancelike, a condition known as "catatonia."

Most delusions, hallucinations, and movement disorders experienced by people with schizophrenia are a direct outgrowth of the brain's inability to interpret and respond appropriately to stimuli. Although the responses of people with schizophrenia to their delusions and hallucinations often look illogical to the common observer, they are logical outcomes given what their brains are experiencing. When functional magnetic resonance imaging scans of people with schizophrenia who experience persistent auditory hallucinations were compared with scans from people without schizophrenia, scientists found that auditory hallucinations are associated with activation of an area of the brain at the junction of the superior temporal gyrus and the inferior parietal lobule, especially on the right side. This area, often referred to as the temporoparietal junction, contains one of the brain's two auditory areas. Its association with auditory hallucinations is consistent with other evidence involved in causing the symptoms of schizophrenia, again confirming that schizophrenia is a brain disease.

Negative symptoms of schizophrenia are disruptions to normal emotions and behaviors. They include flat affect, reduced pleasure in everyday life, difficulty sustaining everyday activities, and not speaking. Cognitive symptoms include the inability to understand information or make decisions, trouble focusing or paying attention, and problems using new information.

As you can see, schizophrenia may present itself in many ways. Joe's experiences were hardly unusual.

Another Way for Brains to Break

Schizophrenia is just one way for brains to malfunction. Sharon's illness had a very different beginning. Let's take a look.

"Mrs. Lopez is such a stupid asshole." Tears filled Holly's brown eyes. She slammed her backpack on the floor. Although Holly had promised her mother, Sharon, that she wouldn't wear the Justin Timberlake "Put Your Filthy Hands All over Me" T-shirt to school, she'd done it anyway.

Sharon looked out the open living room window and breathed deeply. Even the sweet smell of the purple hyacinths in her garden could not soothe her unease on the warm mid-May afternoon in 2007. Sharon grabbed her hair, twisted it, and held it on top of her head. She hated confrontations with Holly.

"You've been butting heads with that Spanish teacher since September. I thought we'd solved this problem. Why don't you get it? You can't keep talking back to her."

Although Holly had seen little of her father since Sharon had left him when Holly was 3 years old, Holly had inherited his stubborn, intimidating nature and tendency to rage. Sharon knew that the only way to get Holly to cooperate with Mrs. Lopez was for Sharon to back off. And so, in November, Sharon had said, "If you want to keep acting like the class clown and pissing Mrs. Lopez off, you're on your own. When you want my help and you're ready to behave, let me know."

For weeks the struggle between Holly and Mrs. Lopez had continued. Then, one afternoon in December, Holly pulled out her cell phone and called Sharon from a stall in one of the school bathrooms. She was crying.

"Mom, please help me. I want this stuff with Mrs. Lopez to stop. I'll do anything you say."

Sharon arranged meetings with the guidance counselor and the assistant principal. She hired a Spanish tutor. Holly stopped fooling around in class, and Mrs. Lopez stopped criticizing her.

For five months, life was manageable. But now Holly's belligerence had returned with a vengeance.

"Mom, why don't *you* get it? Mrs. Lopez won't stop picking on me. She hates me. She's always wagging her finger at me. Do something to make her stop!"

"She'd stop if you'd behave yourself. How many times do I have to tell you to stop cracking jokes and rolling your eyes? Show her some respect. Apologize for whatever you did and move on. The school year is almost over."

"I'm never going to apologize to that bitch," Holly growled. Digging through her backpack, Holly retrieved a sheet of paper. "By the way, Mom, here's my stupid progress report. You have to sign it." Holly threw the paper at Sharon's feet and stomped upstairs.

Sharon bent down, picked up the progress report, and braced herself. She knew that Holly was barely passing Spanish. Sharon's heart sank as she learned that Holly also was failing math.

Sharon hired a math tutor. She stopped asking Holly about the Spanish teacher, but she did not stop worrying about her daughter.

Days after Holly returned her signed progress report to school, Sharon began experiencing unfamiliar physical symptoms. Exhausted, she'd fall asleep by 10:30 at night and waken, filled with worry, at 3:30 in the morning. Equally surprising was that Sharon had lost her usually voracious appetite. Her clothes had become too big for her five-foot-six frame. She'd lost twenty-five pounds in just weeks. At 140 pounds, Sharon weighed less than she had in fifth grade. Merely swallowing had become difficult.

Sharon wondered what was happening to her. She'd been through much worse over the course of her fifty-one years than these struggles with Holly. Yet never had she had trouble sleeping and, despite years of dieting, never had she lost so much weight in so little time.

When Sharon was 12, two neighborhood boys had lured her into the apple orchard behind the school. They'd stripped off her clothes, held her down, and called her a slut. The boys were all set to rape her, but they were frightened off by the footsteps of a passerby, and Sharon was able to escape. Though Sharon endured weeks of taunts from the two boys, she told no one—not her parents, not her sisters, not even her best friend—what had happened.

Eight months later, just before Sharon turned 13, her mother died of cancer. As a young child, Sharon had recognized that her mother hadn't wanted a third daughter. Sharon's mother always had claimed that Sharon's older sisters needed her more. Sharon had longed for her mother to put her arms around her and say she loved her. How many times had Sharon tried to grab her mother's hand, only to be told "Stop hanging on me" and brushed away. When her mother died, Sharon realized she would never get the motherly affection she'd craved. But while her mother's death saddened Sharon, it hadn't broken her.

That June, when seventh grade had ended, Sharon's father sold the family's sprawling home in Winnetka, Illinois, and moved with Sharon to a two-bedroom high-rise apartment in Peoria. Sharon longed for her older sisters—Mindy recently married and Karen in college—who both remained in the Chicago area. She missed her friends and her relatives. The only connection to Sharon's old life was Kitty, her 2-year-old calico cat.

By August, Sharon's father had stopped coming home at night. He'd spend most of his time with Marcy, a divorcée with two children. Nonetheless, Sharon remained resilient and self-reliant. She would wake herself for school, come home to Kitty, and do her homework. Sometimes Sharon would join her father at Marcy's apartment for dinner, but then she'd go back to the apartment alone, cheered by Kitty's company. Sharon's father said he wanted to move Sharon into Marcy's apartment, but he didn't do it because Marcy was afraid of cats.

Leaving school one warm afternoon in early November, Sharon noticed her father sitting in his royal blue Grand Prix. *How odd*, thought Sharon. *Dad only picks me up from school when I have a doctor's appointment or when it's really cold outside.* Opening the car door, Sharon knew something bad had happened. The somber look on her father's face was the same look he'd had the morning he'd told Sharon her mother had died.

Sharon steadied herself and asked, "Dad, what's wrong?"

"Sharon, a pipe burst in the apartment and there was a big flood."

"Oh, no! Is Kitty okay?"

"Honey, Kitty died," her father said. Sharon sobbed. Her father hugged her.

When Sharon stopped crying, her father said, "You can't go back to the apartment. It's a total loss. Marcy says you should come stay at her apartment. There's a couch in the living room you can sleep on."

"I don't want to live with Marcy," Sharon said. "She doesn't like me. And I don't want to sleep on her dumb sofa. It's in the living room. I wouldn't have any privacy." Sharon thought about the bedroom with red carpet and white curtains that she'd shared with her sister Mindy when their mother was alive. Could life get any worse than being relegated to sleeping in Marcy's living room?

That Valentine's Day, nearly one year after Sharon's mother had died, Sharon's father married Marcy. Despite all the adversity and turmoil, Sharon remained stable, grounded, and strong. But that was a long time ago.

Now Sharon tried to make sense of the physical symptoms she was experiencing. Sharon had always been a problem solver, a trait that drew her to the field of social work. She'd gravitated to geriatrics when she realized that helping older people and their families figure out how to adapt to the challenges of dementia and physical declines was gratifying. But try as she might, Sharon could not make sense of her aches and pains, tiredness, sleep disturbances, and weight loss, and so she made an appointment with her family doctor. The doctor said that Sharon was depressed and prescribed Wellbutrin, an antidepressant.

It wasn't long before Sharon convinced herself that her problem was the result of her having failed Holly. A single mother for over a dozen years, Sharon had all but resigned herself to living without a man. But two years ago, Sharon had met Lennie and fallen in love. She wrote poems to Lennie and sent him funny cards. At Sharon's initiative, she and Lennie developed new passions—wine tasting, bird watching, concerts. The sex was great too. Thinking that Holly would require less of her energies once she entered high school, Sharon had actively nurtured the relationship with Lennie. Now, Sharon believed that she'd indulged herself at Holly's expense.

With the aid of the math and Spanish tutors, Holly passed both classes and went to the sleepaway camp she'd enjoyed during previous summers.

Holly's crisis had passed, but Sharon felt no relief.

Sharon went back to her family doctor. The doctor changed Sharon's medication to Lexapro, an antidepressant and anti-anxiety medication that he said would give her some relief. It did not. As the summer progressed, so did Sharon's symptoms. Her hands tingled. Her mouth was dry. She felt a tightening around her biceps, as though rubber bands were wound around them. The doctor prescribed Ambien, a sleeping aid. The Ambien helped Sharon sleep, but it did not make her body stop hurting, so the doctor switched her medication back to Wellbutrin.

Days after leaving for camp, Holly called home. She said she'd forgotten her hairbrush and asked Sharon to send it to her.

Sharon didn't know what to do first. Panicking, Sharon telephoned her niece. "Holly forgot her hairbrush. What should I do?"

"Aunt Sharon, just go to the store, buy an envelope, put the hairbrush in it, go to the post office, have it weighed, and send it to her."

Of course, Sharon knew what she needed to do, but even the smallest tasks had become overwhelming. She was exhausted all the time. It didn't make sense that such a mundane task could be so intimidating. Somehow, Sharon forced herself to send the hairbrush to Holly.

Thinking that a vacation might help, Sharon and Lennie went ahead with plans they'd made to hike in Acadia National Park, a place Sharon had always wanted to visit. As they approached the summit of Cadillac Mountain on the Fourth of July weekend,

Sharon sighed and said, "Okay, this is nice. Can we go down now?" Sharon had never experienced such flat affect and such intense anxiety. There was no place where she felt calm. She was usually the one who would gush nonstop about a beautiful view. Lennie said, "Honey, I'm frightened. I've never seen you so sad." Sharon turned and walked down the mountain.

Returning home, Sharon felt broken and empty. It hurt to walk. Even the smallest tasks, like opening the mailbox, were overwhelming. She couldn't eat. She couldn't sleep. She couldn't make decisions. She couldn't watch television. She couldn't stand it when Lennie touched her. Every day dragged on with no relief. Each night Sharon went to sleep with the hope that by morning she would return to her normal self. After all, her worries about Holly were over. But it did not happen.

Sharon was terrified. Never had she felt so powerless. Sobbing, she told Mindy, "I feel like I'm sinking in quicksand and I can't climb out."

Sharon wondered why these awful symptoms had surfaced now but never before. She had not felt this way when, six months after her wedding, her first husband had told her that he was in love with a woman he'd met at work and that he wanted a divorce. Yes, she was brokenhearted and grieved when she realized that her second marriage, to Holly's father, was doomed by his dependence on heroin. But she had not stopped eating or sleeping. She had continued to function. Now, she could not.

Toward the end of the summer, knowing that Holly would soon be home from camp, Sharon confided to Mindy, "I can't live like this. I can't stand living in my body. I can't read. I can't pay my bills. I can't even shop for groceries."

Mindy made Sharon an appointment with a psychiatrist who diagnosed Sharon with major clinical depression. The psychiatrist put her back on Lexapro, increasing the dosage that the family doctor had prescribed.

Hearing the psychiatrist's diagnosis, Sharon wondered whether her depression was related to the depression her father had experienced when he had lost his job at age 62 or to his suicide attempt four years later. Sharon remembered how much weight her father had lost, how he'd stopped shaving, eating, and taking his medications. Did depression go even further back in her family? Sharon thought about when she had been a newly minted, 24-year-old social worker. She'd helped her family negotiate nursing home care for her father's mother, who was so depressed she couldn't get herself out of the bathtub.

Now, barely able to function, Sharon kept pushing herself to go to work while hiding her illness from her boss and coworkers. The staff at the clinic where Sharon worked asked her why she no longer joined the group for lunch. Her coworkers asked Sharon why she was uncharacteristically quiet in meetings. They made comments about her sharp weight loss. But no one, not even the supervising psychiatrist who met with Sharon every Wednesday morning, asked her whether she was depressed.

One night, while Mindy cooked dinner, Sharon scrolled through the pictures on her phone. Sharon sighed, "It's so strange that the people at work can't see how sick I am. Why can't they see my pain?"

"Sharon, I don't know why you're so surprised. You've gone out of your way to hide your depression from them," Mindy said.

Looking at a photo of herself and Holly taken during Visiting Day at camp that summer, Sharon froze.

"On my gosh, Mindy. Look at this picture. Remember how awful I felt on Visiting Day? I didn't want to go to camp. I could barely get out of bed. You kept saying how upset Holly would have been if I didn't go, so I forced myself. Look at this picture. Even I can't see how sick I was. All my pain is invisible."

In the middle of July, Sharon was given additional work responsibilities. She had to lead more family meetings. She had to supervise a social work student. She had to write more reports.

Sharon trudged on. Meeting with her psychiatrist at the beginning of September, Sharon worried about how much longer she could survive. Her new responsibility supervising a social work student meant she had to make lesson plans, create spreadsheets monitoring the student's progress, develop learning objectives, and submit monthly reports. She had to attend a weekly class too.

The walls of Sharon's dark tunnel closed.

A week after her appointment with the psychiatrist, as Sharon's family readied to celebrate Rosh Hashana, the Jewish New Year, she was making other plans.

Sharon was not going to hide. She wasn't going to settle. She began to formulate a plan that would solve all her problems.

She was going to kill herself.

Depression

Depressive disorders—including the major depressive disorder Sharon experienced and persistent depressive disorders, known as dysthymia—are very different from sadness. Sadness is a normal human emotion. Sadness generally follows an upsetting event. We feel sad about something—the death of a friend, the disappointment of not getting a promotion, the hurt of being betrayed by a spouse. Over time, sadness fades. We adjust to the loss, the disappointment, and the hurt. Depression, on the other hand, is an abnormal emotional state, an illness that affects thinking, emotions, perceptions, and behaviors. Unlike sadness, depression often occurs in the absence of difficult events or loss. Like Sharon, people who are depressed feel sad about everything. Their energy is sapped. They experience no joy, pleasure, or satisfaction. People who are sad can be cajoled by friends to "get over" it. When people who are depressed are told to "snap out of it" or "it's all in your head," they only feel worse. That's because people who are depressed need medical treatment.

The physical symptoms Sharon experienced—pain, fatigue, weight loss, and insomnia—are common in people with depression and are often the reason people seek out medical help. A World Health Organization study of people meeting the criteria for depression found that 69 percent of patients reported physical symptoms as the sole reason for their doctor visit. Because patients complain of physical ailments, depression often is not diagnosed, as doctors look to other illnesses for cause. Research also finds that the greater the number of physical symptoms a patient complains about, the more likely that patient is to have depression. The more painful the physical symptoms are, the more severe the depression. In addition to her physical symptoms, Sharon's extended depressed mood, diminished interest in daily activities, feelings of guilt, indecisiveness, and plans to kill herself were hallmarks of major depressive disorder. Approximately 7 percent of people in the United States suffer from this illness.

What if an algorithm existed that would identify people at risk for experiencing the onset of major depression? Then, people could be treated before they felt as devastated as Sharon did. That was the goal of a team of Canadian scientists. Following more than 20,000 people in the United States for three years who were free of depression when they were recruited, the scientists identified unique risk factors for the onset of depression. These included being a woman, having annual personal income under $13,000, experiencing previous suicide attempts or thoughts of suicide, presence of depression in biological relatives, depressive and anxious symptoms, role impairment due to emotional problems, traumatic experience, childhood maltreatment, and experiencing racial discrimination. For Sharon, being a woman, the depression her father and paternal grandmother had experienced, her worrying, the attempted rape, and the rejection by her mother made it likely that she would experience an onset of major depressive disorder. What these factors could not predict, however, is when the illness might strike.

There is some evidence to suggest that the sleep disturbance Sharon experienced might have been the best clue to predicting her depression. It is also possible that the sleeping problems were early symptoms of depression. Indeed, while the sleep medication Sharon's doctor prescribed did help her sleep, it did not alleviate her depression.

Although predicting whether an individual will attempt suicide or succeed in killing themselves is difficult, people who are depressed often consider ending their lives. Like Sharon, people who are depressed think about giving up when obstacles seem unbeatable. They want to end their excruciating anxiety and pain. They have lost hope. They don't want to be a burden on others. In short, they believe that death is a better option than life.

Still Another Way for Brains to Break

The onset of Michelle's illness, in July of 1989, came as a surprise to her, as well as to her four children and her husband.

"Amy, Carrie, wake up. We're going to have a midnight tea party!" Michelle flicked on the light in the bedroom her daughters shared and playfully roused the girls.

Eight-year-old Amy rubbed her eyes and groaned. Her 7-year-old sister Carrie sprang out of bed. Carrie had gushed when she'd told her friends about her mother painting the full-wall mural in the Catholic school's cafeteria depicting the amusement park at Mesker Zoo. Leading from the stairs to the cafeteria, Michelle had drawn a bear, a squirrel, a raccoon, and a blue bird, their heads bowed in prayer as they gazed at the Holy Bible on a table. A rosary dangled from the raccoon's pocket. Michelle often did projects with her kids. With Michelle's help, Carrie had made the gingerbread house that had won Mrs. Ballard's second-grade homeroom award last Christmas. Earlier this summer, Michelle had organized water balloon fights and games of neighborhood flashlight tag at dusk. Yes, hosting a midnight tea party was something Michelle would do.

Michelle led her daughters into the kitchen. They paraded past the built-in china cabinet where Michelle's brass candlesticks, her brown ceramic pot, and the topper from her wedding cake were displayed. The small stand near the window where Michelle kept her plants was empty. Carrie said, "Mommy, what happened to the plants?"

When they reached the kitchen table, Carrie laughed. "Mommy, what are your silly plants doing here?" Michelle had carefully placed the plants next to the yellow and orange tea party cups she had given to Amy and Carrie last Christmas. Today, unlike other tea parties Michelle had planned for the girls, there were no tiny peanut butter and jelly sandwiches or pink sugar cookies.

"Drink up girls," Michelle said, tipping her blue and white gardening can over the plants, flooding them with water.

Amy stood silently by the table, her brown eyes widening. As the water filtered through the plants and collected as a black liquid in the saucers under the plants, Carrie said, "That's icky. I'm not drinking it."

Michelle carefully lifted one of the saucers to her lips, raised her pinky finger, and sipped the murky mess. "It's delicious girls. Try it!"

Amy lifted a saucer, brought it to her lips gingerly, and sipped. She wrinkled her nose and curled her upper lip. "Yech, that's gross!" Amy sputtered, spitting the plant water across the table.

Michelle said, "I know what we should do, girls. Let's go out-side, take off all our clothes, and make a rainbow with our clothes!"

Barefoot, Michelle raced to the front door and opened it. Even in the early morning hours, she could feel the humid air typical of Indiana at the end of July.

"Mommy, I'm tired. It's dark and scary outside," Carrie said. "I don't want to make a clothes rainbow." Carrie flashed Michelle the grin that always melted Michelle's heart and convinced her to do whatever Carrie wanted. "I want to go back to bed."

"Mom, stop being so weird. You're scaring me and Carrie," Amy said. "When's Daddy coming home?"

"He'll be home in the morning, around 8:00," Michelle answered. Tim was working the twenty-four-hour shift at the Evansville Fire Department.

Something was different about Michelle. For days, she hadn't eaten much. She hadn't brushed her hair either, and now a brown tangled mess swirled around her face. She'd been wearing the same white T-shirt and beige shorts for three days. Instead of sitting and reading a book at the playground like she usually did while the kids were playing, yesterday Michelle had swung from the top of the jungle gym. She'd never done that before. That afternoon Michelle had told Carrie, Amy, and their 11-year-old brother Matt to string pumpkin seeds with needle and thread in preparation for "the end" and "a return to the time of Adam and Eve." Amy and Carrie had said the project was fun. Matt had just rolled his eyes.

For almost a week, Michelle had been having trouble sleeping. In fact, for the past three days, Michelle hadn't slept at all. Even though Michelle often felt exhausted, there also were times when she had strange bursts of energy.

Michelle had come to believe that the late-night television commercials were sending her private messages. When a commercial for Zest soap promised to make users "zestfully clean,"

Michelle's ego swelled, for she was zestful. When a commercial for Clorox 2 said "Momma's got the magic," Michelle believed she was magical. The high was short-lived, however. Once the burst ended, Michelle was left confused and agitated.

Despite Michelle's best efforts to keep the girls awake, Amy and Carrie went back to bed.

Michelle wandered aimlessly around the house. As she roamed, she picked up a hand towel, dish, and pair of scissors, adding them to the spatula, spoon, and sock already in her arms. She felt lost. Her aimlessness frightened her.

Hours passed. Hoping that watching the sunrise would calm her, Michelle went outside to sit on the front porch. As she stared into the sky, Michelle saw the rising sun transform into a butterfly flapping its wings.

Shortly before 7:00, Mary Ellen, the mother of Matt's friend Jeff, drove by and rolled down her window.

"You're up early this morning," Michelle said.

"Just running over to Walmart to get a water bottle for Jeff. He's so excited about Boy Scout camp. Is Matt all packed? Does he need anything?"

Michelle realized that she'd forgotten to help Matt prepare for the trip, but she wasn't about to let Mary Ellen know. Without missing a beat, she said, "Matt packed his stuff last night. He's ready."

Mary Ellen drove down the street. As Michelle turned to go back into the house, she saw a man wearing a trench coat walking toward her. He hoisted a long shotgun on his right shoulder. Panicking, Michelle ran inside and slammed the front door. She woke Matt, Amy, and Carrie and told them what she'd seen. Matt raced to the living room window.

"Mom, did you really see a man with a gun?" Matt asked. "I don't see him."

Michelle didn't answer. She'd forgotten about the man with the shotgun and had started frantically moving the furniture in the living room. "Matt, help me move the couch," Michelle pleaded. "The world is going to end. The devil is coming. We need to get ready quickly!"

The doorbell rang. Amy opened the door. Michelle heard a man say "Morning. What seems to be the problem here?" Michelle lowered her end of the couch and wiped the sweat from her forehead. She saw a police officer standing in her living room. "There's no problem, officer. We're just moving some furniture."

"We got a 911 call from this address. Who called?"

"I don't know," Michelle said. She looked at Matt, Amy, and Carrie.

"Um, I did," Amy said in a soft voice.

"What's wrong?" asked the policeman.

Amy said nothing.

"Matt, quick, help me move the coffee table. I told you, the devil's coming." Michelle said.

"Little girl, why did you call 911? Did something bad happen?"

Amy was silent.

"Did someone hurt you?"

Nothing.

"Honey, I can't help you if you won't tell me what the problem is."

He waited.

"Mommy woke us up in the middle of the night and we had a tea party. Mommy and Amy drank icky plant water," Carrie said to the policeman.

"Ma'am, do you need help?" the officer asked looking at Michelle.

"Yes, help me move that bookcase. It's too heavy for Matt."

The officer turned to Amy. "Sweetie, there's nothing I can do if you won't tell me what the problem is. I'm going to have to leave now, but if something bad happens, call 911 and I'll come back."

When Tim came home a half hour later, Amy ran to the door. Before her father had both feet in the house, Amy cried, "Daddy, Mommy woke us up in the middle of the night and we had a weird tea party and she said we should take off all our clothes and make a clothes rainbow and she said she saw a man with a gun across the street and she said the world is going to end so she made Matt help her move all the furniture." Amy stopped long enough to take a breath. "And Daddy, Mommy said you're the devil. It's not true, is it?"

Tim hugged Amy. He looked at the jumble of tables and chairs in the living room. Then he looked at his 31-year-old wife, the woman whom he had known for sixteen years and been married to for eleven.

Since they'd married, Michelle had been the bedrock of the family. Her strength and ability to know what to do in difficult situations had saved the family more than once. Earlier that year, when Andy, the youngest of Michelle and Tim's four children, had flipped hot turkey juice from the roasting pan on himself, burning his thighs and knees, Michelle calmly had held the bawling baby's legs under the cold water of the bathtub faucet. For two weeks, Michelle had slept in Andy's hospital room. Each day she had distracted Andy from the pain, encouraging him to play with the Barrel of Monkeys toys while he received whirlpool baths.

Shortly after Andy had come home from the hospital, as Michelle was reading to the kids before bedtime, she heard a faint clicking sound coming from the wall. When she pulled back a corner of the wallpaper, she saw a swarm of termites. Although the repairs cost the family nearly all of their savings, Michelle had remained steadfast.

Just two months ago, Tim had been stricken with meningitis. The doctors told Michelle that Tim could die. Michelle massaged the pressure points on Tim's feet, prayed for his recovery, and nursed him back to health.

"Michelle, honey, what's going on?" Tim asked gently, following Michelle into their bedroom.

"What are you doing here? You're the devil. Get away from me!" Michelle yelled. She flung the applesauce snack pack she'd been eating at Tim. He ducked as the pale-yellow mush flew across the room. The applesauce slid down the bureau.

"Kids, come here," Michelle commanded as she raced into the kitchen. The children followed obediently. Stretching her arms around her four children, Michelle shouted at Tim. "Get away from my kids. Don't hurt my children, you devil."

Carrie said, "Mommy, why are you yelling at Daddy?"

"Michelle, calm down. You're scaring the kids. It's me, Tim."

"Jesus, I denounce the devil. I'm ready to return to the days of Adam and Eve." Michelle howled.

Michelle continued screaming at Tim. The children watched in terror. Just days ago, when the family had gathered for dinner to celebrate her thirty-first birthday, she'd cleaned the house and shopped for dinner. She'd made a big fuss about the pictures the kids had drawn, and she'd thrown her arms around Tim and kissed him when she saw the ruby earrings he'd picked out for her.

Michelle's father had a long history of too much drinking, verbal abuse, and religious hyperactivity. One day, he'd loaded up the car and driven to Minnesota. There, he had been arrested for boisterous behavior. He'd kept a Bible next to his ashtray on the kitchen table and would read scripture aloud, repeating the same verse over and over, his voice growing louder with each repetition. Like Michelle, her father also had shouted about the devil. Ultimately, Michelle's father had been diagnosed with manic depression. For years, he'd been stabilized on a drug called lithium.

Had Michelle inherited her father's illness?

"Michelle, please stop. You're scaring the kids," Tim said.

"The world is ending. The devil is here!" Michelle yelled.

Carrie started crying.

"Michelle, stop it. The kids are terrified," Tim shouted. "Matt, take the girls and Andy to the safe zone. Right *now!*"

Matt picked up Andy and raced out the front door to the fence between their house and the neighbor's house, the place his parents had taught him and the girls to go in case of fire. Amy and Carrie followed him.

With the children gone, Michelle calmed down a bit. For seconds, there was silence. Michelle and Tim stared at each other.

Suddenly, the whistle of the 8:15 train filled the room. Living just two blocks from the train tracks, Michelle had grown so accustomed to the whistle that blew four times a day that often she wouldn't even notice it. But now, the train's whistle was a menacing screech, a signal that the devil had come to get her and all the other lost souls.

"Tim, this is the end. Come back to the days of Adam and Eve with me. Let's take our clothes off!"

Michelle began dancing around the house. She ripped off her T-shirt. Tim grabbed her.

Even though Tim was almost a foot taller than Michelle and outweighed her by nearly fifty pounds, he was no match for Michelle's energized state. Michelle screamed and darted out the back door.

She ran to the neighbor's yard. Tim ran after her. Michelle took off her shorts and jumped onto the neighbor's patio table. She waved her arms and seductively swayed her hips like a stripper on a dance floor.

"Michelle," Tim yelled. "Put your clothes back on."

Instead, Michelle removed her bra. She continued dancing and screamed, "I'm free. I'm free!"

The neighbors peered out their back door.

"Michelle, put your clothes back on, *Now!*"

Something about the tone of Tim's voice made Michelle freeze. She stopped dancing. She stared into the sun.

"Please call an ambulance. I need help." And then came her blood curdling scream, *"Help me!"*

Bipolar Disorder

A manic episode, like the incident Michelle had shortly after her thirty-first birthday, is the hallmark of Type I bipolar disorder. People experiencing a manic episode have an inflated sense of self-esteem. They do not sleep much. They talk nonstop. They are very distractible. They are irritable and have high levels of energy. Type I bipolar disorder, Type II bipolar disorder, and cyclothymic disorder were once known collectively as "manic depression," the diagnosis given to Michelle's father and my mother. In 1980, the term "manic depression" was officially changed in the *Diagnostic and Statistical Manual of Mental Disorders* (*DSM-III*) to "bipolar disorder." This change better reflected clinicians' understanding about the symptoms required for diagnosing an episode of illness. It also better distinguished unipolar depression from bipolar depression, the latter diagnosis used when there was any evidence of mania in addition to the depression. The rapid shifts in mood Michelle experienced, fluctuating from irritability to euphoria, are called lability. Although the mean age of onset for Type I bipolar disorder is 18 years old, it can occur from childhood through old age. Many people in the midst of a manic episode do not think that they are ill or in need of treatment. Michelle's insight and call for help, along with her moments of lucidity during the manic episode, show the complexity of this illness.

The strongest risk factor for Type I bipolar disorder is a family history of bipolar disorder, which Michelle had. That history was helpful for rendering a diagnosis because, without this knowledge, some of the experiences Michelle had—especially the tea party, seeing the sun turn into a butterfly, and envisioning the man with a gun—might have led to a diagnosis of schizophrenia. In fact, schizophrenia and bipolar disorder are often mistaken for one another. The positive symptoms of schizophrenia, such as delusions of grandeur, hallucinations, and paranoia, can look like mania. Negative symptoms of schizophrenia, including apathy, emotional withdrawal, low energy, and social isolation, resemble depression. Some scientists have suggested that schizophrenia and bipolar disorder should be thought of as being on a continuum, with schizophrenia being primarily a thought disorder and bipolar disorder being primarily a mood disorder. The significant overlap of abnormalities in the brains of people with schizophrenia and bipolar disorder also suggests that they may represent a continuum of psychosis; yet, at the same time, there are enough notable differences that make this conclusion premature. Indeed, a third diagnosis—schizoaffective disorder—is used when characteristics of both schizophrenia and bipolar disorder are present. Not only are the symptoms of schizophrenia and bipolar disorder similar, but so too are many of the medications used to treat these disorders.

Bipolar disorder and depression can also be confused. As we'll see in later chapters, accurate diagnosis of these conditions is especially important because effective treatments for bipolar disorders and depression differ. During the fall of 1966, when my mother's agitation and feelings of worthlessness frightened my father, he took her to the doctor. My mother told the doctor she felt sad. She said she felt hopeless and that she got no pleasure from any of her usual activities. In six weeks, she'd lost more than twenty-five pounds. She couldn't sleep, and she couldn't concentrate long enough to read a newspaper article. These behaviors led my mother's psychiatrist to diagnose depression.

By the summer, though, my mother's crippling depression was replaced by hypomania. She'd spend her days alone, reading books about the economies of foreign countries, playing the piano, and trying to reinvigorate her career. She didn't sleep much. She was irritable. She said she had a lot on her mind.

Hypomanic episodes can last for weeks or even months and typically do not involve psychotic symptoms. Hospitalization is not likely. In my mother's case, hypomania lasted from June through August for years. Sometimes people in the grip of a hypomanic episode are more talkative than usual. Sometimes they experience racing thoughts. And sometimes people engage in behaviors that have painful consequences—they go on expensive shopping sprees, make foolish business investments, or act in sexually promiscuous ways—although my mother did none of these.

Today a person like my mother, someone experiencing recurring mood fluctuations of crippling depressive episodes and at least one hypomanic episode, would most likely be diagnosed with Type II bipolar disorder.

The distinction between Type I bipolar disorder and Type II bipolar disorder is that people with Type I bipolar disorder experience full-blown mania that often results in hospitalization. People with depression and hypomania are diagnosed with Type II bipolar disorder. However, if they experience a full-blown manic episode, the diagnosis changes to Type I bipolar disorder. While the hypomania of Type II bipolar disorder is less debilitating and less likely to require hospitalization than the full-blown mania of Type I bipolar disorder, this does not make Type II bipolar disorder a milder form of bipolar disorder. People with both Type I bipolar disorder and Type II bipolar disorder experience depressive episodes. However, compared to people with Type I bipolar disorder, people with Type II bipolar disorder spend, on average, more time in the depressive phase of their illness. Although Type II bipolar disorder can begin in late adolescence and throughout adulthood, the average age at onset is in the midtwenties, slightly later than onsets of Type I bipolar disorder, but earlier than for major depressive disorder. My mother was 43 when she experienced her first depressive episode, and she was 44 when her hypomania caused her psychiatrist to change her diagnosis from depression to manic depression. As was true in my mother's case, Type II bipolar disorder most often begins with a depressive episode and is not recognized as Type II bipolar disorder until a hypomanic episode occurs.

The onset of my daughter Sophie's bipolar disorder had a much different look. For years, Sophie had chronic fluctuating mood disturbances with numerous periods of hypomanic symptoms and some periods of depressive symptoms. From the time Sophie was 8, I don't recall that there ever was a time of more than two months when she was symptom-free. Because Sophie's hypomanic symptoms were short-lived—usually lasting for several hours, but never longer than a day or two—and her depressive symptoms were neither severe nor pervasive, she was diagnosed with cyclothymic disorder. With cyclothymic disorder, a person's mood swings between periods of mild depression and hypomania. The lows never reach those experienced by people with depression, Type I bipolar disorder, or Type II bipolar disorder, and the highs never reach the mania of Type I bipolar disorder. I'd always wondered whether Sophie's plans to run away with a pervert she'd met on the internet—behavior that frightened my husband and me into taking her to the emergency room—qualified as a full manic episode, but her doctor didn't seem to think so.

Although Sophie's symptoms of bipolar disorder became evident when she was 8, Michelle's when she was 31, and my mother's when she was 43, illnesses on the bipolar disorder spectrum can begin both much earlier in life and much later. My friend Tina's labor lasted only five hours. The baby kicked Tina's pelvic floor so violently that her coccyx broke. Baby Jimmy's unusual behavior continued after his birth. He didn't sleep more than two hours at a time until he was 3-and-a-half years old. As first-time parents, Tina and her husband consulted one specialist after the next, looking for both an explanation and a solution to Jimmy's inability to sleep. Jimmy didn't have allergies. He didn't have colic. One doctor shrugged his shoulders and said, "He's just wired." Jimmy went from crawling to running. He spoke in two- to four-word sentences when he was 1 year old. At age 4, before he started day care, Jimmy had taught himself to read and use the computer. *Was this evidence of a very bright child?* Tina wondered. Staff at Jimmy's day care could not handle him. They often called Tina to pick him up early. By the time Jimmy was 7 years old, he'd been diagnosed with severe attention deficit hyperactivity disorder, Type I bipolar disorder, and obsessive-compulsive disorder.

Because the age of onset of bipolar disorder illnesses can vary greatly, some have speculated that bipolar disorder may be a developmental disorder. Contrasting the clinical features and outcomes of three groups of people—those with symptom onset prior to age 21 (early), those with onset between ages 21 and 34, and those with onset after age 34—scientists found that people in the early-onset group were the sickest. More recent evidence suggests that children like Jimmy who experience the onset of bipolar disorder very early have the most severe form of the illness.

Genes, Environment, or Both?

The serious mental illnesses experienced by Joe, Sharon, Michelle, and my mother seemed to come out of nowhere. One day Joe was a typical 17-year-old boy playing basketball, Sharon was a middle-aged woman parenting a teenager, and Michelle was a young mother busy entertaining her four children during summer vacation. And then, like the flip of a switch, everything changed. Joe was aiming a shotgun at his beloved grandmother, Sharon was making plans to kill herself, and

Michelle was dancing naked on her neighbor's patio furniture. The month before my mother became sick, my family had moved from Detroit to the suburbs. My mother had very competently packed and unpacked our belongings, set up our new house, and gotten my brothers and me situated in our new schools. And then, suddenly, she could not even get out of bed.

For my daughter Sophie, the lines between normal and not normal were blurred. With children, it is often difficult to tell whether behaviors are due to a mental illness or to a developmental hurdle. That's why serious mental illnesses are often not definitively diagnosed until early adulthood. In hindsight, I trace the beginning of Sophie's illness to age 8, but there was no clear marker for that. Perhaps Sophie's mental illness started years earlier, but she was not formally diagnosed with bipolar disorder until she was 16. In Jimmy's case, his illness seemed evident from birth.

We do not have a specific formula for identifying people who will develop a serious mental illness, but we do know that genes and environment both play critical roles. Serious mental illnesses are highly heritable. The child of a person with a serious mental illness is more likely to develop that same illness or another serious mental illness than the child of parents without these illnesses. I learned years after adopting Sophie that her birth mother had bipolar disorder. Joe developed the schizophrenia his mother had suffered, Sharon's depression was similar to her father's and paternal grandmother's depression, and Michelle, like her father, had bipolar disorder. Of course, having a parent with a serious mental illness does not guarantee that a child will have the illness. Joe, Sharon, and Michelle all had siblings who did not have the same illnesses. My mother bore three children, and neither my brothers nor I have developed bipolar disorder. To my knowledge, my mother's parents and her sister did not have a mental illness. Significant research now focuses on identifying the gene or set of genes that may lead to serious mental illnesses, but, to date, no gene for schizophrenia, depression, or bipolar disorder has been discovered. Rather, these illnesses are considered to be polygenic disorders, meaning that several genes likely interact to increase vulnerability.

While many researchers continue to search for so-called "insanity genes," others have looked to environmental causes. There is good evidence that people exposed to traumatic experiences—childhood abuse, extreme violence, or significant loss—are at higher risk than others for developing a serious mental illness. In my mother's case, I've often wondered whether she would have developed manic depression had her own mother not died when my mother was 3 years old or had my mother had a loving stepmother rather than the abusive one she did have. Similarly, the rejection Sharon experienced from her mother and/or the other significant losses she experienced early in life may have been contributing causes to her depression.

In addition to trauma, stress can contribute to the onset of a serious mental illness. Major stressors can be both positive and negative and include death of a loved one, medical illness, relocation, starting college or a new job, inheriting a large sum of money, and having a baby. Minor stressors include meeting deadlines and relationship conflict. In the year before the onset of Michelle's illness, her 2-year-old son Andy was severely burned, her house was infested with termites, her husband Tim nearly died from meningitis, and her father was hospitalized for severe mania. While the conflict Sharon had with Holly may have looked ordinary to some, to Sharon it was serious. A woman whose own mother had rejected her, Sharon had made being a good mother to Holly her highest priority. When Sharon was unable to solve Holly's problem with the Spanish teacher, she blamed herself, perhaps igniting her depression.

But experiencing a significant trauma or stress does not guarantee that a person will become psychotic. Plenty of people who are abused as children, have serious health conditions, or experience parental death do not develop a serious mental illness.

The diathesis-stress model best explains the relationship between stress and the onset of serious mental illness. *Diathesis* is the Greek word for "vulnerability." In this model, vulnerability is the predisposition an individual has for developing an illness. Diathesis can stem from genetics, biology, or psychological makeup. Diatheses are largely stable, but not unchangeable, over a person's life span. Stress, on the other hand, is external to the person and can include a discrete event such as a divorce or death in the family, a chronic experience such as a long-term illness or ongoing marital problems, or daily hassles, such as demanding school assignment deadlines. Stress disrupts a person's psychological equilibrium.

According to the diathesis-stress model, all people have some level of diathesis for any given mental illness. Individuals have unique points at which they will develop the illness, a point that depends on the interaction between their vulnerability and the amount of stress they experience. When the combination of predisposition and stress exceeds an individual's threshold, the person develops a mental illness.

Here's another way of looking at the diathesis-stress model. Imagine that each of us is born with a bucket. People with no family history of serious mental illness have a gallon bucket that can hold a full gallon's worth of water. People with a genetic risk for developing a serious mental illness have a half-gallon bucket that can hold only half a gallon of water. Now, imagine that drops of water represent stress. The size of an individual's personal bucket determines how much stress they can hold. From the start, then, people with a smaller bucket are at a disadvantage compared with people who have a larger bucket. Their buckets hold less and get filled faster. When a person's bucket overflows, a serious mental illness ensues.

Stressors can be biological as well as psychological, although little is known about the relationship between biology and serious mental illness. Fuller Torrey, MD, is a clinician and scientist who has long suspected that a virus may be responsible for causing mental illnesses. When Dr. Torrey graduated from McGill University Medical School in 1963, Sigmund Freud's contention that mental illnesses such as schizophrenia and bipolar disorder were caused by bad parenting prevailed. Yet logic and Dr. Torrey's medical training convinced him that these illnesses were brain disorders that couldn't be cured on the analyst's couch.

From 1977 to 1986, Dr. Torrey was on the clinical staff of St. Elizabeth's Hospital in Washington, DC, where he treated people with severe psychiatric disorders. From 1986 to 1992, Dr. Torrey studied the brains of identical twins and found that the brains of people with schizophrenia have clear structural abnormalities, just like other neurological diseases such as epilepsy. The twin study ended the debate over whether schizophrenia is a biological disorder or the product of misplaced Oedipal issues. It took mental illnesses off the couch and into the lab. Now Dr. Torrey spends his time studying whether exposure to viruses and other infectious agents may cause serious mental illnesses.

Wanting to better understand how a virus could cause serious mental illnesses, I asked to meet with Dr. Torrey. He was then 78 years old and had published twenty books and more than two hundred scientific journal articles about serious mental illness. Before my visit, I read Dr. Torrey's book *Surviving Schizophrenia: A Family Manual*. In the preface to this book, Dr. Torrey mentions his younger sister Rhoda, who died in 2010 after having suffered with schizophrenia for fifty-three years. Details about her were scant. I knew it would be easy to get Dr. Torrey talking about his research, but I wondered whether he'd be willing to talk about Rhoda. Knowing how my experiences with both my mother and my daughter had shaped my career, I wondered what Dr. Torrey's experience had been.

On a warm December day, I took the train from Philadelphia to Washington, DC. I met Dr. Torrey at his office in the Stanley Medical Research Institute. I started our conversation by asking him what gave him the courage to do the work he's done. Dr. Torrey smiled and said, "I haven't followed the path I was supposed to follow for a long, long time. I was supposed to be a country doctor. In medical school at McGill University, I realized that the brain is the most interesting part of the body by far. The heart and the liver are pretty boring, actually. In fact, virtually all of the body looks kind of lackluster until you get to see the brain. I think I would have gone into psychiatry even if my sister hadn't developed schizophrenia."

The opening I'd been hoping for.

"Tell me about your sister," I urged.

"Rhoda was two years younger than me. She was perfectly normal, a typical 1950s teenager, until her senior year of high school. She was interested in clothes and boys, probably in that order. She was a pretty quiet, shy kid. But the summer before she was to start college—she had just turned 18—she developed acute psychosis. She was confused, had delusional thinking, and heard voices in her head."

"What happened to her?"

"Rhoda's was a very classic kind of schizophrenia story. She was given Thorazine, and she recovered reasonably well from her first break. She went to a trade school instead of college. Then she had a second break. She recovered much more slowly from that second break and tried to kill herself. She recovered only modestly, and then, when she was 21, she had a third break. Rhoda suffered through electroshock therapy and insulin coma therapy—the few treatments available at the time—but nothing worked."

"It must have been very difficult for you and your parents," I said.

"My dad died when I was 6; Rhoda was 4. Mom took Rhoda to the best psychiatrists on the East Coast. Rhoda saw Lawrence Kolb, chairman of the Department of Psychiatry at Columbia University Medical Center and director of the New York State Psychiatric Institute. She saw Erich Lindemann, chief of psychiatry at Massachusetts General. Rhoda was hospitalized at several of the best private hospitals—Silver Hill in Connecticut and Brattleboro Retreat in Vermont. Still, she never got well. She ended up in the state hospital about ten miles away from where I grew up in upstate New York for nearly twenty-five years."

"In the 1950s, when Rhoda got sick, psychiatrists were saying bad parenting caused mental illness. They were mostly blaming the moms, right?"

"Right. In Boston, Erich Lindemann and his team said the reason Rhoda got sick was because my father had died very young and that my mother wasn't able to take proper care of Rhoda. I remember thinking even then that it seemed like a really silly idea. But my mother, who always deferred to important specialists, said, 'Whatever they said must be true.' Despite all our discussions, Mom died in 1983 believing she'd done something to cause Rhoda's illness."

"Did Rhoda ever leave the state hospital?"

"She left when the state hospital closed in 1985 and lived in the community for about ten years in a group home in Rome, New York. She probably functioned there as well as she ever did after her illness began. She had a boyfriend and a reasonable life. Initially, she responded well to clozapine, but it didn't last long. She had a lot of side effects. She drooled. She couldn't hold her urine. As she aged, she lost some of her vision. She was a heavy smoker and she developed COPD. She lived in various group homes, in nursing homes, and then she spent several years in Utica State Hospital before she died in 2010. She lived to be 70. Sad life. A wasted life. I've taken care of a lot of patients over the years and I'd say my sister was probably amongst the very sickest."

I saw the pain in Dr. Torrey's eyes.

"Tell me a little about this place—the Stanley Medical Research Institute," I said.

"Back in 1988, out of the blue, I got a phone call from Ted Stanley. He said he had a son Jonathan who'd been diagnosed with schizophrenia. Hoping to learn how to help his son, Ted had read my book *Surviving Schizophrenia*. He said he wanted to come to Washington and meet me. So I said, 'Yes, I'd be happy to.' Mr. Stanley suggested we meet at a nice restaurant. I didn't really know of any nice restaurants, but I found one in Georgetown. Mr. Stanley said, 'I'd like to meet your wife too.' I thought that was a little unusual. My wife is an economist with a life of her own. Usually, she'd do her social things and I'd do mine. Since this invitation sounded a little different, my wife agreed to come along."

I took a sip of my water and waited for Dr. Torrey to continue.

"After we ordered our dinners, Mr. Stanley said he'd like me to help him plan some research. He said he was thinking about a study costing between $50,000 and $100,000. I told him I thought I could help him. As we talked, it was clear to me that he was trying to figure out who I was—was I stable or some kind of kook? As we finished dessert, Mr. Stanley said, 'What we're really thinking about is more like a million dollars.' At first, I didn't say anything. A million dollars was a lot of money. I knew I could put his money to good use."

"That was quite a dinner," I chuckled.

"That was just the start. Since the Stanley Medical Research Institute began, it has provided $550 million for studies about the causes and treatment of schizophrenia and bipolar disorder in 30 countries."

"How did Mr. Stanley make his money?"

"He co-founded the Danbury Mint and made a fortune selling collectibles. He started selling medals commemorating the Apollo 11 moon landing and expanded into jewelry, coins, commemorative stamps, decorative plates, and other collectibles. His company has annual sales of about $350 million."

"And his son Jonathan? What happened to him?"

"When Jonathan was a junior in college, he became very sick. He was visiting a friend in New York and suspected secret agents were following him. For three days, he raced through the city's streets and subways without food or water until the police found him penniless in a deli perched naked on a plastic milk crate. When Ted got to the hospital, Jonathan was in a straitjacket. Turned out that Jonathan had bipolar disorder. He's done beautifully on lithium. He's a guy who went from psychotic to normal with some pills. Got a law degree, and worked at the Treatment Advocacy Center for several years. He's semi-retired in Florida now."

Before visiting Dr. Torrey, I learned that in addition to funding research on the causes and treatment of serious mental illness, the Stanley Medical Research Institute maintains a postmortem repository of brain tissue from people with schizophrenia, bipolar disorder, and depression and from people without these illnesses. Much of what we've learned about the relationship between viruses and mental illnesses has been supported by the Stanley funds. I wanted to understand this better.

"I'm fascinated by your work on viruses and mental illness. How did you come up with the idea?" I asked.

"Actually, as far back as 1845 scientists thought that an infectious agent might be the cause of some forms of insanity. When I resurrected the idea in 1972, most of my colleagues thought *I* was crazy. What really happened was that I started thinking like the anthropologist I'd trained to be while I was finishing my psychiatric residency at Stanford."

"Tell me about that," I urged.

"First, for a long time, we've known that viral encephalitis and some other infections have symptoms that look a lot like schizophrenia. Many people with schizophrenia report that their disease set in after signs of a viral infection. I figured that couldn't be a coincidence. Second, when my sister started hearing voices, she looked physically sick. She and many of the people who were my psychiatric patients over the years looked like they had a physical disease."

I thought about some of the people with schizophrenia I'd known. Many of them had looked gaunt and pale.

"Third, there are some areas of the world that have much higher rates of schizophrenia than other areas. Northern Europe has more than Southern Europe. In the highlands of Papua New Guinea, there are no cases of schizophrenia."

"But couldn't that be explained by genetics?" I asked.

"It could, but schizophrenia turns up in clusters in many of the same environments that breed influenza. Like the flu, schizophrenia is most prevalent in poor urban areas in cold climates where crowded households are hotbeds of infection in wintertime. Ireland, for example, has one of the highest rates of schizophrenia in the world, while in the tropics, schizophrenia is virtually unheard of. And there's also good evidence that a disproportionate number of people with schizophrenia are born in the winter and spring. If it were purely genetic, the genes would express themselves throughout the year in a fairly regular pattern. I figured that viruses must be involved because of the seasonal patterns."

Dr. Torrey's excitement about his work was clear.

"Do you know what the virus is?"

"For the past several years, my research has focused on *Toxoplasma gondii*, a parasite carried by cats. My colleagues and I published several papers showing that, if your family owned a cat when you were a child, you have an increased chance of developing schizophrenia as an adult."

"Are all cats infected?"

"No. Only cats that eat a mouse or rat or bird that is infected become infected. It's mostly outdoor cats. Cats are infectious for about two weeks, when they are weaned from their mother and just starting to hunt. Infected cats excrete millions of oocysts, infectious parasites that complete their life cycle on the cat's gut. Where do cats poop? In dirt or sandboxes. They love sandboxes. The oocysts can remain viable for at least two years in moist soil."

"So, kids get infected when they play in the sandbox?" I said.

"Exactly. Little kids play in the sandbox and put their hands in their mouth."

"Fascinating."

"I also realized that the rise of schizophrenia that began in the late 1900s coincided with the beginning of people keeping cats as indoor pets. Before that cats were kept out in the barn." Watching the passion in Dr. Torrey's eyes as he talked about his research made me believe in what he was saying. I wondered whether this work had any connection to Rhoda.

"Was your sister exposed to a cat when she was younger?"

"She was," he said.

"But you were too, right?"

"Butterball was her cat. I had little to do with her."

"Her cat."

Dr. Torrey nodded in agreement.

"Rhoda loved that cat. She and her best friend Diane used to dress it up. They played with that cat all the time. And they loved playing in our sandbox. I'll tell you something I've found surprising. Not only did Rhoda develop schizophrenia, but so too did Diane."

"Amazing. Was Butterball an outdoor cat?"

"Oh yeah. There was a field behind us. We didn't have Butterball for too long. Maybe a year or two. She got sick. Although most cats don't get sick with *Toxo*, Butterball had seizures. Eventually she was put to sleep because there was clearly something wrong with her."

"Very powerful evidence."

"The story gets even better. We've got some preliminary evidence suggesting that having a dog in childhood protects people from developing schizophrenia."

"I can explain that one," I said. "A dog will chase away the cats."

Dr. Torrey smiled.

Between 1995 and 2019, Dr. Torrey and others have done research examining the role that dog and cat ownership in childhood has on development of serious mental illnesses. Some of this research finds that people who have a pet cat during infancy and childhood develop schizophrenia later in life, while other studies do not find this. In their most recent study, Torrey and his team found that exposure to a pet dog during the first twelve years of life was associated with a 25 percent decreased likelihood of having a subsequent diagnosis of schizophrenia. Exposure to a pet dog was not associated with a subsequent diagnosis of bipolar disorder. In this study, exposure to a pet cat was not associated with subsequent diagnosis of schizophrenia or bipolar disorder. Similarly, some research suggests that children born of mothers who had inflammation during the early months of their pregnancy may have an elevated risk for developing a psychotic disorder in adulthood.

Serious mental illnesses are most likely the product of interactions between genes and environments. Recently a large team of scientists created an environmental risk score that included an individual's ethnic group, urbanicity, paternal age, birth weight, cannabis exposure, and childhood adversity. They combined this information with a genetic risk score based on the individual's genome sequence and created algorithms that tested the interactions between genetic and environmental factors. The algorithm enabled the researchers to differentiate between people with and without a psychotic disorder. More-over, the research revealed that the higher the risk score, the more severe the psychotic symptoms.

Helping People as a Serious Mental Illness Develops

Given what we know about the onset of serious mental illness, what can we do to make life better for people as these illnesses unfold?

The unpredictable onsets of serious mental illnesses, in terms of both who will become affected and at what point in a person's life they will become ill, make it imperative that we increase awareness about these illnesses. Schizophrenia, depression, and bipolar disorder can no longer remain illnesses understood only by psychiatrists, psychologists, and social workers. The gatekeepers of our medical system—pediatricians, primary care physicians, nurse practitioners, and family doctors—must develop a basic understanding and awareness of the warning signs of these illnesses. When I told Sophie's pediatrician about her symptoms, the doctor was sure Sophie had ADHD.

Teachers, school counselors, and sports coaches also need to be educated. And, of course, family members, who first spot the signs of the disease, need to be made aware of the warning signs.

The National Alliance on Mental Illness has free programs called "Ending the Silence" that are ideal for students and school staff. The fifty-minute program for students includes warning signs, facts, and statistics about how to get help for themselves or a friend. The one-hour presentation for school staff members includes information about warning signs, facts and statistics, how to approach students, and how to work with families.

A good time to educate the public about serious mental illness starts in middle school. Most middle schools have health units targeting topics such as safe sex, AIDS, smoking, alcohol and drugs, and healthy eating. Facts about cancer, heart disease, and diabetes are also taught in middle schools, yet there is a deafening silence about mental illnesses. In middle school, my daughter Sophie was cutting herself. One of her friends attempted suicide. They were not alone. The 2010 National Comorbidity Study Adolescent Supplement found that just over 20 percent of children between the ages of 13 and 18 had been diagnosed with a seriously debilitating mental disorder. Of course, this doesn't include the countless others who have not received a diagnosis but who have a mental illness.

Education about mental illnesses should start in middle school and continue throughout high school because half of all people with serious mental illnesses experience onset by the age of 14. High schools are an ideal place to screen students for mental illnesses and direct students to places in the community where they can get help. This, of course, requires training for school faculty and staff, who often know of students who need help but do not know how to help. Educating high school students about mental illnesses would strengthen the natural support system already existing in these schools. At this age, kids are more likely to turn to other kids than to an adult when they have a problem. When my daughter was in high school, her boyfriend threatened to kill himself. He'd had a fight with his mother, grabbed his army knife, and ran away. Readying to harm himself, he phoned my daughter to say goodbye. Because Sophie was frightened, she told me what was going on, and we were able to get help for the boy. Not all troubled high school kids are as lucky. How empowering it would be for high school students to know how to help a peer who discloses depression, suicidal thoughts, or hallucinations. If we can help high school students understand that mental illnesses are brain disorders, not character flaws, we will be taking a step in the right direction toward preventing needless suicides and other suffering.

At Palos Verdes High School in California, Principal Charles Park saw a 30 percent increase in the number of students reporting suicidal thoughts over a four-year period. Also rising was the number of kids looking for emotional support. His response was a student wellness center offering sessions on yoga, meditation, and other stress-relief programs. Monthly programs focus on topics that include drug and alcohol use, stress, and anxiety. Creating a space within the high school that is calming, safe, and predictable gives students a place to start difficult conversations before they are in acute distress.

Although we have much to learn about the onset of serious mental illnesses, there are clues that help identify people likely to be at risk.

First, we must be aware of the genetic predisposition underlying serious mental illnesses and maintain vigilance. While most children whose mother or father has schizophrenia or bipolar disorder will not develop a mental illness, many will.

Second, we can heighten awareness regarding the importance of behavior changes. Changes in visible behaviors—inability to sleep, grades dropping, failure to complete work assignments, withdrawal from or inability to get along with friends and family—represent signs that a serious mental illness may be brewing. Similarly, the onset of risky sexual activities, irresponsible use of alcohol or drugs, and rash spending sprees signal that there may be a serious problem.

While there may be many clues that serious mental illness is looming, it is important to understand that the first indications are usually invisible to all but the person developing the illness. These changes often are so frightening that people try to hide them from others. Months before Joe pointed a gun at this grandmother's chest, he was aware of the battle ensuing in his head between good and evil, his conversations with God, and his belief that he was God—but he told no one. For weeks, Sharon was aware of her loss of appetite, tingling hand, dry mouth, and tight biceps—but she kept these symptoms to herself. Michelle felt that the television ads were sending her messages—but she didn't even tell her husband.

Certainly, it is understandable that people are frightened by the early indicators of serious mental illness. Hearing voices that others do not hear is terrifying. People fear not being believed and worry about being labeled "crazy." Having racing thoughts all night rather than getting a good night's sleep is alarming. Not being able to sleep at night is upsetting. Yet concealing the initial indications of serious mental illnesses will not make the illnesses go away. It only makes things worse.

CHAPTER 3

Crisis Care

LIKE ALL THE stories in this book, this one is true.

On November 18, 2013, a man, concerned that his 24-year-old son Gus was in crisis, secured an emergency custody order to have Gus taken to the hospital for a psychiatric evaluation. Years earlier, Gus had been diagnosed with bipolar disorder. He'd attempted suicide twice. Over the past few months, Gus had gained weight as he had gotten sicker and more delusional. Gus hadn't bathed in days. He'd let his beard and hair grow long. He barely spoke. Now, Gus sat on the front porch of his father's house strumming his banjo, willingly waiting for the sheriff to take him to Bath Community Hospital in Hot Springs, Virginia.

The man thought about what he'd read in Gus's journal the night before. Gus had described the man as a dog and himself as God.

At the hospital, Gus paced. He stared. He paced some more. He said, "Why the hell is everyone out to get me?" Gazing into his father's eyes, Gus said, "Where's my real dad?" Gus insisted that he'd been tortured and starved for his entire life.

After six hours, a caseworker, saying that Gus was not suicidal, readied to send him home. Worried that her son would harm himself or someone else, Gus's mother begged the caseworker to hospitalize him. Seeking to appease her, the caseworker searched for but was unable to find an available psychiatric bed in all of Virginia, and so he sent Gus home.

The man knew this was not a good idea. He told his ex-wife not to worry; he would take care of Gus. The man's stomach turned as he thought about how he would keep Gus and himself safe that night.

At home, Gus retreated to his journal. He wrote furiously. When the man was ready to call it a day, he said good night to Gus and locked his bedroom door. Gus had never caused the man harm, but there was something about the look in Gus's eyes that frightened him.

Several hours later, the man was awakened by the rattle of the doorknob. Gus was trying to get into his room. The man thought about calling the police, but he knew that if he did, they would handcuff Gus and take him to the police station. He didn't want his son to spend the night in jail, and he didn't want Gus to have an arrest record. The poor kid had enough problems.

"Gus, go to sleep," the man said. "We'll talk in the morning."

The man pulled the covers over his head and went back to sleep.

Early the next morning, the man woke, showered, and went to feed the animals on his farm.

On his way back to the house, the man saw Gus walking toward him. He waved and said, "G'morning Gus. Sleep well?"

Gus said nothing.

The morning was still. The man saw that Gus had a knife in his right hand and a rifle slung over his shoulder.

As he approached his father, Gus raised the knife and stabbed the man.

The man cried out, "Gus, I love you. Why are you doing this?"

Gus stabbed his father thirteen times. The man's eye, back, face, arm, and chest were bloodied. His right ear was severed. A chunk of his tongue was chopped off.

At last, Gus stopped. He walked into the woods, saying nothing.

The man stumbled off and made it to a secondary road where he was rescued by a passerby.

In the woods, Gus shot himself to death with the rifle.

The man whose mentally ill son was turned away at the emergency room was Virginia senator Creigh Deeds.

If a psychiatric hospital bed cannot be found for a state senator's son who agreed to seek help in the midst of his crisis, what hope is there for the rest of us?

Was it always this difficult to get care in the midst of crisis? How did we get to this point? What can we do about it?

A Look Back

In colonial America, where the population was widely dispersed and treatments for mental illness nonexistent, a person like Gus who was in the midst of a crisis would have been confined to a small space within his family home at public expense. By the early eighteenth century, growth in the general population was accompanied by an increase in the number of people with mental illness. The informal manner in which the colonialists had provided crisis care no longer worked. Almshouses, funded by the community, sprang up—first in Boston, and then in other large cities. They provided food and care to a diverse population, including the poor, the old, and people with mental illness.

As the population grew, almshouses were unable to keep pace with the growing number of people with mental illness. Why weren't these sick people hospitalized? Because public hospitals did not exist in the United States until 1751. Thomas Bond, a colonist studying to become a doctor, traveled abroad to learn his profession. Impressed with the benevolent model of care in English and French hospitals, Bond decided to build a public hospital in Philadelphia. With Benjamin Franklin's help raising funds, Pennsylvania Hospital became the first private American hospital, serving the sick, the injured, and those with mental illness.

Even once there were hospitals, very few people with mental illness were hospitalized. Between 1752 and 1754, 18 of the 117 people admitted to Pennsylvania Hospital suffered from mental illness. These patients were housed in the basement of the hospital, shackled to the walls. It was the only way hospital administrators knew how to keep the patients safe. People with mental illness cared for at Pennsylvania Hospital in its first few years were, like Gus, people in crisis. One woman had murdered her infant. A farmer had burned down his barn to get rid of rats. Mental illness, like physical illness, was viewed as purely bodily in origin. As a result, bloodletting and purges were used to relieve pressure on the brain or to remove blockages believed to cause mental illness. Patients with mental illness did not stay long in the hospital; more than 80 percent were discharged within a few months. The Quaker tradition of helping the less fortunate guided the efforts of Bond and Franklin, yet the public regarded people with mental illness as curiosities. Hoping to quell the throngs of Sunday gawkers who disturbed the patients, Pennsylvania Hospital began charging an "admission fee" in 1762 to minimize the number of people coming to stare at and taunt the patients.

The first public hospital built exclusively for people with mental illness, The Public Hospital for Persons of Insane and Disordered Minds, was established in 1773 in Williamsburg, Virginia. Like at Pennsylvania Hospital, restraints, bleedings, and plunge baths were used to calm people in crisis. Admission was limited to two groups of people, those considered danger-ous and those considered curable. The hospital had twenty-four isolation cells. Each had a stout door with a barred window that looked onto a dim central passage. A mattress and chamber pot were the sole furnishings. An iron ring in the wall attached to a chained shackle fettered the patient's wrist or leg. Between 1773 and 1790, 20 percent of the patients were discharged from this facility, pronounced as cured. However, because diagnosis of mental illness was primitive and treatments nonexistent, it is likely that being discharged had nothing to do with being cured.

The Growth of Private Asylums

The early private and public hospitals led to the development of private asylums. The word "asylum" means "refuge, protec-tion, sanctuary." This is the experience the Quakers hoped to create when, between 1813 and 1822, they established The Asylum for Persons Deprived of the Use of Their Reason (Friends Hospital), The Asylum for the Insane (McLean Hos-pital), and The Hartford Retreat for the Insane. Based on the philosophy of Philippe Pinel, a psychiatrist in charge of the first Parisian asylums, mental illnesses were believed to be curable if identified and treated early. Lacking medications, "moral treatment"—removing people from the rigors of urban life and providing them with a restful sojourn in a quiet, pastoral setting—was considered the only humane response.

Consistent with this philosophy, Friends Hospital was built on a fifty-two-acre farm, ten miles outside of Philadelphia. Like-wise, McLean Hospital was built on a wooded hill on the out-skirts of Boston, where patients skated, skied, rode horses, and played tennis, golf, and croquet on the hospital's lawns. Com-munity and companionship were considered vital, so asylums provided kind, compassionate staff and opportunities to social-ize with other patients. Billiard rooms, bowling alleys, art studios, and gymnasiums allowed patients to exercise and participate in pleasant activities.

Intended to serve the entire community, the early asylums were funded by contributions from affluent elites and supplemented by public subsidies. But still, the nineteenth-century private asylums admitted few patients. McLean, for example, admitted sixty-one patients annually during the first twelve years of its existence. Within the protected structure of asylums, many patients lived through their psychoses, emerging as stabler people. Of the 666 patients discharged between 1818 and 1830, McLean listed 247 as recovered, 96 as much improved, and 91 as improved. Patients were discharged when they could function at a minimally acceptable level in a family and community setting. Although some people were subsequently rehospitalized, many were indeed able to return to life in the community.

The Problem with Private Asylums and the Growth of State Mental Hospitals

Asylums began with an idealistic vision and ended as a social malady. By the 1820s, private hospitals faced serious financial problems. They could not meet growing demand as population expansion, unemployment, widening class distinctions, and immigration of minority ethnic populations increased poverty, disease, and crime. The hope that private hospitals could serve the needs of the entire community was destroyed.

A new model was needed to provide care to the growing number of people in crisis. Mental illness became the responsibility of the states. However, because most states lacked resources and saw their primary function as protecting both individuals and communities from behavior that was obstructive or dangerous, the states' goal was providing custody rather than treatment.

States struggled to figure out what to do with people like Gus. Massachusetts, for example, enacted a statute in 1797 and another in 1816 mandating that jails accept "lunatics and persons furiously mad"—people whose behavior threatened the welfare of others. However, when Bible salesman Reverend Louis Dwight found that a man with mental illness had been confined in an unheated room for eight years, he complained to members of the legislature. Dwight pleaded for Massachusetts General Hospital to accept people with mental illness or for Massachusetts to construct a separate institution to treat these people.

Nothing changed until Horace Mann, an educational reformer, proposed that Massachusetts establish an asylum for the insane. As a result of Mann's efforts, the Worcester State Lunatic Hospital was founded in 1833. Like the private asylums, this facility was founded on Pinel's "moral treatment" philosophy. Yet the sheer number of people needing care made it impossible to create a supportive environment. Almost from the day it opened, Worcester State Hospital could not meet the demands placed on it. Between 1833 and 1836, an average of eighty-eight people were admitted annually. In the first year of its existence, over half of admissions came from jails and almshouses, a very different population from that served by the early private asylums. Eager to demonstrate its effectiveness, Worcester State Hospital boasted high discharge rates—between 82 and 91 percent—in each of its first three years. But by 1835, it was clear that Worcester State Hospital was discharging people with mental illness to the local jails. By the end of the decade, patients were returned to jail as quickly as they were sent to Worcester State Hospital.

An Attempt at Reform

In 1841, 39-year-old Dorothea Dix, recently recovered from one of many bouts of depression, visited the East Cambridge Jail near Boston to teach a class to women prisoners. She was surprised to find that many women in jail suffered from mental illness, and she was horrified by the conditions in which the women lived. Over the next two years, Dix, a former headmistress of a Boston school for girls, visited every jail and almshouse in Massachusetts. Then, she developed pamphlets (the only viable means by which a woman could participate in political life) for the legislature, telling lawmakers about the cages, closets, cellars, stalls, and pens in which people lived. She said that people were chained, naked, beaten with rods, and lashed into obedience. In her pamphlets, Dix explained that jails were not the right places for people with mental illness, and she urged the Massachusetts legislature to improve options for these people. Samuel Woodward, the superintendent of Worcester State Hospital, echoed her plea. Woodward admitted that in the ten years since the hospital had opened, sixty-four dangerous patients had been sent from the hospital back to jails. There were as many people with mental illness in jails and houses of correction as there had been before the hospital was established.

The Massachusetts legislature responded by adding beds to Worcester State Hospital. By 1846, however, the facility had deteriorated so much that the hospital's board of visitors noted that if patients were not mad when they came to the hospital, they soon would become mad. The legislature authorized the opening of new hospitals in Taunton in 1854 and Northampton in 1858. But even with these additions, overcrowding persisted.

A Good Idea Gone Bad

Dix's success in Massachusetts launched her career as an apostle for asylums. Her vision was that large-scale institutions would assume functions once the purview of the family. Thus, the 1840s and 1850s became decades of asylum building. On average, more than one new state asylum opened each year. Spurred by the early Quakers, the founders of asylums believed that "moral treatment"—treatment directed to the whole individual—was the only humane response to mental illness.

The first state hospitals, carefully documented by architect and photographer Christopher Payne in his book *Asylum: Inside the Closed World of State Mental Hospitals*, were palatial buildings, with high ceilings, lofty windows, and spacious grounds. Though Dix was the catalyst for the initial wave of asylum building, Thomas Story Kirkbride provided the blueprint for asylum expansion. As superintendent of Pennsylvania Hospital, Kirkbride had come to believe that a well-designed and beautifully landscaped hospital could heal mental illness and that a peaceful environment filled with structured regimens would enable patients to recover and reenter the outside world. Physically, Kirkbride's asylums were designed like a formation of birds in flight—each had a central administration building flanked symmetrically by linked pavilions stepped back to create a shallow "V." This layout facilitated segregation of patients according to gender, degree of affliction, and social class. The most disturbed patients were housed in the outermost wards, while people who were better adjusted lived closer to the center, along with the staff. The stepped arrangement of the wards made the hospital easier to manage and provided an abundance of natural light, which Kirkbride believed had a healing quality. Many of the asylum landscapes, designed by Frederick Law Olmsted, became prototypes for public parks. As visitors to the asylums never got beyond the public lobbies of the administration buildings, these spaces and landscapes presented to the public a positive image of asylums. The rural settings afforded privacy and land for farming and gardening. As part of their therapy, patients often worked on hospital farms that produced their own food. They also worked in the kitchens, laundries, and gardens, which provided opportunities for learning vocational skills and skills of daily life. These hospitals provided control and protection for patients, both from their own impulses and demons and from society's ridicule, isolation, and abuse.

Yet state asylums were plagued by problems almost from the start. They were expensive, and taxes could not cover their costs. Asylum directors were not medically trained, and many were dishonest. Despite this, state asylums continued to be funded and built because the number of people in the community who needed care continued to grow. State asylums promised to treat and cure mental illness, ultimately saving money, but in reality these asylums neither treated mental illness nor saved money. By the end of her career, Dix was responsible for founding or enlarging over thirty mental hospitals in the United States and abroad.

The number of asylums grew quickly, as did the number of beds in these hospitals. In 1824, there were only eight asylums in the United States, each with an average of 116 beds. As long as asylums remained small, superintendents were able to manage the care and treatment of patients. By 1860, there were forty-one asylums with an average of 386 beds each, and by 1890 there were sixty-six asylums with an average of 802 beds each. From the very start, the population of people with mental illness far exceeded the number of available beds. With treatments limited to insulin shock therapy and bloodletting, few people got better. Not surprisingly, discharge rates fell. By the end of the nineteenth century, "moral therapy" was regarded as a failure. Most patients remained in asylums for decades and died there. Every asylum had its own graveyard.

As the number of patients increased, hospitals grew in size and complexity. Large numbers of patients, combined with inadequate funding and staffing, caused state hospitals to fall short of their original ideals. By the end of the nineteenth century, asylums had become places of squalor and neglect. Many were run by inept, corrupt, or sadistic bureaucrats, a situation that persisted through the first half of the twentieth century. Therapeutic goals were replaced by goals of order, efficiency, and custodial care. During this time, the population of people with mental illness living in poorhouses, almshouses, and jails also soared, largely because hospitals discharged patients who failed to improve. Mentally ill people had no place else to go.

First-Person Stories: Nellie Bly and Clifford Beers

By the late 1880s, New York newspapers were filled with chilling tales about brutality and patient abuse at the city's psychiatric hospitals. Elizabeth Cochrane Seaman, who used the pen name Nellie Bly, was a 23-year-old journalist who convinced her editor to allow her to feign mental illness in order to get herself committed to Blackwell's Island, New York's most atrocious psychiatric hospital. She wanted to see what was really going on there. Dressed in tattered secondhand clothes, Nellie stopped bathing and brushing her teeth. Hoping to convince the authorities she was a lunatic, she practiced making faraway expressions in front of the mirror. She wandered the streets, posing as Nellie Moreno, a Cuban immigrant.

Nellie had perfected her role so well that, during a single night in a cheap boarding house, Temporary Home for Females, No. 84 Second Avenue, she frightened the residents and convinced them she was crazy. The matron of the house called the police. Bly was hauled off to the Essex Market Police Courtroom, where a judge pronounced her insane and ordered her to Bellevue Hospital's psychiatric ward. There she was diagnosed "delusional and insane." A few days later, Nellie was sent to Blackwell's Island.

Opened in 1839, Blackwell's Island (now known as Roosevelt Island) was built as a state-of-the-art institution committed to moral and humane rehabilitation of its patients. When funding got cut, Blackwell's Island became a warehouse, staffed in part by inmates of a nearby penitentiary.

Taking careful notes of her own experiences and those of her fellow inmates, Bly documented life on Blackwell's Island. Then, once her editor freed her from Blackwell's Island, Nellie Bly wrote a series of tell-all articles about life in a mental institution. These articles became the source for Bly's best-selling book, *Ten Days in a Madhouse*. Bly's writing reveals "oblivious doctors" and "coarse, massive orderlies who choked, beat, and harassed" patients. Bly writes of her surprise to find many patients who looked and acted sane. Some were immigrant women, confined because they could not make themselves understood. Bly writes about a disoriented young girl who was beaten by the nurses, held naked in a cold bath, and thrown on her bed because she refused to cooperate with the staff. She describes rancid food and dirty linens. She tells how ice baths were a daily occurrence and how morphine and chloral were used to sedate difficult patients. Although these were standard treatments for people with mental illness, Bly was convinced that what passed for treatment was, in reality, punishment. According to Bly, the endless enforced isolation the women experienced was not because they were a menace to other people but because the staff were mean and vindictive.

In 1900, Clifford Beers, a 24-year-old clerk in a New York City life insurance company, did not need to feign mental illness. Over the course of three years, the man who would become a leading advocate for reforming the way people with mental illnesses are cared for gained entry into not one but three psychiatric hospitals.

As a student at Yale University, Beers had experienced frequent bouts of anxiety and depression. He feared developing epilepsy and a brain tumor—conditions that killed his older brother. As a tax collector in New Haven, Beers experienced snapping nerves and bouts of depression. On June 23, 1900, Beers had terrifying sensations at work, rendering him helpless. He couldn't speak, his hands shook, and his vision blurred. In his memoir, Beers says that his brain "felt as though pricked by a million needles at white heat." Distraught, Beers went home, where his persistent dread of developing epilepsy spiraled. During a four-day frenzy, he contemplated ways to kill himself—should he die by drowning, overdose on drugs, or sever his jugular vein? While his family ate dinner, Beers dropped feetfirst from his fourth-floor bedroom window, his fingers clinging to the window sill. Letting go, his heels struck the ground, crushing one heel bone and breaking most of the small bones in the arches of his feet.

At Grace Hospital, recovering from these injuries, Beers experienced hallucinations and delusions for the first time in his life. He saw a man standing outside his second-story window. He knew he'd been placed under arrest and was expected to confess to a crime. After a month, Beers's feet had healed, so he went home to convalesce. However, his delusions and hallucinations continued. He smelled burning human flesh. He saw handwriting on his bedsheets. His brother George was out to get him. There was a detective under his bed who pressed pieces of ice against his injured heels at night.

Knowing that Beers needed more help than they could provide, his family had him admitted to Stamford Hall, a small private asylum. Each night, during the eight months he was there, his hands were shackled. Frequently the attendants overpowered him and tied him down. A doctor, angry that Beers refused to answer his questions, seized Beers by the arm and jerked him from the bed. Yet even in the midst of this turmoil, there were kindhearted people. One attendant, who had quit Stamford Hall because he was disgusted with its care, offered and then provided care for Beers in his own home for three months. But even with compassionate care from this man and his family, Beers's delusions and hallucinations continued.

Beers knew he needed to be in an asylum but wanted to be in a place where he would be treated with respect. In his autobiography, *A Mind That Found Itself*, Beers wrote, "It is the even-going routine of institutional life which affords the indispensable quieting effect—provided that routine is well ordered, and not defeated by annoyances imposed by ignorant or indifferent doctors and attendants."

Beers was admitted to the Hartford Retreat in June 1901, a facility he describes as one of the best psychiatric institutions in the country. He walked its beautiful grounds and within a few weeks experienced contentment that he said was "due directly and entirely to an environment more nearly in tune with my ill-tuned mind." For fourteen months, Beers read and kept to himself, talking with staff and residents only when it was absolutely necessary.

But Beers was not cured, not by a long shot. He still believed that his relatives were not his relatives, that detectives were pursuing him, and that a criminal trial was impending. Believing that a date for his trial had been set, Beers redoubled efforts to kill himself. He considered death by hanging but decided he'd rather plunge a sharp weapon into his heart. However, when he found a six-inch knife lying on the ground, Beers convinced himself that the detective who had been watching him had planted the knife, and so he tossed it aside.

Beers abandoned his plan to kill himself and instead spent his days dreaming up ways for his brother George to prove that he really was his brother. On August 30, 1902, George passed the test. He appeared at Hartford Retreat with Clifford's passport, just as Clifford had requested. Convinced that he had found the family lost to him, delusions about his family lifted. Beers writes, "My mind seemed to have found itself."

While reestablishing the relationship with his family marked a turning point for Beers, it did not restore his health. He says, "The pendulum had swung too far." All of a sudden, the man who hadn't spoken for months did not stop talking. His mood became elated. He slept for only two or three hours a night. He planned vast, vague humanitarian projects; he interpreted the most trifling incidents as messages from God. He wrote letters so long that when spread on the floor they spanned a distance of a hundred feet. He told the hospital's superintendent what workers were doing wrong, and he refused to cooperate with hospital rules.

In September of 1902, Beers spoke rudely to his physician. In retaliation, the doctor transferred Beers to the violent ward, a place with wooden floors and bare walls. Heavy benches lined the perimeter of the common room. When Beers's requests for paper and pencils were refused, he threw a dining room chair through a window. Surprisingly, within days, he was transferred back to his original ward.

Believing he was now in charge of the hospital, Beers fought with the attendants and the doctors. Lacking effective ways to help Beers, the doctors put him in seclusion, removing his books, writing, and drawing materials. Angry, Beers kicked the door. When that failed to generate attention, he threw his shoe at the ceiling light, smashing it. Attendants charged into the room, threw Beers on the bed, and choked him. Hours later, hoping again to call attention to himself, Beers made a noose with his suspenders and feigned suicide. Taunting the attendants, Beers admitted to his ruse and threatened to really kill himself with a piece of glass from the broken light that he'd hidden in his mouth. After yet a third fight, Beers was restrained for fifteen hours by an angry physician who adjusted the straitjacket so that Beers could barely breathe. The pain was awful.

For twenty-one days, Beers was confined in a room with padded walls that was twelve feet long, seven feet wide, and twelve feet high. Food was passed to him through a small opening. It was so cold Beers could see his breath. When Beers refused medication, one attendant held him down, another held the medicine and funnel, and the doctor poured the medicine into his mouth.

Although Beers's family was not able to see him, they were told about his manic state, the need for restraints, and the use of seclusion. His brother George decided that Clifford should be transferred to yet a third psychiatric institution, this one a public institution—the Connecticut State Hospital. At this time, moves from private hospitals to state hospitals typically were made when patients were particularly troublesome. Connecticut State Hospital housed 2,300 patients and had a view of a beautiful river and valley. Beers was allowed to write, draw, and walk the property.

However, Beers soon became bored and began talking non-stop about his plans for reforming mental hospitals. If patients in private hospitals were being abused, he reasoned that surely those in state facilities must also experience abuse. Beers resolved to inspect every ward within Connecticut State Hospital. He barricaded himself in his room and threatened to stay there until the governor of the state, the judge who committed him, and his brother arrived.

The staff burst open the door and carried Beers to the violent ward. They stripped Beers to his underwear and thrust him into a bare cell, forcing him to sleep on the floor for three weeks. He was hungry and cold. He couldn't sleep because the hallway was always noisy. He was denied a bath. When Beers taunted the attendants, their response was to kick or choke him, stopping only when Beers feigned unconsciousness. Beers saw other incoherent and delusional patients treated similarly. During this time, Beers's delusions of grandeur continued. He was going to fly to St. Louis to receive a $100,000 reward for developing an efficient airship. He was going to revitalize New Haven, turning churches into cathedrals.

In March 1903, after nearly four months in the violent ward, Beers calmed down and was transferred to a ward where he had a room to himself with a bed, chair, and wardrobe. He was discharged from Connecticut State Hospital on September 10, 1903.

Despite all the brutality Beers had been subjected to over the course of three years, he said, "Should my condition ever demand it, I would again enter a hospital for the insane, quite as willingly as the average person now enters a hospital for the treatment of bodily ailments." Beers knew how desperate he had been for help and how vulnerable people with mental illness are. But he also knew that abusive behavior on the part of hospital staff is unacceptable.

Although Nellie Bly's exposé and Clifford Beers's memoir generated attention, the abuses and squalor persisted as the number of people with mental illness continued to grow. Asylums expanded in number and size. Some asylums, immense to begin with, began to resemble small towns. Pilgrim State on Long Island, for example, housed more than 14,000 patients by 1954.

Another Good Idea Gone Bad: Deinstitutionalization

By the mid-twentieth century, 322 state and county hospitals contained more than 558,000 inpatient psychiatric beds. Growth in the number of people with mental illness was not the only problem for asylums. In the era before Social Security and Medicaid, state hospitals became the dumping ground for older people suffering from dementia and for people with neurological conditions, epilepsy, syphilis, and developmental disabilities. It was virtually impossible for asylums to provide good care.

The 1950s brought the emptying of state psychiatric hospitals. Commonly referred to as "deinstitutionalization," the movement was driven by complex, interwoven factors, including widespread recognition that the asylums were filled with abuse; the emergence of psychiatric medications, making it possible to stabilize people and allow them to live safely in the community; financial incentives that encouraged treatment outside of institutions; and the growing belief that patients would be better off cared for in small, community-based settings. The possibility that hospitalization need not be custodial or lifelong emerged. Mental illness could be transformed and a hopeless population of asylum dwellers reduced if a short stay in the hospital could address crisis situations and be followed by a return to the community where people could be maintained on medication and monitored in outpatient clinics.

The Community Mental Health Act, signed into law by President Kennedy in 1963, supported the deinstitutionalization goal. This act provided $150 million of funding over four and a half years and promised to create a network of 1,500 community mental health centers across the country where patients could get care while living in the community. But just twenty-two days after Kennedy signed the act, he was assassinated. Deprived of Kennedy's stewardship, the country never established enough community mental health centers to accommodate the number of people with mental illness. Deinstitutionalization began as a trickle in the 1960s and became a flood by the 1980s—even though it had become clear by then that releasing mentally ill patients before they were stabilized created more problems than it solved. When President Reagan cut federal funding for mental health, people with serious mental illness started roaming every major US city. No city had the infrastructure to deal with the hundreds of thousands of mentally ill patients who had been turned away from the state hospitals.

Joe, Michelle, and Sharon

Much can be learned about crisis care in twentieth-century America from the experiences of the people you met in chapter 2—Joe, Michelle, and Sharon.

When we left Joe and his grandmother in the last chapter, Joe, believing his grandmother was Satan, was pointing a gun at her chest.

Joe pulled back the hammer with his thumb, cocking the shotgun, and Grandma reached her hands toward Joe, pleading, "Joe. Don't. You've never been mean to me." Joe released his grip on the trigger and slowly and carefully depressed the hammer, uncocking it. Grandma cowered as Joe removed the shell and put it in his pocket.

Joe watched his grandmother. Seconds passed. Neither of them moved. Then, Joe turned, walked out of his grandmother's bedroom, went downstairs to the kitchen, and put the gun away.

Joe and Grandma sat quietly in the kitchen. The crisis had passed. Joe was exhausted. When Uncle Fred came home from the bar, Grandma told him what had happened. Fred looked at Joe quizzically, but Joe had no explanation for his behavior.

In a soft voice, Grandma said, "Joe, I think we need to take you to Middletown." Fred sadly nodded in agreement. Joe gazed at the floor. The fear he'd had since his mother had been taken to Middletown State Hospital years ago—that he would inherit her mental illness—had become a reality.

As Fred drove them to the hospital, he and Grandma talked quietly. Joe sat silently in the backseat.

Joe spent that night in a large room filled with twenty patients, all of whom were sleeping when he arrived. Joe tossed and turned. He struggled to figure out what was real and what was not.

Within a few days, Joe was treated with Thorazine and moved to a smaller room with two beds. Several of these smaller rooms were connected by a hallway that was not far from the large room holding the newly arrived patients and a lounge area. Off the lounge was an open-air smoking room enclosed by chicken wire. From the smoking room, Joe could see the hospital's rustic grounds, where he would be free to walk once he became more lucid. Joe had become one of the hospital's four thousand patients.

Joe's initial feelings of being trapped in a strange, sinister place gave way as he saw that the hospital was clean and well staffed. The orderlies were retired New York City policemen; nurses and student nurses were kind and compassionate.

During the two and a half months that Joe spent at Middletown, he found camaraderie among the patients. They walked the grounds and threw footballs during the day; in the evenings, they played pinochle. Chaperoned excursions included a visit to the World's Fair in New York City. As Joe talked with the other patients, he learned that there were many reasons people were there. An older man named Ray had signed himself into Middletown hoping doctors could stop his sexual attraction to other men. Barry, just a year older than Joe, talked of drug-induced trips he'd experienced. Tony believed that miracles would happen when he made love to the sexy Italian actress Gina Lollobrigida. A boy about Joe's age had epilepsy. A 14-year-old boy was easily agitated and often had to be restrained by the orderlies.

Joe was assigned a soft-spoken psychiatrist whom he saw once a week. Although the doctor tried to get Joe to explain what he might have been thinking the night he held the gun to his grandmother's chest, Joe found it difficult to answer. He was shy, fearful, and quiet around strangers. It was hard for Joe to describe the bizarre thoughts he'd had. Yet Joe knew that the doctor held total power over him and that he would never leave the hospital unless the doctor said he could.

In addition to Thorazine, Joe was given fifteen electroconvulsive shock treatments over the course of three weeks. Joe noticed short-term memory loss immediately after each treatment but found that his memory returned to normal soon after the treatments ended.

In May 1964, when Joe was released from Middletown, he believed that the shock treatments had cured him and his troubles were behind him. Joe was wrong. He did not take the Thorazine as it had been prescribed because it reminded him that he had an illness. Besides, side effects from the medicines hampered Joe's athletic abilities. It wasn't long before Joe's psychotic thoughts returned, but he refused treatment and, because he was now older than 18, he could not be forced to return to Middletown. Joe worked a series of menial, low-paying jobs and drifted along, trying to keep his psychosis at bay.

Joe's second hospitalization, in 1968, also lasted for about two and a half months. This time the New York City policemen who had served as orderlies were no longer there. They had been replaced by drugs used to chemically restrain patients. Wards previously open were now locked. Group therapy had replaced individual therapy.

In 1979, when Joe had his third crisis, things were much different.

Joe had told Molly about his mental illness soon after he met her, but it hadn't stopped her from marrying him in 1975. Although Molly had not witnessed Joe's previous psychotic breaks, she recognized this break before Joe was willing to admit it. Desperate to get help for Joe, Molly went to the police. She didn't know where else to turn. The police said that nothing could be done unless Joe committed a crime. Frightened, Molly left Joe and moved in with a friend.

Joe wandered the streets of Tucson, where he and Molly had moved shortly after they had married. He believed himself to be many people, angels, and gods. When he decided that the girls in his Playboy magazine centerfolds were alive and trapped on the pages, he freed them by cutting around their images with a razor blade. Believing that a demon was hiding in his golf bag, Joe tore the golf bag apart, took it outside to the concrete landing at his front door, doused it with lighter fluid, and set it on fire.

Police called to the scene put Joe in handcuffs and took him to the Pima County Jail. There he was stripped, body cavity searched, and put in a cell, where he fell asleep. When Joe awoke, he hollered, took off his pants, and tried to pry open the cell door. The guards put him in restraints. The next morning, Joe was fingerprinted, charged with arson, and taken to the psychiatric ward of the local hospital. When doctors determined that Joe was not a danger to himself or others, he was returned to the jail. There he was kept in solitary confinement in a small cell with a steel door. Meals were delivered through a small opening at floor level. For nearly a month, Joe was given liquid Thorazine and bounced between the jail, where he spent twenty-one days, and the psychiatric ward, where he spent five days. The felony arson charges were dropped when Joe promised the judge he would take his medications.

Joe's experiences were typical of the way people with serious mental illnesses were treated at this time. In the span of just fifteen years, society's response to Joe's psychiatric crises had morphed from a compassionate two-and-a-half-month stay in a state hospital to a callous twenty-one-day jail stay combined with a five-day stay in a psychiatric hospital.

A decade later, here's what happened when Michelle needed crisis care.

It was July of 1989 when Michelle ran out of her house and danced unclothed on her neighbor's lawn furniture. Hearing her husband Tim's pleas for her to stop, she screamed, "Please call an ambulance. I need help." Tim convinced Michelle to put her clothes on as he led her back inside their house. The neighbors watched.

A policeman and two ambulance attendants responded to Tim's 911 call. Although Michelle had asked for help, when the rescue workers tried to help her, she became combative. In the chaos of the moment, Michelle broke the glass on her kitchen china cabinet. She grabbed the police officer's glasses and flung them across the room, sending them crashing into the stove. The ambulance attendants knocked Michelle to the floor, strapped her tightly to a backboard, and took her out to the waiting ambulance.

As the ambulance started to move, Michelle, restrained on the ambulance's gurney, said to the attendant, "Please open the doors and let me free." The bumpy ride upset Michelle, and she screamed at the driver, "What the hell are you doing? Don't you know how to drive this thing?" She lit into Tim as well. As thoughts of the devil and Jesus danced through her mind, Michelle's anger over being restrained grew. The ambulance raced toward Welborn Hospital.

The overhead lights leading from Welborn's emergency room to the psychiatric ward were harsh. In the psychiatric ward, Michelle felt a sharp pain in her right hip as a needle containing a sedative was jammed in. She fell into a deep sleep.

Michelle awakened slowly. Looking down, she saw that her wrists were shackled with thick brown straps of leather. Her body was stiff and sore. But the hallucinations, the rapid firing of religious ideas, and her fearful anxieties had ended. Once a nurse removed Michelle's physical restraints, she was free to sit in a large, well-lit common room.

Heavily sedated, Michelle slept for much of the next several days. As she improved, consistent with standard practice in psychiatric hospitals, Michelle was moved to a different place in the hospital. On the second floor, Michelle became friendly with some of the other patients. One, a middle-aged man who cried incessantly, was given shock therapy. Within five days, Michelle was well enough to move to the first floor. After she was released from the hospital six days later, Michelle visited her physician on a regular basis—first weekly, then every other week, then monthly, and then every six months. With the help of medication, Michelle's illness was controlled for five years. But she was not cured. Over the next twenty-three years, Michelle was hospitalized seven times, each stay lasting five to six days as her medications were adjusted.

In the fall of 2007, Sharon—the social worker with depression whom you met in chapter 2—had yet a different response to her crisis.

Sharon looked around the festive holiday table. As her family happily chatted with one another, Sharon considered ways to kill herself. Sharon could not stand living with her pain. She decided she would take an overdose of Ambien—the medication her doctor had prescribed to help Sharon sleep. Sharon would refill her prescription the next morning. Between those thirty pills and the fifteen in her medicine cabinet, Sharon figured her life would be over quickly. She would drive to the nearby summer camp, where she knew no one would find her, and swallow the pills.

"Sharon, please pass the brisket," her sister Mindy said.

Sharon thought about how the decision she'd made—to end her life—had brought her a sense of relief. She figured that her daughter Holly would be better off without her. Insurance money would more than compensate Holly's loss. Sharon knew Mindy would take care of Holly.

The next morning, Sharon called her friend Nicole and said, "I'm feeling better." Then, she called her friend Cindy and told her the same thing. Of course, Sharon was not feeling better, but she had made her decision to end her life and she didn't want anyone interfering with her plan.

At 11:00 the next morning, while Holly was watching television, Sharon put Holly's asthma medicine and $200 on the kitchen counter. She stopped at the drugstore and picked up her Ambien. Then, she drove to the camp.

Pulling into what she expected would be the camp's deserted parking lot, Sharon was surprised to see a crew of workmen dredging the lake. With the summer camp season over, the annual cleanup was well underway. The machinery hummed. Determined to complete her plan, Sharon backed up her car and drove to a nearby lake. It was a warm fall day, the leaves just beginning to change colors. Sharon spread a blanket on the ground, swallowed forty-five Ambien pills, lay down, and quickly fell asleep.

By 4:00 that afternoon, as Sharon's family gathered for a second festive meal, they realized Sharon was missing. Mindy called Sharon's cell phone. There was no answer. She called Sharon's friends. No one had heard from Sharon since the morning. When Sharon's nephew tried her cell phone a third time, Sharon answered, her voice weak and disoriented.

"Aunt Sharon, where are you?" he said.

"CVS—the drugstore by the lake," Sharon whispered before dropping the phone and drifting back to sleep.

When Sharon opened her eyes, she was in the intensive care unit (ICU) of the local hospital. Dazed, she said to herself, *Oh shit. I'm not dead. Now things are going to be even worse. I'll get fired. I won't be able to pay my bills. What will happen to Holly?*

Sharon's skin crawled. She was in severe physical pain, the result of too many Ambien.

Sharon was moved from the ICU to a regular room. A "sitter," whose job it was to make sure Sharon didn't try to kill herself again, never left her side. The sitter even followed Sharon to the bathroom.

In three days, Sharon was discharged from the local hospital and admitted to Friends Hospital, the private asylum founded in 1813 as The Asylum for Persons Deprived of the Use of Their Reason by the Quakers. However, the Friends Hospital that Sharon saw as she and Mindy entered the facility was not the Friends Hospital she'd read about in her social work training. Although the grounds were beautiful, the inside of the hospital was old and tired. The furniture was worn. Sharon wondered whether the awful smell came from the patients who looked like street people or from the walls themselves.

When it was time for Mindy to leave, Sharon cried, "Mindy, you can't leave me here!" Mindy realized bringing Sharon to Friends had been a big mistake the moment she walked into the hospital, but she didn't know how else to help her sister. Dejected, Mindy left the hospital.

A nurse took Sharon's shampoo away. She cut the strings off Sharon's robe.

That evening, Sharon sat alone in her room. The mattress was gray. A dresser was secured to the wall. The sole light came from a dim lightbulb screwed to the ceiling. The bathroom was down the hall. Sharon saw other patients walking the hall like zombies. She heard a scream. Terrified, Sharon spent the night dozing and reading a magazine. She wished she could lock herself in the room, but there was no lock on the door.

The next day, after Mindy had spent hours on the phone with the insurance company, Sharon was moved to a different behavioral health facility. While Sharon was not frightened there, she was determined to leave as soon as possible. She resented having to explain over and over—first to the intake worker, then to one nurse after the next, then to the doctor—what had led to her being admitted to the hospital. She didn't think she had anything in common with her 23-year-old roommate or the other patients. The doctor started Sharon on a new medication regimen, and Sharon started to feel better.

To the hospital social worker, Sharon said, "I promise I'll never try to kill myself again. I just want to go home. Yom Kippur is coming up. It's the holiest day of the year for Jewish people. I want to go to synagogue and ask God for forgiveness."

When Sharon returned home after seven days, she flipped through her mail. There, among the credit card bills and junk mail, she was surprised to find a summons ordering her to appear in court. Her crime? "Use of a controlled substance for a purpose other than treatment as prescribed by a physician." Sharon had been cited for ingesting too many Ambien in a public place. When the police who found Sharon in the park had completed their paperwork, issuing this summons was part of their standard operating procedure.

Charges were dismissed, but Sharon did have to appear in court.

Once Sharon was discharged from the hospital, she participated in a full-time intensive outpatient program for two weeks. This was followed by a four-week partial day program designed to teach coping skills.

Today's Mess

What sparked my interest in serious mental illness and led me to spend years doing the research for this book?

Between 2008 and 2011, my husband and I made a half-dozen trips to the emergency room of our local hospital as our daughter Sophie experienced one psychiatric crisis after the next. We made the first trip when Sophie jumped out of her second-story window and gashed her head. She had been sneaking out of the house to meet a man she had met on the internet. We made the other trips because my husband and I were frightened by Sophie's threats to harm herself. We went to the emergency room because, just like Senator Deeds, we did not know where else to take our psychotic child.

There are many reasons why families have trouble getting help for a loved one in crisis. One of the key reasons is the failure to replace closed psychiatric hospitals with the community-based clinics that President Kennedy had envisioned. In 1955, when state hospital beds were the dominant option for people with serious mental illness, the United States had 558,922 inpatient psychiatric beds in state hospitals. In 2014, state hospitals had only 37,209 inpatient psychiatric beds. General hospitals, private psychiatric hospitals, Veterans Affairs hospitals, and other specialty mental health centers had 64,142 inpatient beds. Now, the United States has fewer inpatient psychiatric hospital beds per capita than we had in 1850. Even more troubling, nearly half the psychiatric hospital beds that exist are occupied by forensic patients—people charged with or convicted of crimes. As psychiatric beds have been diverted to the forensic population, fewer beds are left for mentally ill people who have not committed crimes. These people—who, like Gus and Sophie, want help—are forced to wait in loud, chaotic hospital emergency rooms, sometimes for days. Each year, there are an estimated 800,000 emergency room visits in the United States in which symptoms of schizophrenia are the cause and 1.5 million visits where the presented problem is a mood disorder. Sometimes, people like Gus are sent home in crisis, creating life-threatening situations for them, their families, and their communities. Other times, people get treatment only when they get sick enough to commit crimes that send them to jail and then to a forensic psychiatric bed.

In 2015, Arica Nesper and her colleagues were awarded funding from the National Center for Advancing Translational Sciences, part of the National Institutes of Health, to examine the domino effects that ensue when access to inpatient and outpatient resources is restricted. They found that in 2009, Sacramento County eliminated fifty of its one hundred psychiatric beds and closed its outpatient crisis stabilization unit. Over just sixteen months, reduced treatment options in the county of 1.4 million people resulted in the tripling of psychiatric emergencies. The average time psychiatric patients spent in the emergency room increased from fourteen to twenty-two hours. The average number of psychiatric patients held in the emergency room longer than twenty-four hours skyrocketed from 28 to 322 per month. People with serious mental illnesses have fewer and fewer places to go.

Not only did deinstitutionalization increase demand on emergency rooms, but it also created an enormous homeless population. "Sidewalk psychotics" in every major city became stark evidence of inadequate networks of psychiatric clinics and halfway houses. People with mental illness ended up on the streets because there was no infrastructure to care for the hundreds of thousands of people who had been turned away from the state hospitals. The antipsychotic medications that had ushered in the wave of deinstitutionalization turned out to be less miraculous than originally conceived. By 1990 it was clear that the system had overreacted, that the closing of state hospitals had proceeded far too rapidly and without adequate alternatives in place. It was not wholesale closure that the state hospitals needed; it was reform—reducing the overcrowding, increasing the number of well-trained staff, and stopping the negligence and brutality—that was required.

In sum, today's situation is bleak. People with a serious mental illness who are in crisis experience long waits in loud, chaotic hospital emergency rooms. Many are either turned away or hospitalized for just a day or two—not nearly long enough to stabilize them. Some languish in jail. Others roam the streets of our cities, homeless. Clearly, these alternatives are ineffective.

A Path Forward

What should happen when people like Gus, Joe, Michelle, Sharon, and Sophie are in crisis?

Can we learn anything from a past in which people with mental illness were shackled to walls, jailed, and left to roam the streets?

I think we can.

Our past has taught us that people with serious mental illness should not be left to wander the streets. They should not be boarded in emergency rooms. They should not be locked in jail. This only makes things worse for sick people.

Our past teaches us that people with mental illness who are in crisis need care that is kind and effective. Thomas Bond and Benjamin Franklin knew that people with mental illness needed compassionate care. They envisioned the hospital as a sanctuary. But lack of treatment options resulted in patients being chained to the wall. There was nothing else to be done. The "moral treatment" model proposed by Pinel that guided the early private Quaker asylums like Friends Hospital—to provide refuge, protection, and sanctuary—was benevolent. In the absence of effective treatment, removing people from the rigors of urban life and providing them with a restful sojourn in a quiet, pastoral setting was a sound idea. The problem was that these facilities could not provide care to the growing numbers of people who needed it. Dorothea Dix's demand that people with mental illness not be left to rot in jail was kindhearted. However, her vision of compassionate, large state-run facilities was impractical. The deinstitutionalization movement that John Kennedy imagined and initiated was generous. He saw the horrible institutions for the failures they were and wanted to free people from their confines and send them back to their communities. But the failure to provide adequate care in the community made deinstitutionalization a disaster.

The goal of providing compassionate care to people with mental illness who are in crisis is still the right goal. However, the strategies for achieving this goal require rethinking the status quo.

What should we do?

First, we must recognize that when it comes to providing care for people with serious mental illnesses who are in crisis, situations are complex. Complex problems require complex responses. We need an array of solutions capable of meeting the challenges presented by individual circumstances so that care can be tailored to an individual's needs. Health care professionals call this "a continuum of care," a system that guides and tracks patients over time through a comprehensive array of services spanning all levels and intensity of care. We need adequate services in the community, short-term hospital beds, and long-term hospital beds. This is not an either-or issue. Some people in crisis can be managed with community services, others require short-term hospitalizations while medications are adjusted, and still others require care for longer periods of time in protective settings.

When people with mental illness are in crisis—often under the spell of delusions or hallucinations—they need to be in a place where they can't hurt themselves or anyone else. Hospitals are well equipped to serve this function. Hospitals employ health care professionals who can diagnose illnesses, monitor medications and other treatments, and ensure safety until a person is stabilized. This is the role hospitals play when people have health conditions such as stroke, heart failure, and cancer, and it is the role they must serve for people with mental illness.

Just as for patients with strokes, heart failure, and cancer, hospitals must be empowered to care for mentally ill people long enough to ensure that they are stable. While hospitals should not be expected to provide all the care required by patients, they must be enabled to help people through an acute crisis, ensuring that people with a serious mental illness are not a danger to themselves or other people. For many patients with serious mental illness, it takes two to three weeks for antipsychotic medications to reach a therapeutic level. Yet, in 2014, the average length of hospital stays following an acute psychotic episode was only seven days. The current model of very brief hospitalizations does not provide sufficient time to stabilize people in crisis.

In contrast, once the acute crisis passes and patients are stable, hospitals rarely are the best place for people with mental illness. Some communities have transitional facilities that provide a place for people to stay, especially when family or other supports are lacking. In transitional facilities, people can be monitored by nonmedical staff trained to administer medication, provided with transportation, and helped with daily life tasks. Although transitional facilities generally do not have a psychiatrist or nurse on-site, they often have these health care providers on call, available in the case of an emergency, a setback, or a crisis relapse. Transitional beds can serve as a hospital diversion or as a hospital step-down. For most mentally ill people in crisis, stays in transitional facilities should be short-term, typically less than four weeks.

While short-term hospitalization and transitional beds will likely serve the needs of most people with serious mental illness, others will be unable to function in the community, even with supports. This was the situation in which Clifford Beers found himself. For people like Beers, long-term hospitalizations are critical. The past teaches us that such care is best delivered in small, intimate environments—communities that can mimic family care. Overcrowding, understaffing, negligence, and brutality must never be tolerated. Rather, long-term hospital care should be delivered in places that are clean, well ventilated, calm, and quiet—places where people can learn to work and play and where social and vocational skills can be practiced. Staff and administrators must be compassionate, well-trained professionals dedicated to helping people live with mental illness and developing a sense of community. The goal of long-term hospitalization should be to stabilize and reintegrate people into the communities from which they came; long-term hospitalizations should never be life sentences.

For the small group of people with serious mental illness who consistently do not comply with voluntary treatment and have a long history of being homeless, arrested, or violent, assisted outpatient treatment (AOT) is needed. AOT allows judges to order people to time-limited treatment in the community in lieu of incarceration. But judges must follow due process before ordering AOT. This includes a medical examination, a legal hearing, and a thorough assessment of previous arrests, incarcerations, and hospitalizations. AOT plans can include case management services that monitor compliance, supported housing, psychotherapy, and substance abuse counseling. Often, patients need all of these services. Under AOT, judges also order the mental health system to provide the requisite treatment, and patients help develop the treatment plan. While a judge may require a person to take medication, the court order does not allow forcible administration of medicine. People who refuse to cooperate with AOT programs are often sent to prison. AOT programs have been praised for allowing intervention before a crisis rather than waiting until after a crisis occurs.

While having all these pieces in place is the first step toward progress, the second step is coordination and integration. If the pieces of the system operate in isolation, people in crisis will not be able to use them. For the system to be effective, well-coordinated links among the components are vital. Warm handoffs—transfer of care between members of the health care team that occurs with the patient and family present—engage patients, families, and professionals, bridging gaps that can occur in even the most comprehensive system. Services must be integrated and complementary so that people do not fall between the cracks.

Models for this kind of comprehensive, programmatic response to crisis have been widely implemented in Australia, Canada, and Europe. In Great Britain, for example, multidisciplinary teams of specially trained staff are available twenty-four hours a day. The teams promptly detect mentally ill people in crisis and initiate treatments, typically using a combination of medication, counseling, and practical help with living skills.

Once people are stabilized, the focus becomes helping them live with the chronic demands of serious mental illness. Preliminary research shows that the model is cost-effective and reduces hospital admissions.

In 2008, the National Institute of Mental Health initiated a research program in the United States known as Recovery After an Initial Schizophrenia Episode (RAISE). RAISE was created to improve the lives of people following an initial onset of schizophrenia through early intervention. As part of RAISE, a comprehensive, multidisciplinary, team-based treatment approach for first-episode psychosis was developed. This program, known as NAVIGATE, helps people access services in the community that can promote management of psychotic symptoms. NAVIGATE is based on the view that recovery from the onset of schizophrenia is possible through the use of carefully monitored medication, family education, individual resiliency training, and supported education and employment.

A large randomized controlled trial involving thirty-four clinics in twenty-one states compared the NAVIGATE program to customary community services, following participants for up to two years. During that time, people receiving NAVIGATE services experienced greater improvement in quality of life and less psychopathology than people receiving customary services. They were also more likely to be involved in work and school than those not receiving NAVIGATE services. Rates of hospitalization were relatively low and did not differ between people receiving NAVIGATE and those receiving customary community services. In short, NAVIGATE looks to be a promising step in the right direction. In fact, a model like NAVIGATE could be adapted beyond first-episode schizophrenia and made available to people with other serious mental illness.

Finally, good crisis care requires that we pay attention not only to people with serious mental illness but also to their families. When individuals with mental illness are in the midst of a crisis, families are often the first to know. Yet most families do not understand these illnesses. Many family members could benefit from learning about what serious mental illnesses are and how they can help when their loved ones are in crisis. As the linchpin of care, families need help negotiating changing roles and securing support for their own well-being during a time that can be extremely stressful.

What to Do When a Family Member Is in Crisis

It may be years, if ever, before optimal crisis care is widely available. Meanwhile, millions of people will have psychiatric crises. What should you do if a family member with mental illness is experiencing a crisis?

The best way to help someone in crisis is to become familiar with the resources available in your community. Because the best time to learn about these resources is before a crisis unfolds, it is important to familiarize yourself with community resources now. Create a crisis plan. Have a list of phone numbers for health care providers and make sure this information is readily available. Know what medications have been prescribed and whether they are being taken as directed. Find out whether there is a mobile crisis unit in your community and whether police officers have been trained to respond to people with mental illness. The biggest mistake most people make is heading for the emergency room of a local hospital. Waits can be long and psychiatric care poor. The chaotic environment of an emergency room can exacerbate a mental health crisis, and unless someone is suicidal, a hospital admission is unlikely.

Next, it is important to recognize the warning signs that a crisis is brewing. Increased stress, physical illness, problems at work or school, changes in family situations, trauma, violence, and substance abuse can lead to a crisis. Often family or friends see changes in a person's behavior that indicate an impending crisis. Warning signs include inability to cope with daily tasks, rapid mood swings, increased agitation, abusive behavior, and decreased interest in school, work, or recreational activities. Some people may lose touch with reality. They may express strange ideas, appear confused, or seem disoriented. They may say they're hearing voices or seeing things that aren't there.

When you see such warning signs, your inclination may be to try to cheer up the person. Don't. Instead, acknowledge their pain and let them talk about it. A comment such as "It sounds like life is really tough now. I'm here for you if you want to talk" is much more helpful than a comment like "It's not so bad. Look at all the good things in your life." Use "I" sentences to let the person know that you're worried and why. For example, "I'm worried about you because you've stopped doing your homework." Avoid "you" comments such as "You don't seem to want to listen to anybody."

As you assess the situation, don't be afraid to ask the person whether she is having suicidal thoughts. Questions such as "Are you thinking about killing yourself?" or "Have you thought about killing yourself?" are appropriate. There is a commonly held belief that asking people about suicide increases the likelihood that they will consider it or attempt it. However, when scholars from King's College in London reviewed thirteen studies published between 2001 and 2013, they found that none of the studies supported this commonly held belief. In fact, the researchers found that acknowledging and talking about suicide may reduce thoughts of suicide and lead to improvements in mental health. If you find that a person is having suicidal thoughts, ask follow-up questions that will give you the answers to what their plans are. It is easier to prevent a crisis when you know the specifics. You will not trigger a suicide just by asking about it.

If someone with a mental illness talks about death (e.g., "It would be better for everyone if I were dead," or "I wish I were dead"), it is important to ask follow-up questions. Answers to questions such as "Have you made a plan?" and "How are you thinking about ending your life?" will enable you to determine whether the person is in danger.

If a family member is in danger of hurting themselves or someone else, emergency assistance is needed. As you seek help, empathize with the person, stay calm, and try to de-escalate the crisis. Keep your voice composed and try not to overreact. Listen to the person and express support and concern. Do not try to argue or reason with the person. Do not try to fix the problem. Offer options, but don't take control. Give the person space, but do not leave them alone.

If you do not believe that the person is in immediate danger and the person has a psychiatrist, therapist, or physician, call that provider. The professional should be able to help assess the situation, offer advice, schedule an appointment, or even have the person admitted to a hospital without having to go first to an emergency room.

If someone is in crisis and you cannot reach a professional, call the National Suicide Prevention Lifeline (1-800-273-8255), where trained crisis workers are available twenty-four hours a day, seven days a week. The call, which is confidential, goes to the nearest crisis center, which can provide crisis counseling and mental health referrals. If your community has a mobile crisis response team, it may be dispatched to conduct a mental health crisis assessment and develop a treatment plan. If the mental health crisis team determines the person to be in immediate danger to themselves or others, the crisis team will refer the situation to 911, and law enforcement will respond. If the situation is not urgent, the team will assess the level of intervention needed and respond accordingly. Alternatively, you can text HOME to 741741—the Crisis Text Line—which provides access to free 24/7 support and information from trained crisis counselors.

If safety is a concern—if you believe that the person is likely to harm him- or herself or someone else, or if serious property damage is occurring—call 911. However, make sure to tell the operator that this is a mental health emergency. Be as specific as you can about the behaviors you are seeing. Instead of saying, "My sister is behaving strangely," say, "My sister hasn't slept in three days, she hasn't eaten in over five days, and she believes that someone is talking to her through the television." Report any threats made, as well as any manic or agitated behaviors. Describe what is going on right now, not what happened a year ago. Alerting the operator that this is a mental health crisis increases the likelihood that he or she will send an officer who knows how to respond to a person in crisis. Be sure to alert the operator if the person has a gun, knife, or other weapon.

When the police officer arrives, provide as much relevant and concise information as possible. Tell the officer about any diagnoses, medications, and hospitalizations, as well as any history of violence. However, know that once an officer arrives on the scene, he or she will assess the situation and determine next steps. The officer—who may know very little about best practices for people with mental illness—will decide whether the person should be taken to jail or to a hospital emergency room.

If the decision is made to take someone with mental illness who is in crisis to the emergency room, be sure to bring a list of the medications and dosages the person is taking. Develop a summary of the person's previous hospitalizations and bring that with you too. Be prepared to wait for hours, perhaps even days. Bringing reading material, music, electronic games, or other distractions may help the person in crisis stay as calm as possible. Emergency rooms are busy places that prioritize life-threatening issues such as heart attacks and strokes over mental illnesses. Bringing someone to the emergency room does not guarantee admission to the hospital. If the person is not admitted and the crisis worsens when you return home, do not be afraid to call the crisis number again. A crisis response team will reassess the situation and make recommendations or referrals based on the current situation. A hospital admission may be more likely on a second visit to the emergency room, especially if the visits are within hours or days of one another.

People with serious mental illness who are in the midst of crisis—like Gus was the day before he shot himself to death—are at their most vulnerable. History has shown us both how families and communities should respond and how they should not.

Now it's up to us to do the right thing.

CHAPTER 4

New Normal

THE AFTERNOON OF my daughter Sophie's high school prom, I took her to our favorite beauty shop so she could have her hair and nails done. The shop was filled with Sophie's friends and their mothers. As the stylists swept hair into braided updos, messy twists, and elegant low buns, the girls chatted about nail polish colors and boys. The mothers wondered aloud where the time had gone as they sipped their coffees.

Watching this normal rite of passage, I thought about all the challenges Sophie and I had faced in the past twelve months. When the doctor had diagnosed Sophie with bipolar disorder in the spring of her junior year of high school, her life changed. Mine did too. We entered a world that challenged us to secure care from competent doctors whom Sophie liked. Our new world defied us to find treatment regimens that controlled Sophie's mania without making her so groggy that she could not stay awake in school. As if these challenges were not enough, I worried about how much to tell people—relatives, friends, the school counselor, even Sophie's younger brother—about her illness.

But those experiences had been mixed with the usual trials and joys of the senior year of high school. We had visited a dozen colleges. Sophie had completed her college applications and was accepted by her first-choice school. She had designed and made her prom dress. She had gotten a part-time job at a grocery store.

So much normal. And so much not.

I smiled and waved as one of the mothers, a long-time friend, walked toward me. Hugging her, I knew that neither she nor any of the other mothers watching their daughters transform into fairy princesses had any idea what hell I'd been through. I had, after all, gone out of my way to hide Sophie's illness. Then I wondered which of these women, all of whom looked quite normal to me, had had their lives turned upside down and their hearts broken by the ravages of mental illness. Mental illnesses are the most hidden of illnesses. What secrets were these women keeping about mental illness? From the statistics I knew about mental illness and secret keeping, I figured that the beauty shop, with about sixty people in it, probably included a few other women whose experiences were like mine. But I had no idea who they were.

Doctors, Drugs, and Disclosure

My family's experiences dealing with serious mental illness are not unique. Once diagnosed, people with a mental illness and their families face three major challenges: (1) finding health care providers, (2) identifying treatment regimens that can quell the symptoms of mental illness, and (3) deciding what to tell people. This chapter explains the history of each issue and offers strategies that people with mental illness and their families may find helpful as they learn to live with a serious mental illness.

Doctors

It's Hard to Find Good Help

When Sophie was 11 and it was clear she was having trouble staying focused and paying attention, finding competent care had been easy. I had told the pediatrician that Sophie could not sit still, that she blurted out whatever she was thinking, and that she could not wait her turn, both at home and at school. The pediatrician diagnosed attention deficit and hyperactivity disorder and put Sophie on Strattera, a selective norepinephrine reuptake inhibitor that improves the way the brain sends and receives messages. However, when Sophie was nearly 13 and I told her pediatrician that Sophie had been cutting her skin, had been pulling the hair out of her head, and had stolen her cousin's cell phone, the pediatrician told me that Sophie needed more help than she could provide. She told me that Sophie should be seeing a psychiatrist, a medical doctor specializing in diagnosing and treating mental illnesses, and she gave me the names of five psychiatrists to call.

Working my way through the pediatrician's list, I came face-to-face with one of the biggest challenges of mental illness— finding good care. The first three psychiatrists I called were not taking new patients. One receptionist offered to put Sophie on her waiting list but told me it was likely that an appointment would not be available for at least six months. I had better luck getting an appointment with the fourth psychiatrist. However, after her first appointment with him, Sophie said he was "creepy" and refused to see him again. I knew that even if this guy were the best psychiatrist in the world, he was wrong for Sophie. If she couldn't trust him, nothing he would say or do would help Sophie. The fifth psychiatrist on the pediatrician's list, Dr. Kane, a nearly 70-year-old woman with a warm Spanish accent, was the winner. Sophie liked her. Dr. Kane quickly put Sophie at ease and added Concerta, a central nervous system simulant often used for ADHD, to the Strattera Sophie was taking.

As we were leaving the office, Dr. Kane told me that Sophie would benefit from talking with a therapist—either a clinical psychologist or social worker. She explained that, as a psychiatrist, she would see Sophie once a month to manage her medications. With the therapist, Sophie would be able to discuss her insecurities and develop strategies to gain control over her impulsive behaviors. I did not understand how this division of labor—where it was the psychiatrist's job to tinker with the chemicals and the therapist's responsibility to counsel the patient—could work. How could separating these intertwined functions help Sophie or any other patient? At best, it seemed an inefficient process; at worst, it was unlikely to help sick people. I was even more skeptical when I asked Dr. Kane for the names of the therapists she usually worked with and she said, "It would be better for you to find someone on your own." Dr. Kane said there would be little if any communication between her and the therapist. She said the insurance company would not pay for it. Of course, doctors deserve to be paid for their time and efforts. But I wondered why insurance companies would not think communication among providers important enough to pay for. I would have looked for another psychiatrist, but I already knew enough about the system to realize I was lucky to have found a doctor who had appointments available and whom Sophie liked.

Mobilizing my resources and capitalizing on my job at a medical school, I identified a dozen possible therapists. I phoned their offices, but one receptionist after the next told me either that the doctor was not accepting new patients or that the next available appointment was more than six months away. None billed insurance. Even though my employer provided excellent health insurance, I would be responsible for paying for treatment and filing paperwork for reimbursement that might or might not be forthcoming. Initial fees for a one-hour consultation in my community ranged from $400 to $700; the cost of subsequent visits for each fifty-minute hour of therapy ranged from $150 to $250. We chose a therapist but quickly stopped seeing her when it became clear that she was unable to keep Sophie from monopolizing the sessions with talk about her desire for a nose job and breast implants instead of explaining why she was stealing things and pulling out her hair. Sophie refused to talk to the second therapist.

Sophie was 13-and-a-half when she scratched "I HATE ME" into her arm and told her friends she was planning to kill herself. Worried, her friends took Sophie to the school counselor, who summoned me to his office. Scrunching his eyebrows, the counselor said, "Sophie really should be talking to someone." I told him I knew that and had been looking for a therapist for months but had been unsuccessful in finding anyone. When I asked him if there was someone he could recommend, he shook his head and said, "No." Dr. Kane added the antidepressant Zoloft to Sophie's regimen of Strattera and Concerta.

At 15-and-a-half, Sophie tied sheets to her bedpost and snuck out of the house in the middle of the night. She returned with a bloody two-inch gash across the back of her head. Dr. Kane added Lamictal, an antiepileptic that she said would help stabilize Sophie's mood, to her medicinal cocktail of Strattera, Concerta, and Zoloft. The doctor said Sophie's behavior suggested she was deeply troubled. She reminded me that her job was to make sure Sophie was properly medicated and that it was up to me to find Sophie a therapist with whom she could discuss her feelings and problems. I had never felt like such a failure. I reminded Dr. Kane of our two unsuccessful therapeutic relationships and asked again whether there was a therapist she could recommend. I wasn't surprised when she had no one to suggest. It was the same thing she had told me months ago.

My husband Josh and I looked for a therapist for nearly six months. Finally, shortly before Sophie turned 16, we found Dr. Shuman. Yet even with weekly therapy sessions and medication, Sophie's impulsive behaviors continued. She had sex with several high school boys, and she often reeked of marijuana. The principal expelled Sophie from school after she had a hair-pulling fight with a girl. Dr. Kane changed Sophie's medications again. This time, she swapped Strattera and Concerta for Vyvanse, a stimulant often used for ADHD, while continuing Sophie on Lamictal and Zoloft. Sophie was taking this medical cocktail when Josh and I discovered her making plans to run away with a 28-year-old man she'd met on the internet who said he was madly in love with her. Then, Sophie was admitted to a psychiatric hospital.

Why Is It So Hard to Find Mental Health Providers?
Psychiatrists are the mainstay for diagnosing and treating serious mental illnesses since they have both the medical training and legal authority to prescribe medications. Yet few psychiatrists are available to people with serious mental illnesses, especially those who receive services in public community mental health centers and those who rely on Medicaid.

Finding a psychiatrist and a therapist for Sophie was difficult because there is a shortage of mental health providers in the United States. Between 2003 and 2013, the average number of psychiatrists per 100,000 people decreased by almost 10 percent. A 2018 report by Merritt Hawkins, a physician search and consulting firm, finds that there are 30,451 psychiatrists in the United States. More than 50 percent of people in the United States live in communities that do not have enough practitioners. Of course, this shortage is not evenly distributed across the country. The top most populous states—California, New York, and Texas—are home to 31.1 percent of psychiatrists. In all of Wyoming, there are only thirty-two psychiatrists.

Because my daughter was a teenager, I was looking for an even rarer bird—a psychiatrist with experience caring for children and adolescents. Like psychiatrists who treat adults, those caring for children and adolescents go to medical school and study four years of general psychiatry. But in addition, child and adolescent psychiatrists must complete a two-year fellowship. There are only 8,300 child and adolescent psychiatrists in the United States, far short of the 12,624 that are needed. In New Jersey, where I live, there are sixteen child and adolescent psychiatrists for every 100,000 children, yet forty-seven child and adolescent psychiatrists for every 100,000 children are needed.

This shortage of psychiatrists is only likely to get worse. Psychiatrists, on average, are among the oldest doctors in the United States. Nearly 60 percent of practicing psychiatrists are 55 years of age or older and will retire in the next several years. Medical training programs are subsidized by the federal government, which established a cap on funding for training psychiatrists in 1997 that continues to restrict the number of new psychiatrists entering the workforce. As such, many retiring psychiatrists will not be replaced. Finding a psychiatrist will only get more difficult.

Other health professionals—behavioral health nurse practitioners; behavioral health physician assistants; clinical, counseling, and school psychologists; substance abuse and behavioral disorder counselors; mental health and substance abuse social workers; mental health counselors; and school guidance counselors—have been trained to provide care to people with mental illnesses but lack the licensing rights in most states to prescribe medications. Some states allow behavioral health nurse practitioners and behavioral health physician assistants to prescribe medication under the supervision of a physician. In New Mexico, Louisiana, Illinois, and Iowa, licensed psychologists (health care professionals with a PhD or PsyD and extensive training in diagnosis, management of mental illness, and psychopharmacology) have the authority to write prescriptions for psychotropic medications. In Colorado, psychiatric nurse practitioners can prescribe medications independently. While diversity in the workforce increases the number of professionals to whom people with serious mental illness and their families can turn, national projections reveal that there will be serious shortages for all of these practitioners by 2025.

Shortages of mental health providers led a group of researchers from the University of Colorado School of Medicine to question how likely a person with depression who wanted treatment and had private insurance would be to secure an appointment with a psychiatrist, a psychologist, or a licensed clinical social worker. Researchers made scripted telephone calls to all behavioral health providers within twenty miles of Denver listed in the online directories of the three largest insurance providers in Colorado. Of all calls made, 11.5 percent resulted in an appointment with a psychiatrist. The likelihood of securing an appointment with a psychologist (43.3%) and a licensed clinical social worker (52.1%) was greater. Another study in which researchers posed as parents seeking care for their 14-year-old daughter in Ohio found that the median wait time for an appointment with a child and adolescent psychiatrist was fifty days, although wait times were as long as 345 days.

Dr. Kane, Sophie's psychiatrist, accepted insurance. I did not realize then how fortunate I was. Between 2005 and 2010, the percentage of psychiatrists in the United States who accepted insurance decreased from 72.3 to 55.3 percent. Fewer than half of all psychiatrists accepted Medicaid, although the numbers were stable over time (49.3% in 2005 vs. 43.1% in 2010). A 2017 report from the National Council Medical Director Institute found that psychiatrists who practice exclusively in cash-only private practices represent 40 percent of the workforce, the second-highest cash-only medical specialty, trailing dermatology. Most psychologists, like the three who treated Sophie and the other dozen I called, do not accept insurance. Mental health professionals who do not accept insurance have made this decision because (1) reimbursement rates offered by insurance companies do not cover actual costs, (2) the time spent submitting bills and waiting for reimbursement is very long, and (3) they believe that it is in patients' best interest for them, rather than insurance companies, to determine the length and type of therapy.

Strategies for Finding a Good Provider

Finding a well-qualified mental health professional is not easy, but it is the key to getting good care. Finding a suitable mental health professional will take perseverance and many phone calls. Most likely, you will need more than one mental health provider, a psychiatrist who can manage medications and a psychologist or other therapist for counseling. Ideally, you will want to find a group of providers working together, but that is very rare.

The first challenge is to identify a professional who has experience caring for people with serious mental illness and is licensed to prescribe medications. Here are some strategies to help you find these people:

- Start with your family doctor, internist, or pediatrician. If you do not already have a diagnosis, these primary care providers can tell you whether the symptoms you or your family member are experiencing might indicate the need to consult a psychiatrist. If your local doctor does suggest that you or your loved one needs a mental health professional, he or she should be able to suggest local people who can help you. If you (or the person with mental illness) were hospitalized following a crisis, talk to the hospital psychiatrist and discharge social worker.

They should be able to refer you to community practitioners.

- Network among family, trusted friends, neighbors, and clergy. Ask them to give you contact information for any people in the medical field whom they know. Ask people in your network about home health aides, pharmacists, lab technicians, emergency medical technicians, physical therapists, occupational therapists, physician assistants, social workers, and nursing assistants, as well as doctors and nurses. Do not forget about medical students and other professionals in training. You never know whom people know. Then, contact these people and ask them whom they would turn to if one of their family members had a serious mental illness.

- If you live near a medical school, call the psychiatry department and ask for a recommendation to one of their doctors.

- If you are a college student, contact the student health center and ask for a referral.

- Find your local National Alliance on Mental Illness (NAMI) group by looking at their website (https://www
.nami.org/find-support/living-with-a-mental-health
-condition/finding-a-mental-health-professional). Call the local NAMI president and ask whether they can recommend a provider. You might also consider joining a local NAMI support group. This will give you the opportunity to meet and network with other people in your community who have had to find mental health providers.

- Find your local Mental Health America affiliate by looking at their website (http://www
.mentalhealthamerica.net/find-affiliate). The contact person should be aware of local providers.

- The *Psychology Today* website is a user-friendly source for identifying local licensed psychiatrists (https://www.psychologytoday.com/us/psychiatrists) as well as psychologists, social workers, and other counselors (https://www.psychologytoday.com/us/therapists). Enter your zip code. You will be able to screen providers by type of insurance accepted (more than forty private insurance companies are included, as are Medicaid and Medicare), diagnoses they specialize in (e.g., depression, bipolar disorder, schizophrenia), and types of therapy practiced. On the site, you will learn about the provider's location, educational background, experience, therapeutic approach, specialty, and cost of services. Some providers include information about other professionals with whom they work.

As you develop your list of providers, make a spreadsheet to help you stay organized. Include the provider's name, phone number, and address. Be sure to keep track of how you found each provider (e.g., from NAMI, your pediatrician, your neighbor's sister). Make note of providers you learn about from multiple sources. This may turn out to be important information, as consensus can build credibility.

Research each provider on websites like ZocDoc and Vitals. Read what other people say, but take both positive and negative comments with a grain of salt, as there are many factors that drive opinions about providers.

Next, call each provider's office. Ask whether the provider is taking new patients, whether he or she accepts your insurance, and how he or she is licensed (psychiatrist, psychologist). Ask whether the provider has experience treating patients with serious mental illness and treating patients your age. Add this information to your spreadsheet.

If the provider is taking new patients, accepts your insurance, and has experience treating people like you, make the first available appointment. This appointment may be months out. However, if you find an earlier appointment with someone else, you can always cancel. Ask to be put on the provider's wait list, should an earlier appointment become available.

Your first visit to a mental health provider is an opportunity to see whether there is a good fit between you and the provider. Be honest about what you are hoping for from the provider. Ask questions, and let the provider's answers guide your next question. Your goal is to be able to make an informed choice and get the care you need. Here are some questions you should consider asking psychiatrists and psychologists:

- Have you worked with people with schizophrenia / bipolar disorder / depression?
- How will we work together to establish goals and evaluate my progress?
- How do you typically work with people like me? How often will we meet? Will it be difficult for me to get follow-up appointments? Can I call or e-mail between appointments if I need to talk?
- What kind of improvements can I expect to see in my health?
- Do you work alone or with other mental health providers? If I need counseling/medication, are there therapists/physicians you would recommend?
- Do you communicate with and include family members in your treatment plans?
- What medications for schizophrenia / bipolar disorder / depression have you found to be particularly helpful?

When you leave the appointment, ask yourself whether you feel comfortable with the provider. Do not be discouraged if the first provider, even someone with a great reputation, does not feel right for you. If this happens, move on to the next person and keep looking. Remember, you are recruiting someone who can help with your treatment long-term.

Here is some additional information I learned along the way regarding paying for mental health care:

- If you are concerned about your ability to meet insurance co-pays or deductibles, let the provider know as soon as possible. Some providers allow payment on a sliding scale or at a discount.

- If the provider you want to see does not accept insurance and you have pretax dollars in your Health Savings Account or Flexible Spending Account, consider using these funds to pay for therapy.

- Visits to a psychologist or psychiatrist may be tax deductible when paid out of pocket. However, this same rule does not apply to a mental health counselor or social worker visits unless you are receiving psychoanalysis. The IRS website shows all currently available tax-deductible medical expenses.

- Some private insurance companies allow you to pay a therapist directly and submit a statement to your insurance for reimbursement. Check with your insurance company.

Finally, family members often accompany the person with mental illness to appointments with health care providers. Sometimes family members fear talking about their loved one in front of that person and so end up not transmitting critical information. Here are some ideas about how family members can make sure health care providers are well-informed and best positioned to help:

- Ask the health provider for a private conversation. The provider may not be receptive to this if time is limited, or if the patient is his or her own legal decision-maker.

- If a conversation is not possible, write the provider a letter. Include details about the patient's past, as well as your concerns. Remember that, while Health Insurance Portability and Accountability Act (HIPAA) laws limit what health providers can tell family members, they do not limit what family members can tell the providers.

Drugs

Treatment, Not Cure

According to Irish lore, there was an enchanted well in Gleann na nGealt. Located deep in the valley west of the village of Camp on County Kerry's Dingle Peninsula, natives called the well "Tobar na nGealt"—"The Well of the Insane." When people who were raving mad drank from the well and ate the watercress growing in its waters, they stopped their wild rants. Locals attributed the well's mysterious healing powers to compassionate fairies. The cure was short lasting, however. By the time people walked from the valley back to their homes in Camp, they were no longer lucid.

In 2012, a team of scientists led by Dr. Henry Lyons of the Tralee Institute of Technology traveled to Gleann na nGealt to learn whether there was more to the well's repute than fairy myth. The well water did indeed have healing powers. Results from dozens of water samples confirmed that the water contained 55.6 parts per billion of the chemical lithium, levels much higher than found in samples from nearby wells. Consistent with more than seventy years of scientific evidence, the scientists concluded that the healing powers of Tobar na nGealt were far more likely due to its water's elevated lithium concentration than to the magic of fairies.

Serious mental illnesses, including schizophrenia, bipolar disorder, and depression, are treatable but not curable. While today's treatments are a far cry from those of the mid-1900s—

insulin coma, convulsive therapies, lobotomies, and sedatives such as barbiturates—their purpose remains the same: to ease the symptoms, not cure the underlying disease. Unfortunately, there are no magic bullets that make these illnesses go away— no penicillin or sulfa that can cure an infection. Moreover, we lack surefire tests to determine whether someone has any of these illnesses—no blood tests, no urine tests, and no X-rays that confirm diagnosis. Treatments used for serious mental illness— whether they be medications like antipsychotics or antidepressants, brain stimulation techniques like electroconvulsive therapy and transcranial magnetic stimulation, or talk-based remedies like cognitive behavioral therapy and psychotherapy— though far from perfect, work for most people if they are used continuously. When people stop treatment, their delusions, hallucinations, wild mood swings, and deep depressions generally come crashing back with a vengeance.

Failure to distinguish treatment of mental illnesses from cure has harmed patients as well as society. In 1951, Henri Laborit, a surgeon in the French navy, hoped to find a drug that would keep his patients from feeling pain while maintaining consciousness, a drug without the dangers of morphine and barbiturates. Experimenting with a surgical anesthetic called chlorpromazine, Laborit discovered that it not only was a powerful anesthetic but also induced a "euphoric quietude." Patients did not lose consciousness; instead, they became sleepy and apathetic and lost interest in what was happening around them. Thinking that the tranquilizer might be beneficial for people with mental illnesses, Laborit urged psychiatrists at Val de Grace, the military hospital in Paris, to try treating their patients with it.

Jacques Lh., a 24-year-old man admitted to the hospital on January 17, 1952, with severe manic agitation, was the first person with psychosis treated with chlorpromazine. No stranger to Val de Grace, Jacques Lh. had a long history as a patient. Each hospitalization brought treatment with electroconvulsive shock, anesthetics such as Pentothal, or insulin injections. However, his remissions were short-lived. Desperate to help Lh., his doctors agreed to try chlorpromazine. Two days after being admitted to the hospital, Lh. received an intramuscular injection of Dolosal, a painkiller with sedative effects, and fifty milligrams of chlorpromazine. He slept at times and was responsive when he was awake. Lh.'s calm lasted eighteen hours. The calm was followed by return to a violent, agitated state that lasted until he received a second injection of chlorpromazine. For twelve days, the treatment continued with similar results. Then, the periods of calm increased markedly and the intervals of agitation became shorter and less violent. Lh. stopped tearing his sheets and trying to burn his blankets. He no longer put flowerpots on his head. He stopped giving passionate speeches about the loss of liberty on Pluto. Twenty days after Jacques Lh. was admitted, the chlorpromazine he had been given made him fit for a normal life. The hospital released him, and he never again presented for treatment at Val-de-Grace. But this does not mean that he was cured.

Physicians using chlorpromazine with other people with schizophrenia reported similar findings. Catatonic patients—who had immobile, unresponsive stupors—responded almost immediately; others took days or weeks to respond. Patients who had been silent for years suddenly spoke. Patients who had been unmoving for decades suddenly started walking. Patients whose screams had once filled the hospital wards calmed and lucidly talked to staff. Scientists shared their findings at meetings and published results in medical journals. In 1952, the drug company Rhône-Poulenc released chlorpromazine as Largactil (meaning "large action"—a drug for many different needs and states) in France.

The United States was slower to embrace the new drug, largely because dominating psychoanalytic beliefs attributed mental illnesses to bad mothering or repressed sexual desires. Most private practice psychiatrists believed that psychoanalysis, not drugs, was the best treatment for mental illness. Unlike psychiatrists in private practice, the state asylum directors embraced the drug, marketed in 1954 as an anti-nausea medicine called Thorazine. The asylum directors watched as Thorazine transformed patients who were wildly psychotic into cooperative patients. Word spread quickly, as straitjackets and lobotomies became unnecessary. By 1964, some 50 million people around the world had taken the drug.

This medication, known scientifically as chlorpromazine and marketed in the United States as Thorazine, was a major advance over existing treatments for serious mental illnesses. Not only did Thorazine revolutionize the atmosphere of psychiatric hospitals, improve staff morale, and create optimism among family members, but it also made it possible for people with these illnesses to live outside a psychiatric hospital. Because care in the community was much less expensive than care in psychiatric hospitals, federal and state governments quickly began shifting funds away from institutions.

However, failure to distinguish Thorazine's ability to treat the symptoms of mental illness from its ability to cure the diseases helped fuel the disastrous deinstitutionalization movement described in the previous chapter. Thorazine was a treatment, not a cure. Once many of the hospitalized people treated with Thorazine were back in their communities, where they no longer followed the strict medication regimens of the institutions, the symptoms of their illnesses returned, just as they had for the Irishmen from Camp who had sipped the waters of Tobar na nGealt. Additionally, many patients had a minimal response to the drug. Others relapsed even after a good response. Some became jaundiced. A number of female patients experienced lactation and false pregnancies. Several patients experienced rigid muscle movements and awkward gaits. This side effect, known as "tardive dyskinesia," ended Thorazine's popularity. Today, Thorazine, the drug once hailed as miraculous, is rarely prescribed.

Serendipitous Findings

Thorazine was not the only psychotropic medication to follow a serendipitous path to discovery. In 1955, Miltown was developed by accident as Frank Belger worked out a method of preserving penicillin. Miltown was marketed as a "minor tranquilizer" and used to treat anxiety among community-dwelling people. That same year, Roland Kuhn, a 43-year-old Swiss psychiatrist working in a psychiatric hospital in the remote Swiss village of Munsterlingen, discovered the antipsychotic effects of chlorpromazine. Working with a drug company that hoped to develop other compounds that would have the antipsychotic effects of chlorpromazine without its side effects, Kuhn tried a new compound that had antihistamine as its base—imipramine. He gave the drug to two hundred patients with schizophrenia and one hundred patients with depression. Although imipramine had little effect on the psychotic symptoms of patients with schizophrenia, Kuhn noted that forty depressed patients responded well to imipramine. Within several weeks, patients "became livelier... more communicative... friendly, content. Patients who had great difficulties in getting up in the morning, get out of bed early with their own initiative.... They initiate relationships with other people, participate in the daily life of the clinic, write letters, and are again interested in family matters." In 1957, researchers noted that patients given Marsilid (iproniazid), a tuberculosis treatment, became excessively happy, and so they began giving the medication to people who were depressed. Scientists did not understand how these drugs worked, but they saw the drugs blunt disturbing symptoms. Even today, new psychotropic medicines follow a similar pattern of development: drugs are discovered, often by chance, and then we figure out who can benefit from them.

When scientists realized that psychotropic medications affected chemical levels in the brain, they began attributing mental illnesses to chemical imbalances. Because Thorazine lowered dopamine levels, researchers hypothesized that schizophrenia was caused by too much dopamine. Because lithium calmed people with bipolar disorder, researchers thought that people experiencing mania might have a deficiency of lithium. Because antidepressants increase serotonin levels, researchers suspected that depression might be caused by too little serotonin. Instead of developing drugs to combat abnormalities, as is typically done, abnormalities were postulated after the fact to explain reactions to drugs. While it is plausible that drugs affecting neurotransmitter levels could relieve symptoms, many scientists have suggested that it is equally possible that the drugs would relieve symptoms even if the neurotransmitters had nothing to do with the illness in the first place.

Some scientists have gone even further, suggesting that psychotropic drugs may cause rather than cure a chemical imbalance. In 1996, Stephen Hyman, former director of the National Institute of Mental Health and a neuroscientist, said, "All psychotropic drugs cause perturbations in neurotransmitter functions." Robert Whitaker, a journalist and finalist for the Pulitzer Prize for Public Service, popularized the idea that serotonin and dopamine may cause, rather than treat, chemical imbalances. His best-selling book *Anatomy of an Epidemic* seeded the argument that people should avoid psychotropic medications at all costs.

We do not understand much about how and why medications soothe the symptoms of mental illnesses. The bigger problem, however, is that we do not understand what causes illnesses such as schizophrenia, bipolar disorder, and depression. Until we understand the cause of these illnesses, it is not likely that we will find cures.

Today's Treatments

Though we lack cures for serious mental illnesses, we are not at a loss for treatments that can help manage the symptoms of serious mental illness. There are antipsychotics like Zyprexa, Risperdal, Seroquel, and Abilify. There are mood stabilizers like lithium, Depakote, Tegretol, and Lamictal. There are antidepressants like Prozac, Cymbalta, and Wellbutrin. And there are antidepressant-antipsychotic medications like Symbyax.

Schizophrenia's delusions and hallucinations are usually treated with antipsychotic medications that reduce dopamine and serotonin levels. Antipsychotic medications are commonly categorized into two classes. First-generation antipsychotics, also known as "typical antipsychotics," were developed in the 1950s. Second-generation antipsychotics, also known as "atypical antipsychotics," emerged in the 1990s. Clozapine (marketed as Clozaril) was the first of the second-generation medications. While clozapine is the only medication licensed for treatment-resistant schizophrenia, there has been increased interest in using clozapine earlier in the disease course, as it is significantly better at treating symptoms than first-generation antipsychotics and some (but not all) second-generation antipsychotics. Clozapine paved the path for medications like Abilify, Zyprexa, Seroquel, and Risperdal. These second-generation medications are called atypical because they do not have the side effects that characterized the first-generation medications, although they do have their own side effects.

Although long-acting injectable (LAI) medications for treating schizophrenia were first introduced in the mid-1960s, they were not well received by either the medical profession or people with schizophrenia. Concern about side effects was widespread. Some psychiatrists did not believe that LAIs alone would deliver an ongoing therapeutic dose. As a consequence, they added oral medications, making it difficult to determine which treatments were effective. When psychiatrists did prescribe LAIs, it was a last resort—after oral medications failed to work. Some patients viewed LAIs as an attempt to impose treatment without regard to patients' feelings or rights.

Yet high rates of nonadherence to oral medications, combined with knowledge regarding the importance of minimizing the severity and frequency of psychotic episodes, led to development of a host of LAIs. Today, five second-generation LAIs, risperidone microspheres (Risperdal Consta), paliperidone palmitate (Invega Sustenna and Invega Trinza), olanzapine pamoate, aripiprazole monohydrate (Abilify Maintena), and aripiprazole lauroxil (Aristada), are approved for the treatment of schizophrenia. These injectables provide dosing options ranging from two to twelve weeks. Consistent evidence indicates that, compared with patients treated with oral medications, patients who received LAIs have a lower risk of disease relapse, lower rates of psychiatric services utilization and hospitalization, and better psychosocial functioning, although they also have higher rates of extrapyramidal syndrome (drug-induced movement disorders such as tardive dyskinesia) and prolactin-related symptoms (e.g., irregular menstrual periods).

Bipolar disorder is treated primarily with mood stabilizers and antipsychotics. Sometimes antidepressants are used, although their safety and effectiveness are controversial. The most widely used mood stabilizers are lithium carbonate and valproic acid (Depakote). Lithium can be very effective in reducing mania and may also prevent recurrence of depression. Depakote is helpful in treating mania. More recently, Lamictal, an antiepileptic drug, has been found to help prevent depression and mania. Antipsychotic medications, including Haldol, Abilify, Zyprexa, and Risperdal, are often used to treat acute symptoms of mania before lithium or Depakote can take full effect (which can take up to several weeks). Latuda and Symbyax are antipsychotic medications approved for use in bipolar I depression. Seroquel, an antipsychotic, is approved to treat bipolar I or II. Emerging evidence suggests that LAI anti-psychotic medications are particularly effective for preventing mania but not depression and for preventing relapse in patients with rapid cycling bipolar disorder. Side effects (including obesity, hypertension, type 2 diabetes, poor bone health, movement disorders, menstrual dysfunction, and sexual difficulties) from LAIs are similar to those from oral medications.

Depression is treated with a variety of antidepressant medications. Doctors often start by prescribing selective serotonin reuptake inhibitors like Prozac, Paxil, Zoloft, and Lexapro—medications that increase the amount of serotonin (a chemical that helps regulate mood) in the brain. A second category of antidepressants, serotonin-norepinephrine reuptake inhibitors like Cymbalta, Effexor XR, and Fetzima, block the absorption (reuptake) of the neurotransmitters serotonin and norepinephrine in the brain, relieving the irritability, sadness, and anxiety of depressive symptoms. Most patients prefer norepinephrine-dopamine reuptake inhibitors such as Wellbutrin, Aplenzin, and Forfivo XL because these medicines usually lack the sexual side effects of other antidepressant medications. Atypical antidepressants such as Trazodone, Remeron, Brintellix, and Viibryd have sedating effects and so are usually taken only in the evening. Tricyclic antidepressants like Tofranil, Pamelor, Surmontil, Norpramin, and Vivactil are usually not a first-line course of treatment because they have more severe side effects than other antidepressants. Finally, monoamine oxidase inhibitors (MAOIs) like Parnate, Nardil, and Marplan are used infrequently because MAOIs break down tyramine, a chemical present in aged cheese, wines, and other aged foods, and elevate blood pressure. Emsam is a newer MAOI administered through a patch that adheres to the skin.

When people have treatment-resistant depression, brain stimulation techniques may be used. Electroconvulsive therapy (ECT; previously known as electroshock therapy) is a noninvasive brain stimulation technique that uses very high current levels to induce controlled, short-term seizures. Treatment lasts an average of one to six seconds, with patients sedated.

Although many people fear even trying ECT, Kitty Dukakis believes that it saved her life. Kitty began swallowing diet pills when she was in high school. In 1988, when her husband Michael lost his presidential bid, Kitty began binge drinking. Intensive rehabilitation programs at Hazelden, Edgehill Newport, Four Winds Psychiatric Hospital, Randolph County Hospital, and Massachusetts General Hospital helped Kitty understand and fight her dependence on amphetamines and alcohol, but they did little to address her underlying depression. Psychiatrists diagnosed depression and bipolar disorder. Kitty tried talk therapies. She tried medications, including Norpramin, Prozac, lithium, Wellbutrin, Effexor, Mirapex, and Zoloft. Directed by her doctors, Kitty tried the medications one at a time and in a multitude of combinations. The drugs had limited benefits and numerous side effects. By 2001, when Kitty was 64, doctors had run out of remedies, and each new episode of depression Kitty experienced was worse than the last one. As a last resort, Kitty agreed to try ECT, a treatment her doctor had told her about three years earlier but which Kitty had refused because having electric current surging through her brain frightened her.

Waking from the anesthesia after her first ECT treatment, Kitty felt so good, so alive, that she told her husband she wanted to go out for dinner to celebrate their thirty-eighth wedding anniversary. Additional treatments have enabled Kitty to keep away the symptoms of depression and rid her need of antidepressants. But ECT does not cure depression; it abates the symptoms. Now in her eighties, Kitty still receives maintenance ECT treatments every few months. Although Kitty has experienced some memory loss, ECT's most feared side effect, she has learned to manage the slight forgetfulness she experiences after each treatment. For Kitty, the memory loss is an acceptable trade-off to the smoldering depression she had not been able to tame. For others, however, ECT can wipe out years of memories. Writer Jonathan Cott, for example, lost fifteen years of recollections. He no longer remembered the murder of John Lennon, books he had written, and friends in his address book. As science progresses, it is likely that new ECT techniques will better protect memory.

Today, transcranial magnetic stimulation (TMS) is the most commonly used brain stimulation technique for people with depression. Nonsedated patients sit in a specially designed chair that holds their head in place while large magnetic coils positioned just above the scalp produce short magnetic pulses. Repetitive transcranial magnetic stimulation is a variant of TMS. With this technique, the speed with which the magnetic coils change polarity increases in microseconds, creating repetitive electromagnetic pulses that provide stronger electromagnetic treatments. To target deeper regions of the brain, doctors use a more direct stimulation method, transcranial direct current stimulation, in which electrodes are secured directly against the scalp. Finally, deep brain stimulation is an invasive and experimental stimulation technique involving surgically implanting parts of the stimulation device into the brain of a fully sedated patient.

Are Some Treatments Better Than Others?

That this wealth of treatments has become available since 1954 is nothing short of amazing. We know that, at least for the short-term, treatment is better than no treatment. But what do we know about how well the different treatments work? Do they all have the same effect?

In 2005, results from a major randomized study of the effectiveness of first- and second-generation medications for schizophrenia were published. Funded by the NIMH, the Clinical Antipsychotic Trials of Intervention Effectiveness (CATIE) study had a novel outcome measure—time to treatment discontinuation. Treatment discontinuation did not mean that patients stopped treatment and left the study; rather, it meant that they and/or their doctors decided to switch or stop the medication to which they had been randomly assigned and try something else, usually because of undesirable side effects. The scientists expected that patients would be more likely to continue treatment using the second-generation medications than the older, first-generation medications. Much to the scientists' surprise, the patients were no more likely to continue treatment with the second-generation drugs than perphenazine, a first-generation drug. The antipsychotic drugs were more similar than different from one another. What differed among the treatments were their side effects. The CATIE study showed that what worked for one person does not necessarily work for another, teaching a very important lesson: treatment for schizophrenia, as well as other serious mental illnesses, must be individualized and closely monitored.

Since the CATIE study, scientists have conducted so many studies seeking to identify the best treatments for serious mental illnesses that they now turn to meta-analyses—the analysis of analyses—to understand options. The conclusion from hundreds and hundreds of studies is that treatment of schizophrenia, depression, and bipolar disorder is more effective than nontreatment.

Existing medications, despite their side effects, are especially effective against the positive symptoms of schizophrenia (hallucinations, delusions, and racing thoughts) but less effective against the negative (apathy, poor social functioning) and cognitive symptoms (disorganized thoughts, difficulty completing tasks, memory problems). A 2012 analysis of sixty-five studies found that 64 percent of people with schizophrenia who were not taking antipsychotics had relapsed, while only 27 percent of people with schizophrenia who were taking antipsychotics had relapsed. This suggests that while taking medications does not guarantee that a person will be symptom-free, failure to take the medications does not necessarily mean that a person will experience symptoms. In other words, taking medication improves the odds of not having a symptom relapse.

Regarding antidepressants, good evidence suggests that all antidepressant medications work about equally well to alleviate the symptoms of depression and to keep the symptoms from coming back. What distinguishes these medications from one another is not their ability to blunt the symptoms of schizophrenia, bipolar disorder, and depression, but rather the side effects they produce.

Side Effects

By the time my daughter Sophie was 16-and-a-half, doctors had prescribed five different medications to treat the symptoms of her mental illness, which grew worse over time. Each medication had its own side effects. Sophie's appetite decreased when she started taking Strattera. She felt dizzy and nauseous when she began taking Concerta. Zoloft made her sleepy. Lamictal made her dizzy, nauseous, and tired. Vyvanse gave her diarrhea, made her jittery, and caused dry mouth. Fortunately, most of these side effects dissipated within a few weeks, as Sophie's body adjusted to the medications and Dr. Kane tinkered with their dosages.

Nothing, however, prepared us for Seroquel, an atypical antipsychotic medication that helps restore the balance of neurotransmitters in the brain. Started during Sophie's weeklong hospitalization when she was 16, the initial dose of Seroquel made Sophie so groggy she could barely lift her head off the table during our visits. Every few days, the staff adjusted the dose until the medicine was able to control Sophie's mania without rendering her a zombie.

Seroquel, however, is associated with major weight gain and metabolic changes. It can lead to high cholesterol, diabetes, and heart disease. Josh and I worried that Sophie, like most teenage girls, would resist taking a medicine that could make her gain weight. Beyond that, we certainly did not want her to take a medication with such serious health risks. Josh slogged through countless research studies, desperate to understand whether there were alternative medicines. He learned that people taking Abilify, another second-generation antipsychotic, usually experienced less weight gain than those who took Seroquel. Once Sophie was out of the hospital, we asked Dr. Kane about the possibility of switching medications. She agreed.

In the end, Abilify controlled Sophie's symptoms. But finding the right mix and dose of medications was not easy. The medications robbed Sophie of the blissful hypomanic euphoria that had heightened her sexuality, energy, and creativity— all symptoms of bipolar disorder. In Sophie's words, "The medicine erases the color from my world." She no longer had the drive to draw, write poetry, or sew. Her passion for reading was gone. Not surprisingly, Sophie learned to hide her racing, impulsive thoughts from Dr. Kane, since reports of these experiences brought an increased dosage of the medication that dulled her even more.

While treating the symptoms of serious mental illness enables many people to think clearly and function in society, existing treatments can also cause harm. Imipramine, for example, can leave the mouth so dry that teeth rot. Antidepressants can leave people sleepy and make it difficult for them to wake. Mixing MAOIs with foods like cheese, chocolate, olives, cured meat, or red wine—foods that contain tyramine—can result in dangerously high blood pressure.

Sometimes the treatments can cause problems that are even worse than the symptoms. Lithium can keep manic symptoms under control, but lithium in excess is poisonous and can cause death. And sometimes medications that have worked for years can stop working or become less effective.

Further complicating matters is the fact that sometimes psychotropic medications diagnosed to quell the symptoms of schizophrenia, depression, or bipolar disorder can trigger new symptoms. For example, bipolar disorder often presents initially with one or more episodes of depression. Antidepressants, however, can trigger mania in some patients with bipolar disorder. This "switching" of mood into mania can be dangerous, and continuing to take antidepressants can make the mania even worse. An analysis that combined results from nearly 100,000 patients with depression treated with an antidepressant found that mood switching occurred in 8.2 percent of people within an average of 2.4 years of treatment. Switching rates were 4.3 times greater among children and teenagers than among adults. Because Sophie's symptoms led Dr. Kane to believe that Sophie had depression, Dr. Kane treated Sophie with Zoloft. After being on Zoloft for about two years, Sophie climbed out her second-floor bedroom window to rendezvous with a pervert she had met on the internet. This likely was Sophie's first full-blown manic episode.

Medications and their side effects are individualized and fluid. As such, constant monitoring—by the person with the illness, the family, and the doctor—is critical, although very difficult.

Are Medications Really Necessary?
Beginning with the first time Sophie's pediatrician suggested that drugs could quell her impulsive behaviors, I worried about the wisdom of relying on medications. What do we really understand about how these medications affect a child's developing brain? Even if the medications helped in the short-term, I wondered about their long-term effects.

Would the side effects be worse than the symptoms?

While there is much about medications that we do not understand, there is little doubt about the importance of beginning treatment as soon as possible. The longer a person goes untreated, the poorer their prognosis. Earlier treatment of first-episode psychosis reduces suicides and increases quality of life, social functioning, and cognitive function. It also decreases schizophrenia's negative symptoms.

People experiencing first-episode psychosis are at risk for a second psychotic episode. Each psychotic episode destroys the brain's gray and white matter. This destruction cannot be reversed. Consistent evidence points to the importance of aggressively treating first-episode psychosis using LAI medications. Yet the common response to first-episode psychosis is to prescribe an oral antipsychotic medication, even though these have high rates of nonadherence. LAIs, the best protection against future episodes, are rarely used after a first psychotic break. They are instead used as a last resort for the sickest patients, after other treatments fail. Reasons for nonuse of LAIs after first-episode psychosis include psychiatrist lack of knowledge, patient and family reluctance, cost, and availability. Yet there is good evidence, among patients who use LAIs and health care professionals who prescribe them, that they are effective.

At the same time, however, we have known for more than a century that approximately one-quarter of people who develop a schizophrenia-like psychosis will recover without treatment and not suffer a relapse. How are the people who recover without treatment different from others? Are there multiple forms of schizophrenia? We just do not know.

Strategies for Finding the Right Treatment
There is no "best" treatment for schizophrenia, bipolar disorder, or depression. The challenge—and it is not an easy one—is to find the right medication or combination of medications that will keep symptoms under control while not causing undesirable

side effects. It is not likely that the first medication the doctor suggests will be the right one for you or your loved one. Moreover, what works for your friend is not necessarily likely to work for you. There are, however, strategies you can use to find treatments that will help. Unfortunately, much of the work is trial and error, so patience and teamwork are critical.

Here are some suggestions to consider:

- Find a competent doctor / health care professional whom you trust and can work with.
- Make sure the doctor knows about all medications, vitamins, and dietary supplements you are taking.
- When the doctor recommends a particular medication, do not be afraid to ask why he or she selected that particular drug instead of others.
- Do not expect the medication to have an immediate effect. Sometimes it takes a month or so for the medication's effects to kick in and alleviate the symptoms.
- Make sure you understand what time of day the doctor wants you to take your medicine. Some medicines work best if taken at night, while others work best if taken during the day. Some medicines should be taken with food; others should be taken on an empty stomach.
- Some medications (e.g., lithium) require you to have frequent blood tests to make sure your kidneys and thyroid are working right. If the doctor orders blood tests, be sure to get them.
- Be an informed consumer. Information about medications changes frequently. Check the US Food and Drug Administration website for the latest warnings, patient medication guides, and newly approved medications.
- Keep a daily record of your medications (dosage, time of day, etc.). Note each day how you feel. Are you tired,

dizzy, nauseous, or restless? Did you develop a rash or facial tic? Is your mouth dry? Do you have diarrhea or constipation? Are you having trouble sleeping? Are your dreams wild? Have you lost or gained interest in sex? Are symptoms of your mental illness worse? Are you thinking of harming yourself? Be sure to monitor your weight at least weekly, since many medications include weight gain among their side effects. Share these daily records with your doctor at every visit.

- Let your doctor know immediately if you think that the medications are doing more harm than good. Sometimes changing the dosage can alleviate side effects, but do not make any changes to your medications without first talking to your doctor.

- Do not stop taking your medicine without consulting your doctor first. Sometimes people feel better and stop taking the medication, only to have the symptoms return. Even if your doctor agrees to eliminate or reduce a medication, you should be vigilant and report any problems you experience or concerns you have to the doctor.

- Therapists, including clinical psychologists and clinical social workers, should be an important part of your treatment team. They can help you solve problems and figure out how to deal with stressful situations.

- Include a family member or friend in your treatment plan. Often the people who are close to you will notice problems before you do. They can help you get the care you need.

Finally, Fuller Torrey's book *Surviving Schizophrenia: A Family Manual* and the NIMH website (https://www.nimh.nih.gov/health/topics/mental-health-medications/index.shtml) provide a wealth of useful information about medications.

Disclosure

Mental illnesses do not exist in a vacuum. They unfold within a social context that includes family members, friends, neighbors, coworkers, and others. However, for people to know that a family member, friend, neighbor, or coworker has a mental illness, they must be told. Unlike a blind person who carries a cane or an amputee who is missing a leg, there are usually no outward signs of mental illness. Unlike other hidden illnesses, such as cancer, diabetes, and heart disease, the ramifications for disclosing mental illnesses can be significant. Decisions about whether to tell, what to tell, whom to tell, and when to tell about your mental illness are personal, complex, and not easy to make.

Stigma

Long ago, the Greeks coined the term "stigma" to refer to the physical mark made by a hot iron, indicating that a person, usually a slave, was inferior. More recently, the term "stigma" has been used to indicate that there is something undesirable about a person and that others should keep away. Erving Goffman, considered by some as the greatest American sociologist of the twentieth century, used the term "stigma" to refer to a "powerful negative social label that radically changes a person's social identity and self-concept." Goffman identified three general sources of stigma: deformities or physical markings, tribal stigmas such as race and religion, and moral or character flaws. Although people with mental illnesses do not bear the physical markings associated with the original meaning of "stigma" and usually don't look different from people without mental illness, in Goffman's model people with mental illnesses have a character flaw.

Knowing a few sociological terms can help explain the stigma of mental illness.

Stereotypes are oversimplified beliefs people have about a group and often result from lack of evidence or experience. For example, news stories about a person with serious mental illness committing a mass shooting contribute to the stereotype that people with schizophrenia are dangerous.

Prejudice is a predetermined judgment about a group resulting from stereotypes. For example, some people are prejudiced against people with schizophrenia, thinking they are scary.

Discrimination is behavior that limits the opportunities of a group of people based on negative stereotypes and prejudices. For example, discrimination results when an employer refuses to hire a person with schizophrenia because the employer believes that people with schizophrenia are dangerous or scary.

Stigma results from negative stereotypes, prejudices, and discrimination. Scientists usually measure the stigma of mental illness by asking people how likely they would be to associate with a person with mental illness and whether people with mental illness should tell others about their diagnosis. Stigma can be public, with negative attitudes and beliefs motivating individuals to fear, reject, avoid, and discriminate against people with mental illness, but it also can be private. This happens when people with mental illness internalize negative stereotypes and prejudices about mental illness and come to believe that they are flawed and less worthy than others.

A Brief History of Mental Illness Stigma

To understand mental illness stigma in the United States, it is helpful to look back to 1951, when the first study of public attitudes about mental illness revealed that among the 3,971 people in Louisville, Kentucky, who participated in the study, about half said they would not tell friends and acquaintances that a family member was mentally ill. A few years later, the first national study on Americans' ideas about mental illness revealed that more than two-thirds of respondents viewed people with psychosis as "dangerous." However, when scientists examined their findings more closely, it turned out that respondents were not worried about physical violence from people with mental illnesses. Rather, they feared that the person with mental illness would be "unpredictable, irrational, and not responsible for their acts. You never know what they are going to do."

Between 1950 and 1996, however, perceptions that people with mental illness are physically violent or frightening evolved. In 1950, 7.2 percent of respondents mentioned violent symptoms when describing a person with mental illness, while in 1996, this increased to 12.1 percent. The relationship between violence and mental illnesses is even stronger when considering people whose mental illness includes psychosis (when emotions and thoughts are so impaired that contact with reality is lost). Among respondents asked to consider mental illness that includes psychosis, the proportion of people mentioning violence more than doubled, increasing from 12.7 percent in 1950 to 31 percent in 1996. These data show that our communities are filled with people who believe that people with mental illnesses are violent.

The Decade of the Brain

On July 17, 1990, President George H. W. Bush designated the 1990s as the "Decade of the Brain." He called for programs, ceremonies, and activities focused on "the three-pound mass of interwoven nerve cells that controls intelligence, the senses, and movement," and he challenged scientists to conquer brain diseases, including Alzheimer's disease, stroke, schizophrenia, depression, and autism. Following this proclamation, funding for scientific research on brain diseases increased, and this research revealed the biological nature of mental illnesses, igniting a new awareness among the public. These efforts helped people realize that mental illnesses have biological roots just like diabetes and heart disease.

A clever analysis of magazine articles shows how public attitudes about depression changed during this time. Examining articles in twenty-nine magazines, including *Essence, Harper's Bazaar, Ladies' Home Journal*, and *Sports Illustrated*, scientists from Canada found that in 1980 authors used the word "depression" to describe a wide variety of things. It was a hodgepodge. Some articles labeled lifestyles and behaviors clearly within the normal range as "depression." Sometimes the same article gave the word "depression" very different meanings. For example, an article published in the August 1980 issue of *Vogue* described depression as "pessimism, anxiety, dissatisfaction, lethargy, crying, irritability and decreased sexual drive." A *Newsweek* article in September 1981 said, "When bonds break—through death, divorce, or children leaving home—women often suffer depression. Some say they would rather kill themselves than live alone." In contrast, articles in these same magazines published after 1990 portrayed depression in terms of biology, biochemistry, genetics, and other biomedical explanations. Depression became associated with a physical problem—sometimes biochemical, sometimes anatomical—related to the functioning of the brain. Typical was an article from 2000 published in *Science News* that said, "Manic depression, also known as bipolar disorder, has a well-deserved reputation as a biologically-based condition. Wayward brain chemicals and genes gone bad seem to bully people back and forth between weeks of moderate-to-intense euphoria and comparable spells of soul deadening depression."

Nationwide studies conducted in 1996 and 2006 also revealed that over time people embraced a more neurobiological understanding of serious mental illnesses. In 1996, 76 percent of the population believed that schizophrenia had neurobiological roots; by 2006, 86 percent of people believed this to be the case. Similarly, in 1996, 54 percent of the population believed that depression had neurobiological roots; by 2006, that number had grown to 67 percent. Beliefs about character flaws and poor upbringing as causes for schizophrenia and depression declined.

The biological basis of mental illness was embraced globally as well. The Stigma in Global Context–Mental Health Study revealed that across sixteen countries in Europe, South America, Asia, Australia, and Africa, 53 percent of people believed that a genetic problem caused schizophrenia; 69.2 percent believed that brain disease caused schizophrenia. This same study found that 44 percent of people believed that genetics caused depression and 49 percent believed that a brain disease caused depression.

Nevertheless, even as public beliefs about the biological underpinnings of mental illness increased, there was little change in their belief that psychosocial stress caused mental illnesses, consistent with the diathesis-stress model of mental illness discussed in chapter 2.

If Mental Illnesses Have Biological Roots, Does Stigma Still Exist?

Many prominent reports suggested that scientific advances during the Decade of the Brain and the public's increased understanding that serious mental illnesses are brain diseases and not willful behaviors would decrease the stigma of mental illness. The 1999 US surgeon general's report, for example, identified scientific research as "a potent weapon against stigma, one that forces skeptics to let go of misconceptions and stereotypes." Antistigma campaigns, built on the premise that neuroscience offers the most effective tool to reduce prejudice and discrimination, flourished. Scientists and advocates believed that as people came to understand the biological roots of mental illness, they would see mental illnesses just like other health conditions, and as a result, negative stereotypes and stigma would diminish and social acceptance of people with mental illness would increase.

The scientists and advocates could not have been more wrong. A nationwide study comparing stigma in 1996 and 2006 found that levels of stigma, high in 1996, remained high in 2006. In 2006, 84 percent of respondents believed that people with schizophrenia were violent toward themselves, and 60 percent believed that people with schizophrenia were violent toward others. In 2006, 69 percent of people said they were unwilling to have a person with schizophrenia marry into their family, 62 percent were unwilling to work closely with a person having schizophrenia, 52 percent were unwilling to socialize with someone with schizophrenia, 45 percent were unwilling to have a neighbor with schizophrenia, and 35 percent were unwilling to make friends with a person having schizophrenia.

Stigma was not subsiding; in fact, when measured in terms of willingness to have someone with schizophrenia as a neighbor, it was getting worse. After all, in 1996, 34 percent had been unwilling to have a neighbor with schizophrenia.

Stigma regarding depression, although slightly less than that for schizophrenia, also did not change over the ten-year period. In 2006, 70 percent of respondents believed that people with depression were violent toward themselves; 32 percent believed that they were violent toward others. In 2006, 53 percent of people said they were unwilling to have a person with depression marry into their family, 47 percent were unwilling to work closely with a person having depression, 30 percent were unwilling to socialize with someone with depression, 20 percent were unwilling to have a neighbor with depression, and 21 percent were unwilling to make friends with a person having depression.

Internationally, trends are similar. Data from the sixteen-country Stigma in Global Context–Mental Health Study revealed that a majority of respondents believed that people with schizophrenia were violent toward themselves and others. Across the sixteen countries, 68 percent of people were unwilling to have a person with schizophrenia marry into their family. More than one-third of respondents were unwilling to work closely with a person having schizophrenia, were unwilling to socialize with someone with schizophrenia, were unwilling to have a neighbor with schizophrenia, and would not make friends with a person having schizophrenia. The international data likewise found high levels of stigma regarding a person with depression.

Together, this research suggests that understanding that serious mental illnesses have biogenetic roots decreases perceptions that people with these illnesses are to blame for their behaviors. However, biogenetic explanations increase beliefs that people with mental illness are dangerous and should be avoided. Other evidence shows that the nature of the biogenetic cause can also influence stigma. One review found that believing that brain disease causes mental illness was associated with increased social distance, but believing that biochemical imbalances or genetics cause mental illness was not.

American children, as well as adults, have stigmatizing beliefs about people with mental illness. Further, beliefs about the cause of illness influence the stigma experienced by people with mental illnesses themselves. Recently, a systematic review of studies of stigma experienced by people with mental illness revealed that when people with mental illness believe that their illnesses have a biological basis, they too report more pessimism regarding recovery, higher levels of self-guilt, and increased stigma toward other people with mental illness.

Stigma is alive and well, making the challenges of living with a serious mental illness even harder.

What Do We Tell People?

Back to my story. While finding mental health providers was taxing and identifying a treatment regimen that worked was puzzling, deciding what and how much to tell people about Sophie's illness was what kept me awake at night. I could not tell anyone how I worried that this illness might keep Sophie from going to college, having a successful career, and marrying. Josh and I worried that people would think us bad parents. My son refused to invite friends to come to the house, fearing they would shun him if Sophie had one of her rants while they were visiting.

When the pediatrician diagnosed Sophie with ADHD and we needed to make decisions about medications, I called my brother Ben, a physician. Although this medical problem was far afield of his expertise as a nephrologist, he read the literature, consulted with his colleagues in psychiatry, and gave me a thoughtful explanation about the medications and treatment plan that they believed would be most effective.

I have always known I can count on Ben. Yet despite Ben's knowledge of medicine and my close and trusting relationship with him, I did not tell Ben that Sophie had gotten into a hair-pulling fight with a girl in school or that she had pilfered money from me. Even once Sophie's doctor prescribed medications that would quell these behaviors, I did not tell Ben about the treatments Dr. Kane prescribed, the diagnoses of bipolar disorder and borderline personality disorder, or the psychiatric hospitalizations.

It was not just Ben I did not tell about Sophie's illness. I did not tell anyone.

Why? Maybe it was my desire to avoid facing the reality that Sophie suffered from a serious mental illness. Maybe it was to protect Sophie from the stigma of mental illness and enable her to have some semblance of a normal relationship with other people. I did not want anyone to think that Sophie was a bad person, and I did not want people to exclude or fear her. I also did not tell people because I worried that they would think that Josh and I were bad parents. I did not want Sophie's brother to be shunned.

Hiding Sophie's mental illness was not the first time I had hidden mental illness.

For nine years, beginning when I was 12, my mother's moods had varied with the seasons. But in the late 1960s and early 1970s, no one talked about mental illness. Not a single doctor or social worker ever talked to my brothers or me about mom's illness. Maybe they talked to my father, an engineer at Ford Motor Company who did his best to keep his family together. Although no one ever told me not to talk about my mother's illness, somehow it just became our family secret. When my mother was hospitalized, we told people she had had a "nervous breakdown," and even then we did not share details about her incessant crying and suicide attempts.

Secrets about my mother made me lonely. I hurried home from high school every afternoon, rather than getting involved in sports or other activities. I never invited friends to my house because I did not want them to see my mother's strange behaviors. How would I ever explain her pacing and crying?

My mother killed herself during final exams week of my senior year in college. Although my mother's death brought me much sadness, it also brought relief. It meant I no longer had to worry about her. I no longer wondered whether she would kill herself. I no longer was constantly on edge, waiting for that phone call to tell me she had taken an overdose of pills and was again in the hospital. However, I did not understand so many things about my mother's suicide. What had made her sick in the first place? She had been fine, at least to my knowledge, until she was 43. Why did she get sick then?

With my mother's suicide, I could no longer hide her mental illness. I had to tell my college friends about why she had killed herself. They were supportive and kind. My professors understood and excused me from finals. However, this compassion did not stop me from keeping the secret of my mother's illness from everyone else. During the next ten years, I got a master's degree in psychology and then a PhD in human development. I told friends who entered my life after my mother's death that she had died in a car accident on an icy road. I extended our family secret about my mother's mental illness to her suicide.

Why did I do this? The truth is, I could never figure out how to explain my mother's death to my friends. There never seemed to be the right time to say, "My mother suffered from manic depression and she killed herself." I could not tell this to someone with whom I was beginning a relationship. It was much too personal. As friendships blossomed and I shared concerns about boyfriends and worries about work, my silence about my mother persisted. I knew I was hiding. My stomach squirmed each time I told my made-up story of her death. But when I imagined conversations in which I told the truth, I fell apart. I do not know whether I worried more about how difficult it would be for me to say the words or about how difficult it would be for others to hear them. I did not want pity, and I did not want them to think poorly of my mother or me. Should the floodgates open, I knew that the pain would be intolerable. And so, I hid the truth.

In 1985, when I knew that I had a future with Josh, I also knew I had to tell him about my mother's mental illness and her suicide. For days I worried about what to say and whether this would be a deal breaker. My ten-year silence was broken as I sobbed, searching for the right words to tell him. He held my hand, looked into my eyes, and made it easy. He married me anyway. Yet even this did not free me to share my secret with friends. I figured Josh responded the way he did because he was in love with me.

I kept my mother's illness and suicide a secret for nearly four decades. I kept my daughter's mental illness a secret for a decade. I feared that people would think less of my mother and my daughter because they suffered from mental illness, but I also feared that they would think less of me. When I was a child,

I thought that my family was the only one dealing with mental illness. As an adult, particularly one with a PhD in psychology, I was acutely aware that that was not true. Yet even as an adult, I managed to convince myself that my family was the only one. My daughter was the only kid who had multiple stays in a psychiatric hospital. My daughter was the only one cutting herself and saying, "I'd rather hurt myself and bleed than feel nothing." Because I believed that I was the only one dealing with these horrible things, and because I did not want people to think poorly of my daughter or of me, I continued to hide.

Because I did not tell anyone about the struggles I had, no one could help me.

Stigma's Long Arm

Stigma surrounding mental illness is not limited to those who suffer from one. Like an infectious disease, stigma can spread from people with a stigmatized condition to people who associate with them. In 1963, Erving Goffman, the sociologist whose thinking about stigma has guided the field for more than half a century, suggested that people related to a stigmatized person (such as family members) share some of the discredit of the stigmatized person. Stigma, he said, spreads out in waves, its rippling effects having greatest intensity among people who are closest to the person diagnosed with mental illness. According to Goffman, "courtesy stigma" or "stigma by association" happens when society loses respect for a person because that person has an association with a stigmatized person. Like stigma, courtesy stigma can lead to social isolation, decreasing social support.

One of the first studies about courtesy stigma found that wives of men admitted to a state psychiatric hospital worried that people would mock their children because of their husbands' hospitalization. More recent studies find that between 25 and 50 percent of family members believe that the mental illness of a relative is shameful and should be hidden. Nearly half of parents and spouses of patients with serious mental illness admitted for the first time to a psychiatric hospital concealed the hospitalization from friends and relatives.

Serious mental illnesses threaten families in ways that other illnesses do not. Shame is forty times more prevalent in families of people with mental illness than in families of people with cancer. Stephen Hinshaw, an eminent scholar, says, "The predominant coping mechanism for families in response to the mental disorder of a child, spouse, or other relative has been one of secrecy and concealment." Feelings of blame and shame lead to social avoidance. Three large studies reported that between 20 and 30 percent of family members had strained or distant relationships with extended family and/or friends because of their relative with mental illness.

Many people hide the fact that someone in their family has a mental illness because they believe that the mental illness is a character flaw or a sign of weakness. One study reported that nearly half of family members of a person with mental illness agreed with the statement "Most people look down on families that have a member who is mentally ill living with them." More than 70 percent of people disagreed with the statement "Most people believe that parents of children with a mental illness are just as responsible and caring as other parents."

Families hide for good reason. Studies of public attitudes find that people believe that family members, especially parents, are responsible for their child's mental illness. Typically, incompetent parenting skills are blamed. The public blames siblings and spouses of people with mental illness for failing to help the person with mental illness adhere to treatment. Moreover, the public believes that a parent's mental illness contaminates their children. In many ways, the genetic attributions of mental illness spurred by the Decade of the Brain made courtesy stigma worse.

Fighting Stigma

Ironically, the Decade of the Brain's emphasis on genetics and biology fueled rather than quelled stigma. Why does stigma continue, and how can we fight it?

Many interventions aimed at minimizing stigma have been developed and tested. Some involve exposing the public to people with serious mental illnesses, using face-to-face interactions or indirect contact via videos. Others are education focused. These interventions provide information, highlight the negative impact that stigma has on people with mental illness, and guide people in effective ways to support and interact with people having mental illness. An analysis of more than sixty studies revealed that, while both contact interventions and educational interventions reduced stigma, neither strategy was better than the other.

An analysis of data from more than seventy studies that included over 38,000 people in fourteen countries found that both education and contact had positive effects on stigma reduction for adults and adolescents with a mental illness. However, contact, especially face-to-face contact, was more effective than education at reducing stigma for adults, while education was more effective for adolescents. Perhaps adolescents have less firmly developed beliefs and so are more responsive to education. Alternatively, perhaps millennials who are more open, confident, and willing to discuss their own mental health are more tolerant of others. A study of more than five hundred junior and senior high school students in Ottawa integrated a mental health module into existing courses and found that increasing knowledge about mental illness decreased stigma.

Some have suggested that stigma continues because the public believes that people with biologically caused illnesses cannot recover. An innovative study using a national sample of adults told some respondents stories about people with schizophrenia and depression who had been treated. Other respondents were told stories about people whose illnesses had gone untreated. Researchers found that public attitudes were more positive when the stories indicated that the mental illnesses were treated, suggesting that treating mental illnesses can decrease stigma.

Another Way to Fight Stigma and Discrimination: Coming Out

Interventions that involve contact with a person with mental illness are a step in the right direction toward alleviating the stigma of mental illness. However, most existing interventions are short-term, are contrived, and lack enough real-life experience to be meaningful.

An alternative model comes from the LGBT community. Once a victim of stigma, the LGBT community has made impressive strides in reducing stigma and discrimination. In 2010, repeal of the "Don't Ask, Don't Tell" policy enabled LGBT people to serve openly in the Armed Forces without fear of reprisal. That same year, the Affordable Care Act prohibited insurers from turning people away because of their sexual orientation. In 2012, LGBT people could not be banned from accessing government housing programs and services. In 2014, the Workplace Discrimination Prevention Executive Order prevented discrimination against any job candidate or employee because he or she is LGBT, and in 2015, same-sex marriage became legalized nationwide.

Much of the progress gained by the LGBT community comes from their willingness to "come out" to their families, friends, workplaces, and schools. This same strategy may be productive for people with serious mental illness, as research suggests that the best way to improve attitudes about a stigmatized population is meaningful contact. When people in the general population interact with someone with mental illness, they become less prejudiced than people without this kind of contact. Similarly, public stigma about family members of people with mental illness should diminish as the public has contact with parents, spouses, and children of people with mental illness.

However, coming out is not an easy decision.

Patrick Corrigan is a clinical psychologist who has set up rehabilitation programs for people with serious mental illness, educated and mentored countless students, and conducted federally funded research. A distinguished professor of psychology at Illinois Institute of Technology, Dr. Corrigan is the author of seventeen books and more than four hundred peer-reviewed articles. He heads the NIMH-funded National Consortium on Stigma and Empowerment. However, Dr. Corrigan does not just study the stigma of mental illness. For Dr. Corrigan, stigma is personal. Living with anxiety, major depression, and bipolar disorder for nearly four decades, Dr. Corrigan has been under the psychiatric care of more than ten psychiatrists. He has taken a variety of medications: some helped relieve his symptoms, while others caused wicked side effects. He has been treated in emergency rooms for depression and anxiety and once was locked in the psychiatric unit of Evanston Hospital.

For years, Dr. Corrigan struggled with what to tell other people about his own illness. Although he had been diagnosed with and treated for mental illness, when the Illinois Department of Professional Regulation's application for licensure asked him in 1990 whether he had ever been diagnosed with a mental illness, he answered "no." He did not tell his colleagues about his illness either because he worried that they would not take his scholarship seriously. He attended conferences about mental illness and stigma, knowing that the issues applied to him, but still only his family and a few close friends knew of his illness.

Dr. Corrigan's understanding of the literature taught him that the most effective strategy for reducing public prejudice and discrimination was having contact with people with mental

illness. He knew, however, that the contact had to be meaningful. And so, little by little, Dr. Corrigan began to share his personal experiences with his colleagues, friends, and broader
community. Since then, Dr. Corrigan's work has centered on
helping people with mental illness decide whether, when, and
how to disclose their illness.

To Tell or Not to Tell: Strategies for Making Disclosure Decisions

Corrigan's program, called "Honest, Open, Proud," helps people
identify the advantages and disadvantages of disclosing their
mental illness, explore ways to disclose their illness, and learn
how to tell their story. He suggests that there are two contradic-
tory yet fundamental rules that should guide decisions about
disclosing mental illness. The first is the Rule of Minimal Risks
with Little Information. This rule counsels caution in disclosing private information because disclosing and then recanting
is harder than letting people know slowly. On the other hand,
the second rule, Delayed Decision Is Lost Opportunity, suggests
that caution in disclosing leads to delay in securing support. By
weighing the costs and benefits of disclosure, individuals must
decide if and when disclosure is right for them.

There are many benefits to disclosing mental illness. Here are
some of the benefits identified by Dr. Corrigan and confirmed
by my own experiences:

- Once you disclose your illness, you no longer have to
  worry about hiding it.
- You may find others who also have a mental illness and
  learn that you are not as alone as you thought you were.
- Future relapses may be less stressful because others will
  be able to help you.
- You are helping eliminate the stigma of mental illness.

On the other hand, the costs of disclosing a mental illness include the following:

- You may lose work, housing, or other opportunities.
- Others may exclude you from social gatherings.
- People might talk about you.
- Future relapses may be more stressful because others will be watching you.

Costs and benefits of disclosing can be short-term or long-term, so thinking through the ramifications of telling is important.

Equally important is recognizing that disclosing mental illness is not an all-or-nothing issue. You may, for example, choose to confide in one friend but not another. You might decide to tell your boss but not your coworkers. Alternatively, you may tell a coworker but not your boss.

Making decisions about disclosing mental illness is a process subject to change over time. When you first meet someone, you may decide not to tell him or her about your illness. As your friendship develops, you may feel more comfortable talking about your illness. Even then, you can disclose your illness slowly, testing the waters and reading responses to your news. For example, you might first tell a friend that sometimes you feel so overwhelmed that you cannot get out of bed and that, at other times, thoughts bouncing around in your head keep you up all night. Depending on your friend's reaction, you might choose to tell her that you were diagnosed with bipolar disorder and that you take medicine for your illness.

There is evidence that disclosing mental illness to a potential employer is not a good idea, as negative attitudes toward job applicants with mental illness are common among employers. However, once a relationship with an employer is established, the costs and benefits of disclosing your mental illness may change.

You are in charge of deciding what you are willing to tell people. You can disclose your mental illness yet retain your privacy. You do not have to share information that you find embarrassing. For example, you might tell your close friend that you have been diagnosed with depression, but not that you were hospitalized six times.

Family Members Coming Out

Family members also need to make decisions about disclosure. When Sophie was 18, she met the love of her life in a psychiatric hospital and moved out of our home. I faced the alternatives of either telling people what had happened or making up a plausible story to explain her absence. I made the decision to tell the truth, to tell my brothers and close friends why Sophie had disappeared from my life and theirs. I wanted the people who are important to me to understand what Josh and I had dealt with for over a decade. I wanted them to know the whole story. However, I did not want to have to tell the story repeatedly. It would have been much too painful and much too exhausting.

That is why I wrote my memoir *Surrounded by Madness*. In the book I show what mental illness can do to a family. I show how when I was a child my mother's mental illness devastated me and how as an adult my daughter's mental illness challenged me. Writing the book was a "coming out" process for me, just as telling his story was for Dr. Corrigan. When I first told close friends of my plan to write a book about the effects of mental illness on my family, I explained that it was a story about being Sophie's mother, still keeping my mother's mental illness secret. Of course, I knew that my story began with my mother's mental illness. As I became more comfortable writing about my mother's illness, I began to talk about it. My friends were supportive and thoughtful when I told them the truth. In return, I learned that some of them also had people in their families who suffered from mental illness—people they had kept hidden from me. When my friend Lori and I put the pieces of our stories together, we realized that her grandmother and my mother could have been roommates at the psychiatric hospital in Detroit. My friend Helen, a psychologist I have known for over thirty years, helped me understand why my mother got sick when she did, something I had struggled to understand for over forty years.

Certainly, there are costs to disclosing and discussing a relative's mental illness. However, mental illness and family secrets are a toxic combination. Living with someone or caring for someone with mental illness is incredibly stressful. People need the support of their family and close friends. Yet, when people hide, getting support is virtually impossible.

Further complicating disclosure decisions is the reality that decisions made by one person in the family are likely to differ from those of others. For example, despite my reluctance to tell people about Sophie's illness, she had no reservations about telling her friends about her illness. Maybe this was because her generation is more open and accepting of mental illnesses. Maybe it was that many of her friends also had diagnosed mental illnesses. When Sophie went to sleepaway camp, I was surprised to see the long line of campers waiting to check their medications with the nurse, each holding a see-through, one-gallon storage bag with vials of medications. Waiting in line, Sophie chatted happily with the kids, comparing diagnosed conditions and medications for ADHD, depression, and bipolar disorder. In other families, people with mental illness—as well as husbands and wives and brothers and sisters—are likely to differ in how much they are willing to disclose.

As such, it is important to weigh the rights and feelings of multiple family members when assessing the costs and benefits of disclosure. When I first thought about writing my memoir, I discussed doing so with my husband, my brothers, and my son because I knew that telling my story also meant telling their story. I could not have gone forward with my memoir if any of these people had objected. Similarly, I shared early drafts of the memoir with them because I wanted to make sure they were as ready as I was to go public with our story. Finally, I changed the names of all characters in the memoir except myself, as my goal was to show what serious mental illness can do to a family, not to harm my daughter.

Concluding Thoughts

Little over a decade ago, it was difficult for NAMI to find celebrities who were willing to go public with their mental illnesses. Patty Duke, one of the first celebrities to speak out about her bipolar disorder, said that as recently as 2006 entertainers risked being blacklisted and denied parts if it were known that they had a mental illness. She felt free to come forward because she had already established a successful career and no longer feared the risks.

Now, it is common for celebrities from the film, entertainment, sports, and music industries to talk about their mental illnesses. Carrie Fisher, Demi Lovato, Jane Pauley, and Mel Gibson are just a few who speak openly about their bipolar disorder diagnoses. Angelina Jolie, Lady Gaga, Jim Carrey, Bruce Springsteen, and Harrison Ford talk about their struggles with depression. Lionel Aldridge enjoyed an eleven-year career with the Green Bay Packers that included two Super Bowl championships before he was diagnosed with paranoid schizophrenia in the 1970s. He hallucinated and heard scary voices inside his head. He lost his family, his job, his money, and even one of his Super Bowl rings. But his life did not end tragically. He got the help he needed and then traveled the country talking about mental illness and recovery. So too have Peter Green of Fleetwood Mac fame and Brian Wilson of the Beach Boys spoken openly about their experiences with schizophrenia. But does knowing that celebrities struggle with serious mental illness decrease stigma and increase help seeking? A study of female students at a small liberal arts college suggests that it does.

In sum, the initial challenges faced by people with serious mental illness and their families once a diagnosis is made—finding health care providers, identifying treatment regimens that can quell the symptoms of mental illness, and deciding what to tell people—are personal, complex, complicated, and fluid. Like many issues regarding mental illnesses, there are no right answers, no one-size-fits-all solution. While this chapter shows some of the strategies for addressing these issues, coping with mental illness is a lifelong battle. And, as you will see in the next chapter, there are many obstacles along the way.

CHAPTER 5

Ongoing Obstacles

ELYN R. SAKS is Orrin B. Evans Professor of Law, Psychology, Psychiatry, and the Behavioral Sciences at the University of Southern California Gould School of Law. A graduate of Vanderbilt University, Oxford University, and Yale Law School, she is on the faculty of the New Center for Psychoanalysis. The John D. and Catherine T. MacArthur Foundation awarded Saks a "Genius Grant" in 2009. These extraordinary accomplishments are even more remarkable because, during her first year of law school, Elyn Saks was diagnosed with chronic paranoid schizophrenia.

One evening, distraught over a grade she had received on the first legal memo she wrote, Saks withdrew to the library. As a classmate approached her, Saks blurted, "What year is this?" "Have you ever killed anyone?" "There's cheese and there's whizzes. I'm a cheese whiz. It has to do with effort and subliminal choice. Vertigo and killing." As Saks continued her wild ranting, her panicked classmate called for help. At the hospital, a doctor convinced Saks to take Navane, an antipsychotic. By the next day, her mind had calmed. Saks stayed on the medicine for ten days and got a lot of work done, but then she decided that Navane made her feel "druggy" and was "not necessary." Without telling the doctor, Saks stopped taking the medicine.

During the second semester, it happened again. Receiving a poorer exam grade than she had expected, Saks curled up in a fetal position on her dorm bed. She moaned and babbled. Certain that faceless, nameless beings were intercepting her thoughts and that daggers were piercing her flesh, Saks managed to drag herself to an afternoon doctor's appointment. Greeting the doctor, she said, "They passed me up. From Jo-Jo. Interdictions are flying everywhere and the other children ate the porridge. No news is good news, bad news brings a flap. Like flipper." Saks was psychotic. The doctor wanted to hospitalize her, but Saks refused. She did, however, agree to resume taking Navane, at an even higher dose than before. Within two weeks, the demons receded and the fog lifted. Saks stayed on Navane for the rest of the school year.

At the beginning of the second year of law school, the doctor thought Saks was doing better, so he decreased the dosage of Navane. Saks began hallucinating, mostly at night, but she did not tell the doctor about the large spiders she saw crawling up her wall. He would want her to take more Navane, and Saks wanted no part of the doctor's medicine. Taking psychotropic medication reminded Saks that her brain was defective, a thought she could not tolerate. She also worried about side effects she had read about but had not experienced—like tardive dyskinesia, a neurological condition characterized by involuntary movement beginning in the face and moving to other parts of the body. Saks thought people were staring at her. She could not concentrate on her schoolwork. But to her doctor, she said, "I think I want to get off my medication now. I don't need it." The doctor, not knowing about the hallucinations, agreed that Saks could slowly taper down the medicine, reducing the dosage by two milligrams a week. Although Saks longed to be completely off the medicine immediately, she agreed to the doctor's plan.

Within three weeks, Saks was visibly fragmented. She struggled to hide the hallucinations and delusions she once so cleverly had kept from the doctor. She felt like she was "going to melt" and "about to be attacked and ripped apart." By the fourth week, Saks's conviction that "the people in the sky poison me. I in turn will poison the world" revealed she was floridly psychotic. She could no longer hide the truth from her doctor. Sure enough, he increased the dosage of Navane. Immediately, Saks started feeling better.

But for Saks, this three-stage pattern—(1) being highly functional and able to write brilliant legal briefs when taking medication, (2) decreasing or stopping the medicine because she did not want to believe she had a mental illness, and (3) becoming psychotic and unable to function—continued for nearly twenty years. Why would someone so brilliant act in such a nonsensical way? Saks explains, "In spite of my history, in spite of all the diagnoses and prescriptions, the frequent delusions and the evil visitations, I still wasn't convinced that I had a mental illness. Nor was I convinced that I really needed medication. To admit to any of it was to admit that my brain was profoundly broken, and I just couldn't do that." She continues,

> My brain was the instrument of my success and my pride, but it
> also carried all the tools for my destruction. Yes, the pills helped,
> but each time I put them in my mouth, it was a reminder that some
> people—smart people I trusted and respected—believed that I was
> mentally ill, that I was defective; every dose of Navane was a
> concession to that. More than anything, I wanted to be healthy and
> whole; I wanted to exist in the world as my authentic self—and I
> deeply believed that the drugs undermined that. And so, I kept
> backing away from them, tinkering with the dose, seeing how far I
> could go before I got burned. And of course, I got burned every
> time—even in my denial, I knew that.

Finally, in her midforties, successful in her career, engaged to be married, and bolstered by long-term friends, Saks acknowledged that she had a serious mental illness and that medicine played a critical role for her. She says, "If I'd had a broken leg and a crutch was required, I'd have used it without ever thinking twice. Was my brain not worth tending to at least as much as my leg? The fact was, I had a condition that required medicine. If I didn't use it, I got sick; if I used it, I got better. I don't know why I had to keep learning that the hard way, but I did."

To this day, Saks continues to be well treated with a combination of medications and talk therapy.

Why Don't People Get Treatment?

In the United States, about half of people with a serious mental illness do not get the treatment they need. Although treatment was available to Saks, for years she refused it. Other people want treatment but cannot get it. What stops sick people from getting treatment? How can we make sure that people are getting—and adhering to—the treatment they need? Understanding the varied and complex reasons why people do not get treatment is critical to developing effective strategies that families and communities can use to help ensure that people with serious mental illnesses get the help they need. To be effective, however, strategies must be responsive to the concerns of the person with mental illness. General, one-size-fits-all responses are doomed to fail.

When People Want Treatment but Can't Get It

The National Survey on Drug Use and Health, our country's primary annual source for information about mental health issues, provides important evidence explaining why people who want treatment do not get it. Researchers asked a sample of these people why they were not receiving treatment. By far, the most commonly reported reason was inability to pay for treatment. More than half of people said they did not have health insurance or the health insurance they had did not cover their treatment. The second most common reason focused on practical concerns. People said they did not know where to go for help, did not have time to go for treatment, or could not get to treatment facilities because they lacked transportation or the facility was too far away. Finally, many people said that although they wanted treatment, they did not seek it because they worried about what other people would think of them. They did not want their friends and neighbors to know about their mental illness. College students worried they might be asked to leave campus. Employees feared that if their boss knew they were receiving treatment they might lose their job. Sharon, the social worker you met in chapter 2, was one of these people. Even though she worked in a helping profession and met weekly with her boss, who was a psychiatrist, Sharon worried that if these people knew she suffered from depression, they might not respect her professional opinions, may not want to work with her, and could take steps to fire her.

Not surprisingly, the reasons people who want care do not get care are complex and not mutually exclusive. Often multiple obstacles stop a person from getting care.

"I Can't Afford Treatment"

Few people can afford the costs of treating serious mental illnesses. The National Survey on Drug Use and Health revealed that among people with a serious mental illness who wanted but had not received treatment in the past year, 52.5 percent said they could not afford the cost, 15.1 percent said health insurance does not pay enough for mental health services, and 11.1 percent said they did not have health insurance that would cover any mental health services.

Mental illnesses are far more common among the poor than the rich. A report from the Centers for Disease Control found that 8.7 percent of people with incomes below the poverty line had a serious mental illness compared with only 1.2 percent of people with incomes at or above four times the poverty level. But it is more than just poverty that is associated with serious mental illness. One of the most consistently replicated findings in the social sciences is the relationship between socioeconomic status (SES) and mental illness. For decades, studies have shown that whether SES is measured in terms of income, education, or occupation, the lower a person's SES, the higher is the risk of any type of mental illness. While we still don't understand whether low SES causes serious mental illness or serious mental illness keeps people from attaining higher levels of education and income, the fact is that many people with serious mental illness are poor, lack education, and do not have resources to pay for medications and other treatments. These problems are even greater for racial and ethnic minority members, who have less access to health services, are less likely to use health care, are more likely to receive poorer quality care, and have higher rates of dropout from care than white people.

To ensure that people are getting all the help paying for mental health care for which they are eligible, it is important to understand some basic information about how Americans pay for mental health care.

FUNDING MENTAL HEALTH SERVICES: PUBLIC RESOURCES

Nearly 60 percent of mental health care in the United States is paid for by public sources such as Medicaid, Medicare, or other federal and state programs. Medicaid is the single largest payer for mental health services, providing health insurance for nearly a third of adults with mental illness. Medicaid is jointly funded by the federal and state governments and administered through the states. People qualify for Medicaid primarily based on their income, although each state sets its own eligibility requirements. States have the option of establishing eligibility based on disability for people whose income is too high to otherwise qualify for Medicaid. The Medicaid website provides comprehensive information about Medicaid eligibility in each state.

In most states, people with a mental illness who are unable to work because of a disability are eligible for Supplemental Security Income (SSI), a federal cash assistance program. To be eligible for SSI, people must have low incomes, possess limited assets, and be unable to work because of their disability. People who get SSI might also be eligible to get other forms of help from their state or county. For example, people may be able to get help buying food through the Supplemental Nutrition Assistance Program (SNAP). In many states, people who receive SSI automatically qualify for Medicaid and do not have to fill out a separate Medicaid application. In other states, SSI guarantees Medicaid eligibility, but to receive Medicaid benefits, people need to sign up for them. In a few states, SSI does not guarantee Medicaid eligibility, but most people are eligible. Information about applying for SSI can be found on the Medicaid website or by calling the local Medicaid office.

People who have worked long enough and paid Social Security taxes may also be eligible for Social Security Disability Insurance (SSDI). The underage children of people who have worked long enough and paid Social Security taxes may also be eligible for SSDI. Eleven categories of mental illness can qualify people for SSDI benefits.

Regardless of the type of disability a person has, in order to receive SSI or SSDI benefits, they must be able to document that they are receiving and complying with treatment. SSI and SSDI can provide a steady income and health insurance for people with serious mental illness, making it possible for many to secure housing, treatment, and other needed supports. The Benefit

Eligibility Screening Tool provides information about whether individuals qualify for SSI and SSDI benefits.

Many people who are eligible for SSI and SSDI never apply for these benefits. Knowing how complicated anything involving the government can be, I wondered about how people with serious mental illnesses and their family members learn about SSI and SSDI benefits. I posed the question to a few Facebook groups that include people with serious mental illness and their families. As I suspected, most people learned about the benefits by chance. Sometimes a social worker mentioned SSI or SSDI during a hospital discharge session. Other times a school counselor suggested it. But mostly, people learned about the benefits from a friend.

Not only do most people not know about these benefits, but studies find that only 10–15 percent of first-time applicants are approved for and receive SSI and SSDI benefits. Denials are most often due to lack of adequate documentation or missed appointments by the applicant. Since the Substance Abuse and Mental Health Services Administration established the SSI/SSDI Outreach, Access, and Recovery (SOAR) Technical Assistance Center and case managers learned how to correctly submit applications, more than 70 percent of applications have been approved. Information about SOAR by state can be found on SAMHSA's website.

The Affordable Care Act of 2010 (ACA) enabled states to expand Medicaid benefits to cover nearly all low-income Americans under age 65. Eligibility for children was extended to at least 138 percent of poverty level in every state. States were given the option of extending eligibility to adults with income at or below 138 percent of the federal poverty level. While the majority of states expanded coverage to adults, some states still do not provide these benefits. Information about whether a state provides expanded coverage to adults can be found on the Medicaid website.

WHAT MEDICAID COVERS

Medicaid offers many benefits to people with serious mental illness. The mandatory benefits that states must provide under federal law include the following: inpatient hospital services, outpatient hospital services, physician services, and transportation to medical care. Optional benefits that states may cover include prescription drugs, clinic services, case management, day treatment programs, rehabilitation services, and inpatient psychiatric service for people under 21. In some states, Medicaid covers services such as personal care, supported employment services, and job coaching that enable people with disabilities to work. A complete list of mandatory and optional benefits can be found on the Medicaid website. Local Medicaid offices can provide valuable information.

MEDICAID ACCESS TO MENTAL HEALTH CARE

Compared with people who are uninsured, people covered by Medicaid have better access to mental health services, are less likely to report unmet needs for services, and are more likely to receive mental health treatment. However, the overall shortage of doctors and other mental health care providers, as well as the relatively small number of providers who accept Medicaid, limits access to health care even though Medicaid will pay for this care.

FUNDING MENTAL HEALTH SERVICES: PRIVATE SOURCES

The ACA changed Medicaid, but it also changed private health insurance, which covers about 40 percent of mental health care. Before the ACA, most private insurance policies did not cover mental illnesses. At that time, a person like my daughter Sophie, who had health insurance when she was diagnosed with bipolar disorder, was trapped in the health plan she had when she was diagnosed. There was no realistic opportunity to be covered by alternative plans. The same was true for a person with schizophrenia, depression, and other mental illnesses. For people who were uninsured at the time of their diagnosis, securing coverage was challenging, expensive, or impossible.

In 1996 and then in 2008, Congress passed mental health parity laws that required large group plans covering mental health treatment to offer benefits comparable to those for medical/surgical care. But there was a huge loophole. The mental health parity laws did not require large group plans to cover mental health. They only required that parity be provided if the company provided mental health coverage.

The ACA, in contrast, stipulated that both private and public health plans must treat mental health services as essential health benefits and that they must do so at parity with general health services. It prohibited coverage exclusions for preexisting conditions and required that prescription drugs, including medications for mental illnesses, be covered.

One of the most important reforms of the ACA for people with serious mental illness was its 2010 mandate that children be covered on their parents' insurance until the age of 26. Despite all the challenges my husband and I had finding good medical care and paying for Sophie's medications and treatments, we were grateful that this change enabled us to continue to use the insurance provided by my employer to pay for the treatments and medications she needed to control the symptoms of her mental illness. Without it, we certainly would have gone into debt. The ability for a parent to insure their child until age 26 is especially important in the case of mental illness because the vast majority of serious mental illnesses emerge in late adolescence and the early twenties. Allowing children to be covered by their parents' insurance until they are 26—along with the expansion of Medicaid and premium subsidies in the health insurance exchanges—has resulted in a sharp decline in the number of young adults without health insurance. According to US Census data, 22.1 percent of people aged 19–25 were uninsured in 2014. That number fell to 13.1 percent in 2016. Being insured, in turn, increased the number of young adults who received outpatient mental health treatment and decreased reports of unmet needs among young adults with serious mental illness.

The ACA has improved the lives of thousands of people with mental illness because it enabled more people to have access to care. Yet a recent comprehensive report found that private health insurers often skimp on coverage for mental illnesses. As such, access to care for mental illnesses remains limited for people with private insurance. Additionally, access is constrained by the cost of co-pays and an inadequate supply of providers, especially for special populations such as children, adolescents, and older people. A study in Denver found that an insured patient had to call seven to ten psychiatrists to find an available appointment. Studies in other regions of the United States report similar findings.

UNINSURED PEOPLE

The ACA extended Medicaid coverage to millions of low-income Americans, yet 27 million people in our country remain uninsured. Most working-age people in the United States obtain health insurance through an employer. A 2019 study by the US Bureau of Labor Statistics reported that medical care benefits are offered to 69 percent of private industry workers and 89 percent of government workers. Yet many workers who are offered health insurance cannot afford their share of the premiums, usually 20 percent of the cost. As a result, these people live without health insurance. Moreover, because health coverage changes with work status, some people become uninsured because the person who carried the health coverage for the family lost their job or changed employers.

While the ACA has helped many people with low and moderate incomes, Medicaid eligibility for adults remains limited in states that have not expanded benefits. Sadly, Texas, where Sophie has lived since she was 18, is one such state. Once Sophie turned 26, my husband and I could no longer cover her medical care using my employer's health insurance plan. Although Sophie was working as a certified nursing assistant in a nursing home, the health plan offered by her employer required co-pays well beyond Sophie's means. Like Sophie, most of the uninsured people are US citizens who have at least one full-time worker in the family with an income that is too high to qualify for Medicaid but too low to make insurance premiums affordable. While most of the uninsured are non-Hispanic whites, people of color are disproportionately more likely to be uninsured than whites. In addition, people who are self-employed and those who are contract workers often do not have adequate insurance.

Lack of health insurance puts people at tremendous social, health, and financial risks. People without insurance are less likely than those with insurance to receive preventive care and treatment for chronic illnesses. Most do not have a regular provider to see when they are sick. They are more likely to be hospitalized for avoidable health problems, and when they are hospitalized, uninsured people receive fewer diagnostic and therapeutic services. Finally, uninsured people face unaffordable medical bills when they do seek care, as hospitals often charge uninsured patients much higher rates than those paid by private and public health insurers. When Sophie, who had neither a primary doctor nor health insurance, experienced severe constipation and stomach pain, she went to the local hospital's emergency room. Tests costing more than $2,000 revealed she was pregnant. Such bills can quickly translate into medical debt since, like Sophie, most uninsured people have little, if any, savings.

STRATEGIES THAT MAY BE HELPFUL WHEN PEOPLE
CAN'T AFFORD TREATMENT

The costs of mental health services and medications are prohibitive. Even though my husband and I had first-rate health insurance, we still paid thousands of dollars each year to the therapists who treated our daughter. Sometimes the medications prescribed by Sophie's doctors were not covered by our insurance plan, and we had to make decisions about whether to pay for the expensive drugs or try a less costly generic.

Here are some strategies that may help cover the expenses associated with mental illnesses, although I caution that the usefulness of any given strategy may change over time and that I am not endorsing any particular strategy:

- Sign up for government benefits either online at the Social Security website (ssa.gov) or by calling 1-800-772-1213. Government benefits include SSDI, SSI, and Medicaid. As indicated above, SSI is based purely on financial need. SSDI is designed for insured workers who have worked long enough and paid Social Security taxes. However, children under 18 can draw SSDI from their parents' benefits. Qualified people can draw funds from the Social Security system even if they've never worked. SSI payments are usually less than those from SSDI, so fill out the SSDI application and see if you are eligible. SSI and SSDI provide monthly benefit payments.

- Apply for Medicaid even if you have private insurance. Medicaid provides health insurance for people with low incomes or special needs. Anyone with a disability meeting the Social Security definition is eligible. In most states, people eligible for SSI are automatically eligible for Medicaid. Medicaid is a benefit, costing nothing to an individual, that can reduce out-of-pocket expenses. More importantly, a host of excellent programs and benefits (described on the Medicaid.gov website) are available only to people on Medicaid. But services covered by Medicaid vary widely by state. To learn about the benefits in each state, start by visiting the Medicaid.gov website (https://www.medicaid.gov/state-overviews/index.html), which provides details on expanded Medicaid benefits for each state. Then, call the local Medicaid office and ask for details. What types of providers are covered? How long can each visit be? How many visits per month are covered? How much are co-pays? Be sure to document the date of the call and the person with whom you spoke.

- Tell your doctor if you are worried about being able to afford your bills and the costs of medications. Sometimes doctors offer sliding scale payment arrangements. Sometimes inexpensive generic medications that are as effective as brand name medications can be prescribed. Sometimes doctors have free samples of medications available to give to patients.

- Private health insurance plans vary widely in coverage. If you are covered by private health insurance, call the company and ask for details about what its policy covers. What types of providers are covered? How long can each visit be? How many visits per month are covered? How much are co-pays? Jot down the date of your call and make sure to get the name of the person with whom you spoke.

- If you are uninsured, you may be able to get some of your medical care from a local free clinic. Free clinics are nonprofit organizations that provide medical care for little or no cost. They may be found in hospitals or stand-alone clinics. To find a nearby free clinic, visit the free clinic finder website maintained by the Partnership for Prescription Assistance (PPA) (https://www.pparx.org

/prescription_assistance_programs/free_clinic_finder).
Additionally, the US Department of Health and Human
Services has a list of Federally Qualified Health Centers
that is searchable by zip code (https://findahealthcenter
.hrsa.gov/). These centers must meet a stringent set of
requirements, including providing care on a sliding fee
scale based on ability to pay. If you are not web savvy, go
to your local library and ask the librarian to help you.

- People who cannot afford prescriptions, either because
  they are uninsured or because they are underinsured,
  should visit the PPA website (https://www.pparx.org
  /gethelp). PPA connects patients with pharmaceutical
  companies. Medications are free or nearly free. After
  people provide basic information about their prescription
  medicines, income, and current prescription medicine
  coverage, PPA matches people with assistance programs
  for which they may be eligible. Make sure, however, to
  speak directly to PPA. There are several companies with
  names similar to "Partnership for Prescription Assistance"
  that charge enrollment and monthly fees.

- GoodRx offers coupons for prescription medications that
  may save you money.

- Walmart has a program through which people can get a
  thirty-day supply of many prescription medications for
  $4 each or a ninety-day supply for $10 each. The program covers most medications commonly prescribed for
  serious mental illness (https://www.walmart.com/cp/$4
  -prescriptions/1078664).

- Medical schools often have programs that train students
  while providing free or low-cost medical care to people
  in their local community. If you live near a medical
  school, give the psychiatry department a call and ask
  whether it has such a program.

Finally, unless you are truly in crisis, avoid going to the emergency room. Emergency room staff generally lack the expertise to help people with serious mental illness, and care in an emergency room is very expensive.

"I Don't Know How to Get the Help I Need"

For many people, the realities of life make the difference between getting and not getting treatment. When Sophie lived with me, I spent hours looking for doctors who had experience treating patients like her and to whom Sophie could relate. I drove her to all of her appointments. When she moved to Texas, Sophie said she could take care of things. But she stopped taking her medication. She had no idea how to find a doctor. She did not drive and, other than by walking, had no way to get to a doctor's office. Sophie was not alone. The National Survey on Drug Use and Health revealed that, among people with a serious mental illness who wanted but had not received treatment in the past year, 32.2 percent said they did not know where to go to get help, 17.4 percent said they did not have time to get to help, and 5.0 percent said they lacked transportation to get to the provider's office.

The following strategies may be helpful when people don't know where to get help or can't get there:

- If you or your loved one is in crisis or needs immediate help, call the National Suicide Prevention Lifeline (1-800-273-8255) or visit its website (https:// suicidepreventionlifeline.org). Trained crisis workers are available to talk twenty-four hours a day, seven days a week. The lifeline provides crisis counseling and mental health referrals. If the situation is life-threatening, call 911 or go to a hospital emergency room.
- If the person with mental illness is not in crisis, talk with your family doctor. He or she may be able to

prescribe medication or suggest mental health providers nearby.

- The SAMHSA Treatment Referral Helpline can connect people with local providers. Call 1-800-662-HELP (4357) or use SAMHSA's Behavioral Health Treatment Locator. Entering an address will identify providers in the area.

- In many areas, dialing 2-1-1 can connect people with local mental health crisis services or enable people to find help nearby.

- Use the *Psychology Today* website to search for mental health professionals in your area. The website can search several criteria, including zip code, city, and provider's name. For each provider listed, you can read about the provider's therapy approach, specialty areas, and information about fees, including whether insurance is accepted and whether sliding scale fees are offered. You'll also find valuable information about each provider's credentials and contact information.

- Talk with a trusted friend, clergyperson, or teacher. Tell the person what is happening and ask for their help. Sometimes this help might be a listening ear. Other times, it might be a ride to the doctor's office or help placing a call to a provider.

Finally, although telepsychiatry and telepsychology—providing mental health care from a distance through technology—is just gaining momentum, in the next few years it is likely to become common for psychiatric evaluations, therapy, patient education, and medication management. In many states, Medicaid already reimburses telehealth care services. What's more, there is growing evidence that telehealth services work. A pilot study in which thirty-eight people with serious mental illness received automated telehealth intervention for six months revealed that psychiatric symptoms decreased and illness management skills increased. Moreover, there were significant decreases in hospital admissions and emergency room visits. A review of forty-six tele-psychiatry studies in twelve countries consistently found that patients view telehealth as feasible and acceptable for illness self-management, medication and treatment adherence, education, and symptom monitoring.

FINDING HELP ON COLLEGE CAMPUSES

The Center for Collegiate Mental Health's 2019 report includes information from 163 college and university counseling centers and describes the experiences of 207,818 unique college students seeking mental health treatment and the perspectives of 4,059 clinicians across 1,580,951 appointments. Depression and anxiety are the most common concerns of students who visit these counseling centers. Nearly 40 percent of students seeking treatment reported suicidal ideation.

Many students, however, do not know that their university has a counseling center. Others do not know how to navigate the center in order to get the help they need. Because many counseling centers charge for appointments, students do not go to the counseling center because they do not want to involve their parents.

Recently colleges and universities around the country have been faced with a new challenge, one rooted in the economics of supply and demand. More and more students coming to college had been diagnosed in high school or middle school with a serious mental illness, including depression and bipolar disorder. Medications and other treatments have enabled these students to attend college. The shedding of stigma surrounding mental illness, more common on college campuses than in the general community, has also caused demand for counseling services to increase.

But providing mental health care is expensive. The rule of thumb is that one counselor is needed for every 1,000–1,500 students. While a small school can easily get by with a handful of counselors, a large school with 50,000 students would require dozens of counselors. Funding is a challenge. Most university counseling centers cannot keep up with student needs. Unless a student is in the midst of a crisis, it is difficult to get an appointment with a counselor. Many students are cut off from services after just a few sessions. Wait times to see a therapist can be weeks long. The consequences of not being seen can be disastrous. Suicides, the second-leading cause of death among college students (after traffic accidents), are at an all-time high.

Some schools have hired additional counselors and added new student fees that directly support mental health service. Other schools have created "caring communities," with websites and educational programming that identify signs of distress and provide guidance to students and faculty who are concerned about a student's well-being. Others have launched online programs whose goal is to build strong communities, enabling people to respond to mental health crises. The Jed Foundation has a number of programs that can help schools evaluate and strengthen their mental health, substance abuse, and suicide prevention programs. It also has information about developing resources and creating partnerships that enable students to access resources. Their suggestions about educating students and communities about when and how to support people struggling with mental illness are first-rate. Finally, in 2002, Alison Malmon, a junior at University of Pennsylvania whose older brother Brian died by suicide after struggling silently with depression and psychosis, launched Active Minds. Active Minds encourages college students who need help to seek help so that tragedies like the one her brother experienced can be prevented. Now on more than seven hundred campuses and including over 600,000 students, Active Minds encourages people to talk about mental illness and suicide so that no one struggles alone.

"I Don't Want Anyone to Know"

For years, Elyn Saks did not tell her parents about her illness or hospitalizations. She says, "I didn't want them to worry; even more important, I didn't want them to think less of me, that I was somehow a weak or crazy failure. I wanted to fix myself, and not have my problems in any way leak into their lives." Like Saks, many people with a serious mental illness who participated in the National Survey on Drug Use and Health worried about stigma. Some said they had not sought treatment because they were concerned that treatment might have negative effects on their job (16.4%). Others thought that treatment might cause neighbors to have a negative opinion of them (15.7%). Some were concerned about confidentiality (15.3%), and some did not want others to find out (12.6%). Consistent with these numbers, a systematic review of 144 studies found that worries about stigma reduce help seeking.

While studying at Oxford, Elyn Saks made friends with three other students. They would cook meals together and spend endless hours talking late into the night. Elyn told her friends that she had intermittently been hospitalized and was in psychoanalysis. She adds, "Nevertheless, there were whole parts of myself I tried desperately to keep hidden. I knew, for instance, not to share my ongoing delusions of evil, in particular the part about my being evil and my total certainty that I was capable of horrible acts of violence. Not that these thoughts were wrong; I believed everyone thought this way, but just knew better than to talk about it, much as everyone passes gas, but not in company."

People with a serious mental illness should reach out to someone they trust and tell them what is happening. The person could be a friend, a family member, a teacher, or a member of the clergy. Sometimes all it takes is talking to one person to help put things in perspective. That person can serve as a sounding board and offer reassurance. Years after she graduated from Oxford, when Elyn was a first-year law student at Yale, she met Steve. From their very first conversation, Elyn knew she would tell Steve the truth about herself. Elyn wanted Steve as a lifelong friend and "didn't believe that could happen unless I revealed the truth about myself and let him 'see' me in full." Steve listened, asked a lot of questions, and became Elyn's lifelong friend. From that point on, whenever Elyn became psychotic, she knew she could call Steve and he would help her through the crisis.

Concerns about treatment confidentiality must be understood in light of the Health Insurance Portability and Accountability Act (HIPAA). HIPAA is a federal law that protects the privacy of individual health information, including information about mental illness diagnosis and treatment. The Office of Civil Rights (OCR) within the US Department of Health and Human Services has enforcement authority over HIPAA. On February 21, 2014, OCR released guidance clarifying how and when health care providers may share an individual's mental health treatment information with others.

Under HIPAA, if the person with mental illness does not object, a health care provider may share information that is necessary or directly related to his or her treatment with that person's family or friends. If the person receiving treatment is an adult who objects to the release of information and is deemed capable of making health care decisions by the health care provider, then the health care provider may not share information with family or friends. However, HIPAA laws do not stop family members or friends from sharing information that they believe is relevant or helpful with a health care provider. Moreover, a provider who receives information from family members or friends of a patient is not required to disclose this information to the patient. If the health care provider determines that the patient does not have the capacity to make health care decisions, then the provider may choose to share information with family, friends, or other individuals involved in the person's care if the provider believes that it is in the person's best interest. If the patient poses a danger to self or others, then the health care provider must disclose this information to the police.

Under no circumstances can providers share information about treatment and diagnosis of mental illness with employers, schools, or neighbors.

When People Do Not Want Treatment

A couple of years after Sophie moved to Texas, she met Mike. Nine years older than Sophie, Mike had grown up in East Texas. Like Sophie, Mike was dependent on methamphetamine. Like Sophie, Mike lived on the street. But unlike Sophie, Mike heard voices and they frightened him. Diagnosed with schizophrenia when he was 9, Mike had taken medications for a few years. But Mike said that the medications made him "feel like a zombie," so he had stopped taking them more than twenty years ago. Many people with serious mental illness say they do not want treatment. Some people do not believe they need treatment because they do not think they are sick. Some people, like Mike, do not want treatment because they dislike the way the medications make them feel. Sadly, like Mike, many people who refuse treatment believe that alcohol or street drugs soothe their symptoms better than prescribed medicines.

"I Don't Need Treatment"

One of the greatest frustrations for people who have not experienced the delusions and hallucinations of serious mental illness is how people who hear and see things that others do not could possibly lack awareness of their illness. In the 2001 movie *A Beautiful Mind*, Ron Howard uses creative cinematography that enables viewers not only to see what hallucinations and delusions look and sound like but also to understand how these psychotic experiences can lead a person to conclude that treatment is unnecessary.

The movie's main character is John Nash, a brilliant mathematician who made groundbreaking contributions to game theory. He identified a powerful tool for analyzing a wide range of competitive situations—from corporate rivalries to legislative decision-making. Nash's discoveries about pure mathematics have been lauded as even more significant. However, after making breakthroughs so important that he would win the Nobel Memorial Prize in Economic Sciences, Nash, at age 30, was diagnosed with schizophrenia.

Early in the movie, Nash is invited to the Pentagon because he has a unique ability to decipher codes. The Department of Defense needs help identifying places in the United States where the Russians had planted bombs. Dialogue among several people in the movie makes it clear to viewers that the visit to the Pentagon is real. However, it also becomes clear that there is a "person" that Nash sees during his visit to the Pentagon, referred to as "Big Brother," that is really a hallucination. Nobody except Nash sees "Big Brother."

One evening, shortly after his visit to the Pentagon, Nash is leaving his MIT lab. He meets "Big Brother," who introduces himself as William Parcher. Parcher tells Nash that he had supervised Oppenheimer's work creating the atomic bomb and says, "I am now increasing your security clearance ... to top secret." Parcher describes a Soviet plan to detonate a bomb on US soil. The agents, he says, are communicating through codes embedded in periodicals and newspapers—codes that John must find and decipher. As part of Nash's orientation to defense work, he (and viewers) watch a technician implant a radium diode above John's wrist. Parcher tells John that the changing numbers on the diode are access codes for drop spots. The scene ends with Parcher saying, "You can tell no one of your work. Just proceed with normal life. Avoid new people. And, assume at all times you are being watched." Viewers watch as Nash's delusions take hold. He believes that he is a spy under constant surveillance. Nash is so certain that a radium diode had been implanted in his wrist that later in the film, desperate to prove to himself and others that he really is a spy, he gouges the skin of his wrist with his fingernails, attempting to dig it out.

Shortly after Parcher recruits Nash, viewers see Nash in his apartment amid a sea of magazines. He circles random words and pictures, slides his work into a top secret envelope, and seals it with wax. Then, in the darkness of night, he walks to a gated abandoned mansion, gains entry via the diode in his wrist, and delivers his report to a rusty mailbox. This scene enables viewers to see that for Nash the delusion that he is a spy for the government is real. We see him walking quickly, constantly looking over his shoulder, worried that he will be caught.

As the film progresses, Nash's job as a secret agent becomes increasingly dangerous. There is a wild midnight car chase. Nash tells Parcher he no longer wants to be a spy, but Parcher threatens to harm Nash's wife if he stops his spy work. At this point, Nash fears his delusions, but he believes they are real and that he cannot escape them. Viewers learn how Nash's delusions and paranoid behavior are understood by other people as we watch him interact with his wife. She says, "What's wrong with you? John, what's going on? Please, you've got to talk to me."

In a scene where John is presenting a guest lecture at Harvard, we see him scrawl mathematical formulas on a blackboard. With suspicion, he watches as a couple of men enter the upper balcony. They are wearing overcoats and hats. Fearful, Nash races out of the room and runs across the quad. The two men give chase. Running down the steps, Nash sees another man standing at the base of the stairway, blocking his way. Nash stops cold. The man at the bottom of the stairs says, "My name is Dr. Rosen. I'm a psychiatrist. I'd like you to come with me, John. Just for a chat."

"And if I say no?"

"I have a court order signed by a judge. I hope we can proceed without any unpleasantness."

"Well, I suppose I don't have much choice." Then, Nash slugs Rosen across the face and screams, "Help me! They're Russians."

In this scene, viewers begin to understand why people with psychosis might refuse treatment. Nash has lost the ability to distinguish the real from the imagined. Because he believes that his delusions are real, he acts on them. Nash was a spy, forced to do a very dangerous job. He no longer wanted to be a spy, but he feared for his life and that of his wife. The treatment Rosen is offering is the last thing that Nash believes he needs.

By enabling viewers to see the world through Nash's eyes, *A Beautiful Mind* shows how psychosis makes behaviors that look alarming to outsiders seem rational and reasonable to the person experiencing the psychosis. It shows the horror of not being able to know what is true and what is not.

Like John Nash, many people with schizophrenia and bipolar disorder and some people with depression experience impaired insight. Dubbed "anosognosia" (the Greek term for "not knowing the disease") in 1914 by the French neurologist Joseph Babinski, lack of awareness is common in people with Alzheimer's disease, Huntington's disease, and other serious mental illnesses. People with anosognosia do not recognize the symptoms of their illness and are unable to attribute consequences and deficits to their illness.

The prevalence of anosognosia is unclear because there is variability in how it is assessed, when it is assessed, and who is doing the assessing. Moreover, good evidence shows that insight exists on a continuum or a set of continua. People can have various degrees of overall insight, insight can vary over the course of an episode of illness, and insight can vary over time. This fluidity has important implications for helping someone with serious mental illness, as it suggests that there are times when a person with schizophrenia, bipolar disorder, or depression may be more aware of their illness than others, providing a window during which they may be more receptive to treatment.

Some scholars have suggested that lack of insight is a feature of schizophrenia but an indicator of illness intensity of bipolar disorder. Between 27 and 57 percent of people with schizophrenia lack awareness of their hallucinations, delusions, thought disorders, and blunt affect. Lack of awareness is less of a problem for people with depression. People with schizophrenia and those with bipolar disorder have similar levels of unawareness of their mental disorder, hallucinations, delusions, thought disorders, and flat affect. Not surprisingly, insight is greater among people with bipolar disorder who are in remission than those who are in the throes of mania or depression. Moreover, insight is more impaired when people with bipolar disorder are manic than when they are depressed.

Lack of insight is often confused with denial, but these experiences are quite different. Denial is a normal psychological defense that may give people hope as they cope with a new diagnosis. Lack of insight, on the other hand, results from physical damage to the brain. Someone with anosognosia, like John Nash, is not simply in denial or being stubborn. On the contrary, their brains cannot process the fact that their thoughts and moods do not reflect reality. Several fascinating studies of people with mental illnesses who had not been treated with medications reveal that lack of insight involves a broad network of anatomical structures within the brain. People with poorer insight have lower gray matter volumes, thinner cortical layers, less white matter, and lower volumes of the right dorsolateral prefrontal cortex. Because these studies included people who had not been treated with medications, it suggests that the illness, and not the psychotropic medications, is responsible for the brain anomalies.

LACK OF INSIGHT AND TREATMENT ADHERENCE

Would anyone take a medication for diabetes or hypertension if they did not believe they had the illness? Probably not. People like John Nash whose mental illness includes delusions—especially those who believe they have superpowers—are among those least likely to adhere to treatment. Why? Because people with superpowers do not need medicine.

Common sense suggests that people who do not realize they are sick are less likely to adhere to treatment than people who do know they are sick. But an important distinction between people with diabetes or hypertension who do not take their medication and people with mental illness who do not take their medication is choice. This choice, whether deemed right or wrong by others, is nonetheless based on the person's subjective appraisal of his or her circumstances. With a mental illness like schizophrenia, nonadherence is not simply a matter of choice, but a complex interplay among choice, lack of insight, and competence.

Surprisingly, while there is strong evidence that poor insight is associated with poor treatment adherence, there is no compelling evidence that medication can increase insight. Psychosocial interventions also have had inconsistent effects.

STRATEGIES THAT MAY BE HELPFUL WHEN YOUR RELATIVE NEEDS HELP BUT DOESN'T THINK HE OR SHE DOES

Lack of insight on the part of people with mental illness is one of the most frustrating challenges for family members. The movie *A Beautiful Mind* shows the frustration Nash's wife, Alicia, experienced as she struggled to understand how her brilliant

husband could not realize how sick he was. With tears stream-
ing down her face, Alicia shows John a stack of envelopes that
John sealed and deposited in what he believed was a secret
mailbox. She says, "None of it's been real, John. They've never
been opened. There is no William Parcher. There is no conspiracy. It's all in your mind. You're sick, John. Don't you understand, you're sick." Like Alicia, family members often are
tempted to explain the benefits of treatment, argue that treatment is important, and beg their loved one to get help. More often than not, these pleas go unheeded—not because the person
doesn't want help, but because they do not believe they need it.

Finally, insight about anosognosia comes from John Nash's
response to his biographer's question about why he believed
that aliens from outer space had recruited him to save the world.
Nash responded, "Because the ideas I had about supernatural
beings came to me the same way that my mathematical ideas
did. So, I took them seriously."

The best advice for trying to help a person who lacks insight
is based on understanding that lack of insight is usually not a
permanent condition. When illnesses are in remission, people
are more likely to recognize they have an illness and accept
help. The best time to establish a treatment regimen is while the
person is in remission, not while in the midst of a psychotic crisis. Use of a long-acting injectable medication should be discussed once a patient having a first-episode psychotic illness
has been stabilized.

Yet certainly people in crisis—when insight is most likely to
be compromised—need help. Xavier Amador, a clinical psychologist, researcher, and author of more than 120 articles
and eight books about serious mental illness, has devoted his
life to helping people with mental illness and their families. Not
only does Amador have professional credentials, but he also has
personal experience helping a loved one with serious mental
illness. In 1981, Xavier's older brother Enrique returned home

after his first hospitalization for schizophrenia. Stabilized on medication in the hospital, Enrique said, "I am not sick. I don't need help." Because Enrique did not think he was sick, he refused to take the medication. But Enrique *was* sick. He *did* need help. Angry shouting matches ensued each time Xavier tried to reason with Enrique.

Nearly twenty years later, Xavier published his book *I Am Not Sick—I Don't Need Help!* In the book, Amador shows that arguing with people with mental illness or trying to convince them that they are wrong about their ideas, especially when they are in throes of a crisis, can only lead to disaster. Instead, Amador offers a four-part communication strategy that he calls LEAP: Listen-Empathize-Agree-Partner. Xavier's book, DVDs, and audio training CDs teach families how to implement each strategy and have enabled many to successfully gain the trust of a loved one with mental illness.

"I Don't Like the Way the Medications Make Me Feel": Creativity and Mental Illness

Many people say that they do not take psychotropic medications because the medications dull their ability to be creative. The links between creativity, mental illness, and psychotropic medications are complex. Before we can understand the effects of medications on creativity, we need to understand the connection between mental illnesses and creativity. But in order to understand the link between creativity and mental illness, we must be clear about how we are defining creativity. To be creative, ideas must both be novel and have utility. People with schizophrenia often have a lot of novel ideas. There are spaceships waiting to take them to a new planet and radio waves delivering important messages. Words are sometimes uttered in combinations so unique that ideas are not understandable. Having novel ideas and developing them into something of value is what makes for creativity. The creative person can manage the flood of ideas, selecting the useful ones and developing them while discarding the others. The person with psychosis is at the mercy of loose associations and disconnected thinking.

The belief that creative people experience psychopathology dates back to the ancient Greeks. Plato suggested that poets, philosophers, and dramatists suffered "divine madness"; Aristotle associated poets with melancholia. The idea of a link between creativity and mental illness was fueled by studying the lives of Vincent Van Gogh, Virginia Woolf, Robert Schumann, Robert Lowell, and Sylvia Plath, all arguably very creative people with diagnosed mental illnesses. And the conviction is a lasting one. Today, the popular media continue to romanticize images of the suffering artist and the mad scientist, invigorated by a new willingness among many creative people, including Demi Lovato, Kanye West, Olly Alexander, Lady Gaga, Beyoncé, Sia, Christina Aguilera, Bruce Springsteen, Kid Cudi, Sinead O'Connor, and Mayim Bialik, to acknowledge and talk about their mental illnesses.

But is it really so? Are mentally ill people more creative than the rest of us? Are creative people more likely to experience a mental illness?

To address this issue, scientists have studied psychiatric illness in creative people and creativity in people with psychiatric illnesses. To study psychiatric illness in creative people, scholars examined the biographies of eminent people. One of the earliest studies examined the lives of eight hundred people regarded as geniuses, including Michelangelo, Luther, Napoleon, Beethoven, and Schopenhauer. The study concluded that it cannot simply be a matter of chance that among geniuses the healthy are a small minority. A study that compared people attending the Iowa Writers Workshop and their first-degree relatives to a matched control group found that 80 percent of the writers had suffered mood disorders and that the writers were four times more likely to suffer bipolar disorder than the healthy controls. Yet another study compared award-winning artists and poets from the United Kingdom to population norms and found that the creative people were six times more likely to be diagnosed with bipolar disorder than other people. In her book *Touched with Fire: Manic-Depressive Illness and the Artistic Temperament*, Kay Redfield Jamison, a psychiatrist diagnosed with bipolar disorder as a teenager, shows how mental illness impacted the work of Ernest Hemingway, William James, Herman Melville, Robert Schumann, Mary Shelley, Vincent Van Gogh, and Virginia Woolf. More recently, Jamison examined the life of Robert Lowell in *Setting the River on Fire: A Study of Genius, Mania, and Character*, showing how bipolar disorder affected his creativity.

While fascinating, these biographical analyses have serious limitations. Diagnoses are not always well documented, and the number of people studied is small. Methods depend on subjective and anecdotal accounts that are not rigorous. Nonetheless, an analysis based on more than thirty studies found that creative people exhibit more mood disorder than noncreative people.

To study creativity in people with and without psychiatric illnesses, scientists usually contrast groups of people using standardized psychological tests and various measures of creativity. Most studies rely on designs that match about fifty people with a diagnosed illness to a like number without the illness. Some studies find that people with mental illness are more creative; others find that they are not.

A study of nearly 1.2 million Swedish people used a different design. Using national registries, scientists matched people who had received treatment for schizophrenia, bipolar disorder, or depression between 1973 and 2003 and their relatives without such a diagnosis with controls who did not have these disorders and their relatives. They found that people in scientific and artistic occupations were no more likely to be diagnosed with a psychiatric disorder than people in other professions. An exception was people with bipolar disorder, who were just slightly more likely to hold scientific and artistic occupations than their peers.

Research consistently finds that creativity does not differ between people with and without serious mental illness. The authors of four major textbooks came to the same conclusion. Some scholars suggest that the question whether there is a link between creativity and mental illness may be too general. Others find that when there are connections between creativity and mental illness, the links tend to be stronger when people experience fewer, less severe symptoms.

Positing that there may be a genetic link between creativity and mental illness, some researchers have taken to studying the unaffected relatives of people with schizophrenia or bipolar disorder. These studies find that relatives of people with bipolar disorder and schizophrenia who do not suffer these mental illnesses have high levels of creativity and are overrepresented in creative professions. Is it possible that the relatives inherited a watered-down version of mental illness that increased their creativity but allowed them to somehow dodge the debilitating characteristics?

Together, these findings suggest that an inverted-U shape characterizes the relationship between creativity and psychosis, with better functioning people who carry the genes for certain mental illnesses tending to have a creative advantage. Either there is a hereditary connection between creativity and mental illness, or milder forms of psychiatric illnesses may enhance creativity. Based on results from neuroimaging and genetic studies, some have suggested that a shared vulnerability model explains the relationship between creativity and psychopathology. Others propose a "mad-genius paradox," suggesting that creative people can be more mentally healthy and highly creative people can be more mentally ill. Particularly gifted people with a history of serious mental illness have their most creative periods at times when they experience either mild symptoms or no clinical symptoms at all. However, it is clear that full-blown bipolar disorder or schizophrenia interferes with creativity. As Sylvia Plath said, "When you are insane, you are busy being insane—all the time....When I was crazy, that's all I was."

TREATMENT AND CREATIVITY

Although the scientific evidence indicates that serious mental illnesses interfere with creativity, it is not uncommon for people with schizophrenia or bipolar disorder to stop taking psychotropic medications because they believe that the medicines hinder their creativity. Collin was one of these people. Collin was 27 when he was diagnosed with Type II bipolar disorder. His mother told me that, as a 5-year-old, Collin was smart, quiet, and funny. Collin loved doing magic tricks, but he was so shy that he would not do them in public—unless he was wearing a costume. When he was 12, Collin started playing guitar. He formed his own band and had a gold record by the time he was 18. Knowing of Collin's struggles with social anxiety and depression, his mother took him to the doctor and made sure he took his prescribed medications. But Collin complained that Prozac, Lexapro, and Paxil dulled his creativity. He told his mother that Depakote made him feel as if he were "walking through butterscotch." He said he could not create or perform when he took these medications, and so he stopped taking them.

Not surprisingly, there is little empirical research to know whether Collin was right about psychotropic medications dulling creativity. Conducting a study that requires people with serious mental illness to stop taking their medications in order to measure whether their creativity changes is not ethical.

What we do know comes largely from anecdotal evidence. And the findings are mixed, most likely dependent on the severity of a person's symptoms and the specific medication or treatment. John Nash, for example, avoided psychiatric treatment, yet the only creative mathematical work he accomplished after his initial psychotic episode occurred during several months when he took trifluoperazine, an antipsychotic. David Foster Wallace, a MacArthur Fellow whose fiction and essays caught the attention of a generation, suffered from recurrent depression. In 2007, he discontinued long-standing treatment with phenelzine (an antidepressant) in part because he thought it was interfering with his ability to finish a novel. His depression relapsed, and he killed himself before completing the book. Similarly, Ernest Hemingway, after what would be the last of several courses of electroconvulsive therapy at the Mayo Clinic before he killed himself, wrote to his biographer A. E. Hotchner, "What is the sense of ruining my head and erasing my memory, which is my capital, and putting me out of business? It was a brilliant cure, but we lost the patient." In contrast, talk show host Dick Cavett told *People Magazine*, "In my case, ECT was miraculous. My wife was dubious, but when she came into my room afterward, I sat up and said, 'Look who's back among the living.' It was like a magic wand."

Finally, a collection of essays edited by psychiatrist Richard M. Berlin shows from insiders' perspectives how psychiatric treatment affected the creativity of sixteen poets. Gwyneth Lewis, J. D. Smith, Jesse Millner, and Renee Ashley, all of whom had severe depression, found that psychotherapy and medication gave them the strength to be creative. Thomas Krampf, diagnosed with schizophrenia, found that an unconventional form of treatment using orthomolecular strategies provided relief, allowing him to write poetry. Ren Powell, diagnosed with bipolar disorder, wrote that the imaginative ideas generated during a manic episode require the clear thinking and craft of stable mental functioning to be transformed into an artistic creation. For more than twenty years, poet Chase Twichell took a variety of medications for depression—Triavil, Elavil, Pamelor, Desyrel, Serzone, Paxil, Zoloft, Buspar, Valium, Effexor, Xanax, Celexa, Lexapro, Wellbutrin, Seroquel, and Klonopin. While the medicines soothed the symptoms of her depression, they also affected her writing. She says, "I can still make the imaginative connections and find the words eventually, but it takes longer and requires far more doggedness than it did before medications. On numerous occasions, I've tried to do without the drugs. . . . Each time the withdrawal was unbearable, but during the brief periods in which I was unmedicated, language came back to me." When Ms. Twichell was in her fifties, a new psychiatrist changed her diagnosis to Type II bipolar disorder and prescribed a cocktail of Celexa, Wellbutrin, and Klonopin. Her moods stabilized, her energy increased, and her creativity flourished.

STRATEGIES THAT MAY BE HELPFUL WHEN CREATIVITY IS OF CONCERN

Romantic notions of the "suffering artist" and "mad scientist" can be harmful for creative people who believe that mood disorder facilitates creativity. When creative people suffer from psychopathology, they may not seek treatment or be noncompliant in treatment, fearing that treatment will negatively impact their creativity. This can create havoc for them and for their family members.

People with concerns about creativity should make sure to discuss their worries with their mental health care provider. The inverted-U-shape relationship between creativity and mental illness suggests that the optimal solution is being on the lowest possible dosage of medication that keeps undesirable symptoms in check and does not hinder creativity. In addition, some medications seem to have less impact on creativity than others. There are numerous medications, each of which has a variety of dosages, so it is very likely that an experienced provider will find the right mix for each patient—one that controls negative symptoms while enabling creativity. However, finding this balance is not easy. It requires patience, good communication between the patient and the provider, and a lot of tinkering. Psychotherapy can be helpful. Regular monitoring of moods provides important feedback to the provider. Several mobile apps, including eMoods, Mood-Log, and Mood, can help monitor moods. Each can be downloaded to smartphones for free, and information can be shared with providers.

Other Things Not to Like about Medications

My daughter Sophie complained that the psychotropic medicines robbed her of her ability to read, to write poetry, and to draw. But she also said that the medicines made her feel lethargic and disoriented. Strattera made her appetite disappear. Even her desire for pizza and hot fudge sundaes disappeared. Concerta made Sophie dizzy and nauseous. Zoloft made her sleepy. Lamictal made her dizzy, nauseous, and tired. Vyvanse gave her diarrhea, made her jittery, and caused dry mouth. Seroquel made Sophie so groggy she could barely get out of bed. Sophie's reactions were common. Side effects of psychotropic medicines are numerous. They include restlessness, dry mouth, dizziness, nausea, diarrhea, constipation, and sexual dysfunction. Sometimes medications can worsen anxiety, depression, or mania. Panic attacks can occur. Medications can spark thoughts of suicide. Weight gain is common; in fact, research finds that weight gain is the health problem most likely to cause nonadherence.

While there is no shortage of things not to like about the side effects of many of the psychotropic medications, a skilled provider who understands a patient's priorities and illness, as well as the advantages and disadvantages of available medications, should be able to find the right combination of medications that will quell the negative symptoms while avoiding nasty side effects. Luckily for Sophie, her doctor was able to reassure her that some of the side effects, such as the dizziness and nausea from Concerta, would dissipate over time. Other times, side effects such as the sleepiness Sophie experienced with Zoloft could be relieved with a lower dose. Still other times, as in the case of Seroquel, the doctor tried a different medication. We found that Abilify calmed Sophie's mania without rendering her unable to function.

"Alcohol and Street Drugs Work Better Than Medicine"

Without medications, guitar-playing Collin became very angry. He put his fist through a glass pane. He threw his telephone across the room. Collin believed that the medications hindered his ability to perform his music, but he also knew that he could not perform without something to dull his pain. He turned to alcohol and soon found that he needed a drink every day in order to play. Embarrassed by this dependence, Collin hid his drinking.

Collin's decision to use alcohol to calm the symptoms of his illness is not uncommon. Nearly a quarter of adults with a serious mental illness meet the criteria for substance use disorder. Relative to the general population, people with serious mental illnesses are 4.6 times more likely to be smokers, 4.0 times more likely to be heavy alcohol users, 3.5 times more likely to be heavy marijuana users, and 4.6 times more likely to use recreational drugs. Among adolescents who had experienced a major depressive episode within the past year, the proportion who used illicit drugs was more than twice as high (33.0%) as that for youth who had not had a depressive episode (15.2%). Adolescents with a past-year major depressive episode also were more likely than those without an episode to use marijuana, nonprescribed psychotherapeutics, inhalants, and hallucinogens.

People with serious mental illnesses who use and abuse alcohol, cannabis, or any other street drugs are less likely to adhere to prescribed medical treatments than people who do not use these substances. Some, like Collin, find that alcohol keeps anxiety and depression in check and heightens sociability. Others, like Mike, use stimulants such as cocaine or methamphetamine. These stimulants spike levels of dopamine, which increases energy, focus, and attention and decreases appetite. Still others turn to opioids like heroin that depress the central nervous system, blunt moods, and help them sleep.

Self-medicating can be tempting. However, it also can be very dangerous. Drinking alcohol and using street drugs can make the symptoms of mental illness far worse. While these substances might temporarily relieve some of the symptoms of serious mental illness, the backlash when the chemicals leave the body can be devastating. Moreover, using street drugs along with prescribed medications changes the way prescribed medications work in ways that are not understood, with effects that are often deadly. Finally, use of illegal drugs creates a host of additional problems, as we will see in the next chapter.

Ongoing Vigilance

Even when people take medications as directed, there can be problems. Vigilant attention to changes in behavior, thoughts, and moods is important, especially during stressful times.

Since her diagnosis of bipolar disorder in 1989, Michelle, the mother of four young children whom you met in chapter 2, had followed doctor's orders. She first took lithium and later switched to Depakote. Both medications relieved her symptoms. By September of 2001, the symptoms of Michelle's mental illness had been well controlled for years.

Overnight, however, the country and Michelle's world fell apart. Planes crashed into the World Trade Center towers. Michelle's daughter Amy had been married for just a couple of years, but her marriage was crumbling. Although Amy had said that her 7-month-old daughter Kassidy could stay with her in-laws in New Mexico for a few months, now Amy had changed her mind. She wanted her baby back. But Amy was working twelve-hour shifts at Luke Air Force Base. It was impossible for her to travel to New Mexico. Amy begged Michelle to help her.

Within a week, Michelle had driven from her home in Indiana to New Mexico, picked up Kassidy, and then continued on to Arizona, where she delivered Kassidy to her mother. Along the way, Michelle had gotten lost several times. She had not slept well in the roadside motels. In Phoenix, Michelle took care of Kassidy while Amy worked. One afternoon, after putting Kassidy down for a nap, Michelle walked into the kitchen and found Kassidy's father, Aaron, sitting at the table.

"Where's Kassidy? I want to play with her," Aaron said.

"She's taking a nap," Michelle replied. Aaron started walking toward Kassidy's room. "I told you she's sleeping. Leave her alone," Michelle said sternly.

"She's my kid and I want to play with her."

"She's a baby, not a toy. Leave her be."

Aaron sat back down at the kitchen table. Michelle washed and dried the lunch dishes, ignoring him. From the corner of her eye, Michelle saw Aaron take a bowie knife from under his pant leg. Glint from the sun hitting the knife made Michelle wince. Aaron stared at the knife. Michelle trembled. Aaron touched the blade with his fingertips. Michelle said nothing. Several minutes later, Aaron put the knife back in its sheath, got up, and left the house.

Sounds of Amy's dog knocking his metal food dish and her hamster squealing and chirping kept Michelle awake at night. Days passed, and Michelle became more and more restless and irritable. There were three bomb threats at the base where Amy worked. Michelle called her husband, Tim, and cried. She told him she could not stop worrying. She said Aaron was the devil. Michelle made cross marks with her fingers in the inside corners of the windows and doors of Amy's house. She removed everything red from Amy's kitchen. Worried that Kassidy had not been baptized, Michelle called her parish priest and asked him how she could baptize the infant. Even as Michelle's illness took hold, she continued caring for Kassidy.

One Sunday afternoon at the end of September, Michelle put Kassidy in the car and drove to Target. Kassidy needed diapers. As she put the diapers in her cart, Michelle started humming. It was what she always did to calm her racing thoughts. Christmas was coming, and Michelle hadn't bought anything for the kids yet. She walked around the store. Putting a small bottle of Vanilla Fields perfume in the cart, Michelle gasped for air. Michelle had been taking medication for bipolar disorder as the doctor prescribed for years, but the stress of traveling to Arizona and caring for Kassidy and the fear that Aaron might hurt her had made it difficult to do anything. Even breathing was hard.

"It's okay, Kassidy," Michelle said. "We'll just go to the pharmacy. They can call the doctor and get grandma her Ativan. Then everything will be all better."

Michelle gave Kassidy a toy to play with and walked to the pharmacy. She broke into tears when she saw the sign that read "Closed on Sunday."

Michelle dug her cell phone out of her purse and called Amy. "Amy," she said, "I'm at Target. I'm afraid to get in the car with Kassidy. I'm sick. I need to go to the hospital."

"My boss won't let me leave here now," Amy said. "Is Kassidy okay?"

"Yes," Michelle said. "What should I do?"

"Call 911." Amy paused. "Maybe I can call Aaron and ask him to take you to the hospital."

The battery on Michelle's phone died.

A Target employee had been watching Michelle. He called 911. Minutes later, fire and ambulance rescue personnel arrived. Just as they were getting ready to load Michelle into the ambulance, Aaron arrived. He said, "I can help her. She's my mother-in-law."

Michelle said, "It's okay. He can drive me to the hospital."

Waiting in a small examining room, Michelle sat in a chair. Aaron sat on the exam table, holding Kassidy on his lap. He played peekaboo with the baby. Kassidy giggled. Without warning, Michelle threw a cup of ice water at Aaron and said, "Stop teasing that baby. This will cool you off."

A nurse whisked Michelle to the psychiatric ward, while a drenched and bewildered Aaron and a laughing baby Kassidy looked on.

Five days later, once the medications took hold, Michelle was released from the hospital.

Concluding Thoughts

Obstacles to treatment are varied and complex. Is there one obstacle that, if removed, would ensure that all people with a serious mental illness would get the treatment they need? The answer is no. Is one obstacle more important than another? The answer is yes. The most important obstacle to treatment is the one that keeps a given person from getting treatment. For Elyn Saks, it was not wanting evidence that her brain was broken. For John Nash, it was not knowing the line between real and not real. For Collin the guitarist, it was fear of losing his creativity.

Among people who want treatment but cannot get it, some cannot afford care. Others cannot find help or get to the help. Still others worry about what people will think. Among people who do not want treatment, some do not know they are ill. Others do not like the way the medications make them feel. Still others believe that alcohol and street drugs work better than prescription medication. While these are the main reasons identified by a host of studies, there are many others.

The strategies provided in this chapter are starting points for coping with these obstacles, but even in the best of cases, as illustrated by Michelle's experience, vigilance must be continuous. Moreover, the demanding nature of serious mental illnesses make its challenges unbeatable by any single individual. Successfully addressing mental illness and its obstacles requires the person with mental illness to partner—with family, with friends, and with providers. Xavier Amador, the clinical psychologist whose brother had schizophrenia and refused help, suggested the importance of listening, empathizing, agreeing, and partnering as strategies for families wanting to help a relative with serious mental illness. These actions can help, both when people with mental illness want treatment and when they do not, but they must be ongoing and responsive to the person with mental illness.

CHAPTER 6

Senseless Suffering

SOPHIE WAS A raging 18-year-old. Furious that her father and I had forbidden her from bringing home the substance abuser she had met on the psychiatric ward, she had feigned suicide and been readmitted to that same facility. At the family discharge meeting, I listened as Sophie told the social worker and psychiatrist that she no longer wanted to live with us, the clueless parents she disdained. Eager to complete the discharge papers, the social worker asked Sophie where she wanted to live. Sophie said she had no idea.

The social worker sighed, stroked his beard thoughtfully, and said, "Sophie, do you know what rock bottom is?"

"No," she muttered.

"Rock bottom is the lowest point a person can reach. It's the point where a person says, 'Hey, something's wrong in my life and I need to do something about it.' What's interesting about rock bottom is that it's a different place for every person. I'll give you an example. For some people, getting a diagnosis of diabetes is enough for them to give up eating sugary foods and start exercising. For other people with diabetes, rock bottom doesn't come until one of their legs has to be amputated. For still others, it happens after their second leg is amputated. Some people never reach rock bottom. Sophie, the cool thing is you get to decide where your rock bottom is."

Sophie glared at him.

I thought about all the times I was sure Sophie had hit rock bottom: when she stole from her cousins, when she got pregnant in high school, when she was expelled from school for fighting with a girl. Each time I thought it couldn't get worse. But it did.

The psychiatrist bit his lip and said, "Until she hits rock bottom, there's not much any of us can do for Sophie. Even Sophie won't be able to help herself until she hits rock bottom."

Believing that people with serious mental illness must hit rock bottom before they can be helped explains why mental illness underlies so many tragedies. It is why people with serious mental illness fill our prisons and wander our streets. As we wait for people with mental illness to reach their rock bottom, too many kill themselves or die by others' hands. Sometimes, they kill other people. Sometimes, they never reach rock bottom. Maybe Adam Lanza hit rock bottom after he slaughtered twenty children between the ages of 6 and 7 and then turned his gun on himself. Maybe he did not.

The idea that we should wait for people with serious mental illness to hit rock bottom is a persistent myth, standing in sharp contrast to what science says. As we saw in the previous chapter, many people with schizophrenia, bipolar disorder, depression, and other serious mental illnesses lack the insight needed to know they are sick. Without this insight, they will never reach rock bottom because they have no rock bottom. They will just keep getting sicker and sicker. Moreover, given the powerful evidence for early and consistent treatment discussed in previous chapters, waiting for people to hit rock bottom before they can be helped might very well be the worst thing we can do. There is no psychiatric condition that benefits from delaying care. Instead, early identification and continuous treatment of serious mental illnesses can alleviate suffering and provide people with the opportunity to lead meaningful, productive lives. The longer we wait for a person with serious mental illness to hit rock bottom, the greater the damage sustained by their brain is likely to be, making it more difficult—or even impossible—to help them.

If the idea that people with a serious mental illness must hit rock bottom before they can be helped is a myth, why does it endure? Why did Sophie's social worker and her Duke-educated psychiatrist insist that she would have to hit rock bottom before they could help her?

The myth persists because requiring people to make independent decisions about their health care is consistent with one of our most fundamental rights—the right of free will. In our society adults have the right to determine treatments they will and will not accept. Allowing, even requiring, individuals to make decisions about the treatments they will accept and those they will refuse—respect for autonomy—lies at the heart of both medical ethics and good practice. Doctors can make recommendations about treatments that may or may not be helpful, but in the end, it is up to each of us to decide whether or not to follow their suggestions. Sophie said she did not want treatment, and because she was 18 years old and did not present an imminent danger to herself or anyone else, she had the right to walk out of the psychiatric hospital and live on the street.

"Until she hits rock bottom, there's not much any of us can do for Sophie."

This chapter shows what happens when we wait for people with serious mental illness to hit rock bottom and recommends evidence-based strategies that can alleviate some of the needless pain and suffering.

Violence

Sunday, January 3, 1999, was a gloomy, rain-soaked day in New York. Andrew Goldstein rose early and listened to Pink Floyd's *The Wall*. He had breakfast at the local McDonald's. Around ten o'clock, he took the subway to Times Square. He spent the afternoon at the Virgin Megastore listening to Madonna and Natalie Imbruglia compact disks at the free listening stations. After eating dinner at a nearby Wendy's, the unemployed 29-year-old who had been diagnosed with schizophrenia ten years earlier entered the subway at Broadway and 23rd Street, heading home. A blonde woman was standing at the end of the darkened platform, about five feet from the tracks. She was leaning against a pole, reading a magazine. Goldstein paced up and down the platform, mumbling to himself. He approached the blonde woman and asked her for the time. She told him it was 5:04, and he backed away. Two minutes later, as the four-hundred-ton N-train roared in, Goldstein brutally shoved the woman toward the tracks. She flew head first under the train, dying instantly, onlookers watching with horror.

Goldstein did not run. Instead, in a calm voice, he said, "I'm crazy. I'm psychotic. Take me to the hospital." Later that night, Goldstein told police that, as the train approached, a spirit had entered him, telling him to push the woman with blonde hair.

The link between mental illness and violence is complex and largely misunderstood. Nearly half of Americans believe that all people with serious mental illnesses are more dangerous than people in the general population. But they are wrong.

To better understand the link between mental illness and violence, we need to take a closer look at the facts. In 1990, the first large study to examine the prevalence of violent behavior in adults with and without diagnosable psychiatric disorders found a significant but fairly modest relationship between violence and mental illness. The twelve-month prevalence rate of violence among people with schizophrenia, bipolar disorder, or major depression was about 7 percent, compared with 2 percent in the general population. But this study also found that, if the risk of violence from mental illness did not exist, 96 percent of all violent crimes would still happen. A more recent survey reported similar patterns, although all rates of violence—2.9 percent for people with serious mental illness compared with 0.8 percent in the general population—were somewhat lower. These data show that people with serious mental illness are about three times more likely to commit violent acts than people who are not mentally ill.

However, once we account for the effects of poverty, previous violence, and substance abuse—conditions that are both common to many with serious mental illness and associated with an increased risk of violence in any population—people with serious mental illness have annual violence rates identical to those in the general population.

Of course, some people with mental illness—people like Goldstein whose psychotic symptoms remain untreated—are more likely to become violent than other people with serious mental illness. Psychiatric symptoms, especially delusions, suspiciousness, and anger, can increase the risk of violence, while treatment can reduce both symptoms and the risk of violence.

The complex relationship between violence and psychosis is highlighted in findings from the CATIE study (Clinical Antipsychotic Trials of Intervention Effectiveness), which identified distinct subgroups of people with schizophrenia who had different levels of risk for violence. Some of the people had a history of antisocial behavior that preceded the onset of their psychotic illness. This group was about twice as likely to have engaged in violent behavior (28.2% vs. 14.6%) as people who did not have an antisocial history. The violent behavior of this group was not only related to their psychotic symptoms but also associated with a history of early life victimization and trauma. For others, psychosis predicted violence. People with delusional thinking, those with suspiciousness, and those who believed that people were persecuting them were approximately three times more likely to commit a serious violent act than patients with mental illness who were not experiencing these symptoms.

There are two circumstances where violence rates among people with serious mental illnesses are much different from those of the general public. One is an active shooting, when an individual engages in killing or attempting to kill people in a confined and populated area—like when James Holmes set off grenades and shot into the audience watching *The Dark Knight* in an Aurora movie theater in 2012. The second is a mass attack, in which three or more people are harmed. A recent FBI report focusing on sixty-three active shooting cases between 2000 and 2013 found that 25 percent of these shooters had a psychiatric diagnosis prior to the shooting. Diagnoses included mood disorder, anxiety disorder, psychosis, personality disorder, and autism. People who knew the shooters and were interviewed after the attacks reported that in the days and weeks prior to the attack the shooters had exhibited a host of concerning behaviors, including unusual sleep patterns, anger, impulsivity, depression, and confused thinking. Similarly, a 2017 Secret Service report of twenty-eight mass attacks found that 64 percent of the attackers had experienced symptoms of mental illness prior to the attacks. Paranoia, hallucinations, delusions, and suicidal thoughts were common; 25 percent of the attackers had been hospitalized for treatment or prescribed psychiatric medications prior to the attacks.

In sum, most violence is unrelated to mental illness. People with serious mental illness do have higher rates of violence than other people. However, when poverty, previous violence, and substance abuse are accounted for and when people are treated for their mental illness, violence rates are no higher than for other people. Although people with serious mental illness are more likely than others to be involved in active shootings and mass attacks, the large majority of people with mental illness are not more violent than other people.

Unlike Goldstein, who did not know the blonde woman he pushed in front of the train, most people with serious mental illness do not choose their target randomly. Rather, between 50 and 60 percent of the victims of violence committed by people with serious mental illness are family members. In comparison, about 16 percent of homicides that are committed by persons without mental illness involve family members. In his book *The Insanity Offense: How America's Failure to Treat the Seriously Mentally Ill Endangers Its Citizens*, psychiatrist and mental health advocate Fuller Torrey chronicles scores of chilling cases in which people in the throes of psychosis killed a family member.

While it is often difficult to know whether a given person with serious mental illness will actually commit a violent act, in Goldstein's case, it was likely. Let's take a look at what happened before Goldstein pushed the blonde woman from the platform.

Goldstein had been an exceptional student, so intelligent that he gained admission to the Bronx High School of Science, one of the city's most elite public schools. In the summer of 1989, just after completing his freshman year in college, Goldstein began having delusions. Convinced that his mother was a monster, Goldstein pushed her into a wall, and he wound up in a psychiatric hospital. Delusions that his neck had disappeared and strange storms were making his body shrink helped doctors diagnose Goldstein as having schizophrenia. His ten-year journey through poorly coordinated services and revolving door care had begun.

In the first of his many hospital stays, Goldstein pleaded for help, saying, "I want to lead a normal life." Doctors prescribed Haldol, and Goldstein improved. But he developed painful spasms, so he stopped taking the medication. By December of

1992, Goldstein's condition had deteriorated so much that he voluntarily committed himself to Creedmoor, a state psychiatric hospital. Hospital notes from his initial days portray a man so paranoid and delusional that he barricaded himself in a nurses' station, believing that the staff was poisoning him with cyanide and that someone with a gun was after him. He attacked two social workers and a nurse. Later, Goldstein settled down; he lived at Creedmoor for eight months and did well.

In an effort to get people out of psychiatric hospitals and into the community, the Creedmoor staff moved Goldstein to its group home on the hospital grounds. There he had more freedom but still had constant supervision and care. Again, he did well. The staff knew that Goldstein could not live on his own. When he went home for a weekend, he stopped taking his medication. Yet regulations mandated that Goldstein had been at Creedmoor long enough, and so he was released from the group home.

In December 1996, Goldstein was living on his own in a squalid basement apartment in Howard Beach, Queens. No counselors or social workers checked up on him. He stopped taking his medicine. He assaulted a customer in a supermarket and ended up in a hospital psychiatric ward, but he did not stay there for long. Over the next year and a half, Goldstein wound up in emergency rooms ten times. He was delusional, begging for help. He told doctors that the earth was running out of oxygen, that he saw people shrinking and growing, and that he was Italian composer Ottorino Respighi. Sometimes he walked to the hospital on his own. Other times he was brought there by police. He attacked a doctor at a clinic, punched a patient in the hospital, and assaulted customers at a fast-food restaurant and a bookstore. He lashed out at women he did not know. He repeatedly begged to live in a group home or psychiatric hospital—someplace where he would be watched so he could not hurt anyone. But each time, the hospital discharged

Goldstein after just a few days. When social workers looked for someplace else where Goldstein could live safely, all they found were long waiting lists. There was no place for him.

Just five months before Goldstein pushed the blonde woman under the train, he had attacked another woman in a Brooklyn subway, but she had fought him off, and he was admitted to Brookdale Hospital. On the second day of his stay, he attacked a nurse and a psychiatrist. Three days later, he lunged from his seat and attacked a social worker. Two weeks later, he punched a therapy aide in the face. Goldstein asked to be sent back to Creedmoor. Creedmoor staff agreed that Goldstein needed hospital care, but they did not have a bed, so Brookdale staff released him to the streets.

On November 24, 1999, Goldstein admitted himself to North General Hospital in Harlem. Asked why he wanted to be hospitalized, Goldstein said, "Severe schizophrenia. Hopefully will cure." He said his delusions were so intense and unbearable that he wanted eyeglasses so he could see the faces of the voices he heard talking to him. Although the nurses' notes on December 11 indicated that he "remained paranoid," he was released from the hospital on December 15. Notes from that day, probably driven more by the hospital's need to free up a bed than by the reality of Goldstein's illness, said he was "stable and improved." He was told to follow up at Bleuler Psychotherapy Center, an outpatient clinic.

Goldstein had been voluntarily hospitalized thirteen times in the previous two years. The 199 days he had spent in emergency rooms or hospitals were not enough to help him. He had attacked thirteen people, including two psychiatrists, a nurse, a social worker, and a therapy aide. He clearly was violent. His housemate said that, a few days before pushing the blonde woman into the train, Goldstein had been acting strangely. He paced the streets and cemeteries of their Queens neighborhood, blanked out in the middle of a sentence, and asked to eat his neighbor's leftover food.

For pushing the blonde woman to her death, Andrew Goldstein was charged with second-degree murder. His lawyer told the jury about the failure of the mental health system to help Goldstein, contending that Goldstein was insane—he did not know right from wrong when he pushed the blonde woman off the platform. The prosecutor argued that Goldstein had acted out of rage and anger toward women. After six days of deliberation, jurors were deadlocked.

Before his second trial, Goldstein's lawyers advised him to stop taking his medication. They hoped this would convince the jury of the debilitating effects his mental illness had and support the claim that he was not guilty by reason of insanity. Judge Carol Berkman said she would allow Goldstein to stop taking his medication as long as he appeared competent to stand trial. If he appeared not to understand his surroundings, she ruled, he would be forcibly given his medication. When Goldstein struck a social worker in the courtroom, the judge ordered that he be offered his medication each day. Goldstein took the medication. This jury deliberated for just ninety minutes in March 2000 and delivered a unanimous verdict rejecting Goldstein's insanity defense. Goldstein was found guilty of second-degree murder and sentenced to twenty-five years to life.

In 2005, the New York Court of Appeals threw out Goldstein's murder conviction, ruling that it had been based on hearsay. A new trial was ordered, but before the trial got underway, Goldstein pleaded guilty to first-degree manslaughter. He was sentenced to twenty-three years in prison and five years of probation, far short of the lifetime he could have spent behind bars had a jury found him guilty of second-degree murder.

One Family Fights to Change Things

The blonde woman Goldstein pushed under the train was 32-year-old Kendra Webdale. After spending a lazy afternoon at home on that soggy Sunday, Kendra headed to the subway, on her way to visit a friend. Kendra had moved to Manhattan's Flatiron District three years earlier from her hometown of Fredonia and was working as a receptionist. She had dreamed of landing a job in the music industry. Kendra loved all that Manhattan had to offer—runs before dawn, researching ideas for her screenplay at the public library, and wandering Central Park. She often took pictures, like a tourist. The third of six children, Kendra was adored by her parents, brother, and four sisters. The close-knit family that enjoyed tent camping, strawberry picking, and just being together was devastated by Kendra's death.

Brian Stettin began work as New York's assistant state attorney general the day after Kendra's death. Charged with reviewing New York's mental health legislation, Stettin learned about how much Goldstein had wanted, but been denied, help. He learned about the huge gaps in the mental health system. Stettin wanted a law that would require people like Goldstein to get help before they harmed someone. Stettin called Kendra's mother, Pat, and asked permission to name the law for Kendra. Although the Webdales knew little about mental illness, they learned quickly and agreed to Stettin's request. They wanted society to pay attention to the needs of people with serious mental illness so that no one else would die because a psychotic person had not gotten the help he or she needed.

Kendra's Law establishes a procedure for obtaining court orders for eligible people to receive and accept assisted outpatient treatment. A person may be placed in AOT only if, after a hearing, the court finds that all seven of the following criteria have been met: people must (1) be at least 18 years old, (2) suffer from a mental illness, (3) be clinically determined to be unlikely to survive safely in the community without supervision, (4) have a history of lack of compliance with treatment, (5) be unlikely to voluntarily participate in the outpatient treatment,

(6) be in need of outpatient treatment to prevent a relapse or deterioration that would be likely to result in serious harm to the person or others, and (7) be likely to benefit from AOT. Goldstein met all seven criteria.

But Kendra's Law does not just require people to get treatment; it obligates state health systems to provide treatment and mandates the state to fund the treatment infrastructure. Under Kendra's Law, the director of community services overseeing the mental health program of a locality must provide or arrange for services and treatment specified in a written plan prepared by a physician. Initial orders for six months can be extended for a year.

Not surprisingly, there was a lot of controversy about a bill that would use a court order to force mentally ill people to get treatment. After all, ours is a society that values the right of individuals to make decisions about their treatment. But on April 28, 1999, another tragedy unfolded. Julio Perez, a 43-year-old with a history of mental illness who lived in a men's shelter for the mentally ill in Upper Manhattan, terrified commuters on a packed rush hour subway platform. He talked to himself. He punched a wall. When someone told him to go away, Perez swung around in a fury and shoved 37-year-old Edgar Rivera into the path of the No. 6 train at the 51st Street station. Rivera survived, but he lost both of his legs. New Yorkers were angry and frightened. There was an outpouring of support for Kendra's Law when New Yorkers saw the pictures photographers had snapped of Rivera leaving the hospital wearing a "Pass Kendra's Law" T-shirt. Governor George Pataki signed Kendra's Law on August 9, 1999; it became effective that November.

Between November 1999 and December 31, 2004, petitions were granted and court orders for AOT were issued for 3,766 people in New York. A 2005 report by the New York State Office of Mental Health revealed that AOT had incredible successes. Over just six months, people receiving the services they needed—case management, medication management, therapy, access to day programs, substance abuse services, and housing support—experienced dramatic improvements in self-care and community living indicators (e.g., ability to access community services, prepare meals, maintain personal hygiene, make and keep medical appoints, manage medication). Their social, interpersonal, and family functioning (e.g., ability to ask for help, effectively handle conflict, and engage in social activities) improved. They were better able to understand instructions, sustain an ordinary routine, and complete tasks. The incidence of harmful behaviors (e.g., suicide attempts, drug and alcohol abuse, physical harm to others, property damage) declined sharply. Longer-term benefits included reduced incidences of hospitalization, homelessness, arrest, and incarceration. Moreover, although about half of AOT recipients reported feeling angry or embarrassed by the experience, the majority of AOT recipients said it helped them gain control over their lives (75%), helped them get and stay well (81%), and made them more likely to keep appointments and take medication (90%).

These findings led New York to reauthorize Kendra's Law in 2005, with a budget of $32 million per year for personnel and medications to handle the AOT population and $125 million per year for enhanced community services. An independent evaluation of Kendra's Law by researchers from Duke University confirmed and extended findings, concluding that the effectiveness of Kendra's Law is not simply a by-product of systemic service enhancements, but rather, at least in part, is attributable to the value of AOT court orders for motivating treatment compliance. In a follow-up study examining the cost of AOT, researchers found that service costs for frequently hospitalized patients with serious mental illness declined 43 percent in New York City in the first year in which participants received AOT after hospital release and then declined an additional 13 percent the second year.

After the Sandy Hook tragedy in 2012, New York revised regulations to allow initial AOT orders of up to a year, with extensions possible. Treatment plans must include case management or other care coordination services. Eligible people who refuse AOT may be held in a hospital for up to seventy-two hours for care, observation, treatment, and determination of whether involuntary admission is warranted.

Today, forty-seven states (all but Connecticut, Maryland, and Massachusetts) and the District of Columbia have statutes authorizing AOT. But AOT varies from place to place. Even within New York, there are regional differences in AOT programs. Many programs are underfunded and underutilized. Mentally ill people still push strangers onto subway tracks—at least fourteen times during 2018. Given this, it is not surprising that the benefits of AOT programs are hotly contested. While the future of AOT is somewhat uncertain, many studies are now examining the conditions under which, and the people for whom, AOT can be most effective.

Meanwhile, in September 2018, 49-year-old Andrew Goldstein was released from prison and entered the mental health system that his actions helped change. Ironically, there is some question as to whether Goldstein now qualifies for AOT. He has been jailed—qualifying him. But for over two decades, he has taken antipsychotic medication, including Haldol, Cogentin, Abilify, and Zyprexa—disqualifying him, as these medications have kept his violent impulses in check.

Court records have been sealed, and it is unclear where Goldstein is now.

Jails and Prisons

In 1939, Lionel Penrose, a British psychiatrist and mathematician, studied patterns of incarceration in eighteen European nations. His research supported his premise, known today as the "Penrose hypothesis," that there was an inverse relationship between the number of people in prisons and the number in psychiatric facilities. It goes like this: when the prison population is large, the asylum population is small, and vice versa. Though the causal relationship underlying the Penrose hypothesis remains controversial, what is clear is that, for most of history, whether people with serious mental illnesses have been hospitalized or imprisoned, they have been mistreated.

In the United States today, people with serious mental illnesses rely more on the criminal justice system than the medical system for treatment. More than three times the number of seriously mentally ill people are in jails (short-term city- or county-level facilities housing inmates awaiting trial) or prisons (longer-term correctional facilities operated at the state or federal levels for inmates found guilty) than in hospitals. More than 40 percent of people with a serious mental illness have been in jail or prison at some point in their life, and more than half of state prisoners and jail inmates have a mental illness. Inmates include people diagnosed with depression (21%), bipolar disorder (12%), and schizophrenia (5%), as well as people not diagnosed but who suffer the symptoms of these illnesses.

Although some people with mental illness—like James Holmes, who killed twelve people and injured seventy others in a Colorado movie theater in 2012—are incarcerated for heinous crimes, most are caged because they commit misdemeanors such as petty theft, trespassing, disorderly conduct, or vandalism.

David was one of these people.

Like all mothers, Anne had dreams for her son. As an infant, David was a delightful, cuddly little guy. By two, he was headstrong. In elementary school, although David was kind, sensitive, and loving, he was also impulsive and obstinate. He challenged everything and everyone. A child psychologist diagnosed ADD and prescribed medication, but the medication made

David nauseous and gave him headaches. It didn't help him focus, so his parents discontinued it.

In high school, David spent hours at the desk in his room, his books open. But he couldn't focus. His grades went from bad to worse. He drank alcohol and smoked marijuana. He skipped classes. When his parents reprimanded him, David got angry and combative. He ignored curfews. One night, after a nasty argument with his parents, David went to a friend's house. He told his friend's parents that Anne and her husband had beat him. The police were called. Anne, her husband, and David were interviewed by a social worker who listened to their stories and easily concluded that David was incorrigible. No charges were filed.

Despite the turmoil, there was much about David that was good. His sense of humor kept his friends and family amused. He worked hard at his golf caddy job, earning a "Caddy of the Year" award.

After high school, David got a job as a contractor's apprentice. He spent money as fast as he made it. He bought a home for himself, his fiancée, and their baby, but he soon found himself alone. His fiancée said he smoked too much marijuana.

David wanted to be a millionaire. He persuaded his parents to cosign a loan so he could start a construction business, and he worked hard for five years. But David's vision and enthusiasm were no match for his lack of attention to detail. His business faltered.

David met and fell in love with Sandy. They got engaged, married, and started a family. During the nationwide recession, David's construction business failed. He started using prescription stimulants, and it wasn't long before he was taking too many of the pills.

During a family vacation when David was in his early thirties, Anne was surprised to see that David never stopped talking. He rarely slept. One afternoon David told Anne that he felt scared. He was short of breath; he said his chest was tight and that his heart was racing. Anne thought that maybe David was having a heart attack, but ten minutes later, as quickly as the symptoms had started, they stopped. Although these symptoms recurred several times during the two-week vacation, David refused to go to the hospital. Years later Anne learned that what David had experienced were panic attacks.

Shortly before David's thirty-fifth birthday, Sandy called Anne. She said David had been pacing all night, praying in strange tongues, and ranting about how President Obama had sought his help to stop a Russian invasion. She said that in his frenzied state David had cut a hole in the basement wall and started a remodeling project, without consulting her.

Sandy and Anne tried to convince David to go to the psychiatric hospital, but he refused. Frightened and worried about her safety and that of her young daughter, Sandy went to court and got a temporary restraining order. A judge ordered that David have no contact with his wife. Not grasping the seriousness of the order, David stopped by his house that evening to get his tools and talk to his daughter. As instructed by the court, Sandy called the police. Twice in that first month, the police jailed David for violating the restraining order and stalking his wife.

David lived with one friend after the next, causing so much chaos in each place that he was asked to leave. When Anne realized that David was living in a rented storage unit, she and her husband flew from their home in California to Missouri to help him.

Things went from bad to worse. Trying to reconcile with his wife, David called her phone frequently. A judge issued a warrant for David's arrest. When David resisted the police, his father was forced to watch helplessly as David was thrown to the ground and subdued.

David agreed to be treated at the psychiatric hospital, and so Anne and her husband bailed him from jail. However, once out of jail, David reneged. He refused treatment. He insisted there was nothing wrong with him. He said, "Mental illnesses aren't real." Desperate, Anne told staff at the emergency room that David was a danger to his family. He was involuntarily admitted to the hospital, diagnosed with bipolar I. A couple days later, while David was still in the hospital, the sheriff served him with divorce papers. Devastated, David called Sandy and begged her forgiveness. He spent eleven days in the hospital, and he was released after being stabilized for only thirty-six hours. One day later, as David and his parents were leaving a medical appointment, the police arrested him. David had disobeyed the restraining order when he called Sandy from the hospital.

Back in jail for four days without the medications he desperately needed, David raged. When his lawyer didn't appear for the arraignment, David cussed at the judge. The judge set bail at $50,000.

Two months later, David was released from jail and his probation was transferred from Missouri to California. He lived with his parents and started seeing a psychiatrist. But having lost his wife and daughter, his business, his truck, and all his belongings, David was inconsolable. He wanted to die. Convinced that overusing prescription stimulants had triggered his manic episode, David thought that, if he stopped using the stimulants, he would get his health back. He was hospitalized twice in two weeks because he was suicidal. When David nearly succumbed to the poisons of carbon monoxide in an attempt to kill himself, he realized he did not want to die. He voluntarily checked himself into a psychiatric hospital for two weeks.

For a while, things got better. David moved in with his brother, sister-in-law, and their three small children. He started seeing a new psychiatrist, but he did not tell the doctor that he'd been diagnosed with bipolar disorder. The doctor diagnosed ADD and prescribed stimulants, the same medication David had abused months earlier.

David got a job as a department manager at Lowe's, where he excelled. The prescription stimulants helped him focus. But when David started taking more of the stimulants than he was supposed to, he became combative. He yelled at his boss and said he was furious that the store was selling "cheap plumbing parts from China." David quit his job, emptied his bank account, and rented a conference room at a local hotel. He called his brother, other relatives, and friends and told them he planned to set up an international foundation that would save the world. He invited them to serve on his board.

With his brother's help, David voluntarily admitted himself to the psychiatric hospital. There he was stabilized on medications. But once again, because the medications made David feel sluggish and because David did not believe he had a mental illness, he checked himself out of the hospital. Homeless, he lived on the streets. He took street drugs that made both his mania and depression worse.

After a few weeks, Anne persuaded David to live with her and her husband. For about a year, David saw the psychiatrist, took his medicine, and did odd jobs. He attended recovery groups and Bible studies.

But then David met a naturopathic doctor who convinced him that if he would lead a healthier lifestyle, he would be fine. David stopped taking his medicine, started running, and took the herbal supplements the doctor recommended. David got more and more agitated and anxious. He talked nonstop. David told Anne he believed that the United States would soon be under martial law. He planned to save Sandy and his children. He would fly to St. Louis to pick them up. Then, they would all fly to London. David fought constantly with his parents. He put his fist through a wall. His parents, fearing for their safety, called the police.

Although David was ill, he managed to comply with his probation order. He saw the psychiatrist each month for the requisite fifteen-minute visits, where he easily convinced the doctor that he no longer needed medication. But David's social worker knew he needed medication and that he was spiraling out of control. Relations worsened between David and his parents. David's pacing, inability to sleep at night, and flight of ideas made his parents edgy. When David had an accident and totaled his car, his parents worried for his safety. When David invited homeless strangers to live in their house, his parents feared for their own safety.

David was court-ordered to get a psychiatric evaluation at a behavioral health hospital. Anne and her husband told the evaluator what was going on at home, and they pleaded with her to admit David to the hospital. Though David told the evaluator about his conspiracy theories and the evaluator recognized he had paranoid ideation, because David did not admit to being suicidal, homicidal, or gravely disabled, he was not admitted to the hospital.

While living in California, David had frequent contact with his Missouri probation officer. She checked in on him and advised him in the divorce and child custody proceedings. After the Sandy Hook tragedy, David's ruminations about a conspiracy theory grew. Concerned that David might become a public safety risk, the probation officer notified officials in California. Anne also worried, and she told the probation officer whenever David stopped taking his medication and his symptoms worsened. The probation officer filed a motion to extradite David back to Missouri, where she believed David would get better care.

Once David was jailed in St. Louis, the probation officer convinced him to waive his rights to a preliminary probation violation hearing. She wanted David to get the treatment he needed. In jail, David waited two months without medication before a bed in the state hospital was available. During the first six weeks of his stay at the state hospital, due process laws prevented David from being forcefully medicated. One night, convinced he was going to die, David called Sandy's phone eight times. He wanted to say goodbye to his daughter. Sandy reported the calls to the police.

Nine months of medication and treatment at the state hospital helped David regain competency. Doctors at the state hospital diagnosed David with schizoaffective disorder—bipolar type and major depression.

Once David was released from the state hospital, he was sent back to the county jail to await his probation violation hearing. But the hearing was delayed for four months. During that time, David stopped taking his medications and attempted suicide several times. When the hearing finally took place, a grand jury charged David with aggravated adult abuse and stalking for the phone calls he had made to Sandy the previous summer when he had been unmedicated.

The judge knew that David needed medical help, not punishment. Although the probation officer had hoped David could live in a group home or a halfway home while serving his sentence, she was unable to find a place for David to live. He had lost his Social Security Disability Insurance benefits and had failed to comply with medication orders. And so the judge sentenced David to prison for three years. Because of David's frequent suicide attempts, he entered the state prison on suicide watch. Depending on his behavior, David was in and out of solitary confinement, where, for twenty-three hours each day, he was in a cell, deprived of phone calls and other human contact. He was handcuffed when guards transferred him from one area of the prison to another. Although David had been referred to the mental health area of the prison, he never made it there.

Four months after entering the prison, David made a rope with his sheets. He hung it from the light fixture. And then, the 39-year-old man hanged himself.

For years it had been clear that David needed help, but he went back and forth between the criminal justice and mental health systems. In the end, David was jailed because he stalked his wife. He killed himself because no one could help him.

David's experience shows how our broken mental health system has seeped into our criminal justice system. Jails and prisons, overcrowded and rife with abuse, have become our psychiatric facilities. Yet jails and prisons lack adequate resources to meet the needs of people with serious mental illnesses. Mental health care in most criminal justice facilities is limited to distributing and managing medications, and even these basic functions often are not done right. A serious shortage of doctors and other mental health providers means long waiting times for psychiatric appointments and therapy sessions that, if they happen at all, last only a few minutes. When hospital units do exist in prisons, there are not enough beds and not enough medical staff. People in the throes of psychosis are put in solitary confinement, as David was, sometimes for days or weeks, simply because there is no place else to put them.

A Yale Law School report found that, in 2014, between 80,000 and 100,000 people were placed in solitary confinement, a number that does not include people in local jails or juvenile, military, or immigration facilities. Nearly half of these people suffered from mental illness. In solitary confinement, where prisoners are confined in cells the size of a closet, deprived of human contact, and exposed to extreme temperatures and poor ventilation, symptoms of mental illness intensify. Suicide by hanging is the leading cause of death in jail, and more than half of all prison suicides occur in solitary confinement.

Not Guilty by Reason of Insanity

If a man with schizophrenia rapes and murders a woman because voices in his head tell him to do so, is he guilty of a crime? Should he go to jail? Should he be hospitalized? The question of guilt when a person is mentally ill has challenged the mental health and criminal justice systems in the United States and elsewhere for more than a century.

The first legal case to address whether a person could be not guilty by reason of insanity involved Scottish wood-carver Daniel M'Naghten. M'Naghten was 30 in 1843 when he shot and killed Edward Drummond, secretary to Prime Minister Robert Peel. M'Naghten said that he had come to London to shoot Peel but had shot Drummond, who had been riding in Peel's carriage, by mistake. M'Naghten's testimony was filled with reports of his paranoia, sleeplessness, and persecution. A medical witness said, "The history of his past life leaves not the remotest doubt... of the presence of insanity.... The act of the prisoner in killing Mr. Drummond to have been committed whilst under a delusion."

When M'Naghten was found not guilty by reason of insanity (NGRI), outcry was widespread. Even Queen Victoria demanded clarification of what the verdict meant. The answer of the judges became the basis for what is known as the M'Naghten rule: "Every man is to be presumed to be sane.... To establish a defense on the ground of insanity, it must be clearly proved that, at the time of the committing of the act, the party accused was laboring under such a defect of reason, from disease of mind, as not to know the nature and quality of the act he was doing; or if he did know it, that he did not know he was doing what was wrong."

While the M'Naghten ruling was important, today, requests for a finding of NGRI and granting of those requests are very rare. On average, fewer than 1 defendant in 100 (0.85%) actually raises the insanity defense nationwide, and the percentage of all defendants found NGRI is only 0.26 percent. When people are found NGRI, they are committed to a psychiatric facility rather than sent to prison. To be released from the hospital, the person must prove to a judge that he or she is no longer a danger to himself or others. Depending on the crime, a person found NGRI may spend far longer in the hospital than he would have spent in prison.

One NGRI verdict that captivated everyday people, as well as legal scholars, involves John W. Hinckley Jr.

On March 30, 1981, Hinckley put a bullet in President Ronald Reagan's chest and gravely injured Press Secretary James Brady. The assassination attempt was designed to impress actress Jodie Foster. Prior to the assassination attempt, Hinckley had fantasized about hijacking a plane or killing himself in front of Foster to win her love. Days after the trial, Hinckley sent a four-page handwritten letter to a *New York Times* reporter that he had intended to read at his sentencing. He said, "My actions of March 30, 1981 have given special meaning to my life and no amount of imprisonment or hospitalization can tarnish my historical deed. The shooting outside the Washington Hilton hotel was the greatest love offering in the history of the world. I sacrificed myself and committed the ultimate crime in hopes of winning the heart of a girl." Just over a year after the shooting, a jury found Hinckley NGRI. He was committed to St. Elizabeth's Hospital, where he was treated for nearly thirty-five years, much longer and probably more effectively than the one- to twenty-five-year sentence he would have served in prison for felony assault or battery. Hinckley was released from the hospital in 2016 with a set of thirty-four conditions, one of which was that after eighteen months he would undergo full psychiatric and psychological evaluations. Today, he is 63. He continues to take the antipsychotic Risperdal and the antidepressant Zoloft prescribed while he was at St. Elizabeth's. Hinckley lives in Williamsburg, Virginia, with his 93-year-old mother and older brother. His doctors agree that he has long been mentally healthy and that his depression and psychosis have long been in remission. Hinckley's case shows that even the most psychotic patients can be helped.

Competence to Stand Trial

Just as the criminal justice system assumes that people are sane when they commit a crime, so too does it require that people be competent when they stand before a judge. A criminal case cannot proceed if the defendant is deemed incompetent. The landmark case of *Dusky v. United States* overwhelmed both the mental health system and the criminal justice system.

Milton Dusky was 33 years old when he was arrested on August 19, 1958. He had no criminal history and a prior diagnosis of schizophrenia. Married with children, he intermittently suffered from visual hallucinations, morbid preoccupations, and depression. He had a long history of alcoholism.

The night before the offense, Dusky drank a quart of vodka and took a handful of tranquilizers. The next day he drove two friends of his son to visit a girl. On the way, they encountered a second girl whom the boys knew. After picking her up, they drove the girl across state lines to Missouri, where the two adolescent boys raped her. Dusky attempted to rape the girl but was unable.

At a competency hearing, Dusky was oriented to time, place, and person. Although he had no memory about the offense, Dusky was tried, found guilty of kidnapping and raping a minor, and sentenced to forty-five years in prison.

In 1960, when the Supreme Court heard his case, Dusky's lawyer argued that he had been too sick at the time of his trial to fully understand what was happening. The Supreme Court ruled in favor of Dusky, making it clear that a defendant must be competent to be tried. But competence meant more than just having an orientation to time and place and having some recollection of the events leading to the charge. Instead, the Supreme Court said that competence means that the accused must have sufficient ability to consult with his lawyer with a reasonable degree of rational understanding and have a sound understanding of the legal proceedings that will ensue. The defendant must understand why he is being charged, the potential consequences of the charges, and the penalty he could face if found guilty. The defendant must have at least a rudimentary understanding of the workings of the justice system. He must, for example, understand what the job of a judge is and what a plea bargain means.

Findings from *Dusky v. United States* make it common for defendants to spend a month or two in jail waiting for a mental health professional to conduct the competency evaluation and make a recommendation to the judge. People found incompetent to stand trial will remain incarcerated until there is an opening at the state mental hospital. There, efforts will be made to make people sane enough to stand trial, a process known as "restoration to competency." But restoration to competency is not the same as adequate and appropriate mental health treatment. The purpose of competency restoration is to allow a person to be processed by the criminal justice system; its goal is to help a person understand his charges and the hearing process and assist his attorney in his defense. Treatment, on the other hand, serves the person with mental illness, enabling a person to thrive. The process of restoration to competency has kept thousands of people stuck in jails or sequestered in state hospitals because they are too sick for their cases to proceed. This, in turn, has created a logjam in our jails and made psychiatric beds for people not convicted of crimes virtually nonexistent.

As Penrose's pendulum has swung toward imprisoning people with serious mental illness rather than hospitalizing them, a new problem has been created. Serious mental illness has become criminalized. Now, many people with mental illness not only bear the stigma of their illness but also endure the stigma of criminal records earned, sometimes for offenses as minor as petty theft, prostitution, or public intoxication.

It Doesn't Have to Be This Way: Decriminalizing Minor Offenses

In April of 2007, 23-year-old Justin Volpe—paranoid, delusional, and high on crack—was arrested on petty theft charges. He was locked in a pretrial detention center cell for forty-six days. His cellmate had stabbed his wife with a pair of scissors. Prisoners screamed around the clock. Justin couldn't sleep. The lights were always on. The guards often beat the prisoners.

Justin was actually a very lucky man. The judge hearing his case in Miami-Dade County's 11th Judicial Circuit Court was Steve Leifman. In 2000, Leifman created the Criminal Mental Health Project (CMHP), a coordinated effort to divert people with serious mental illnesses from the criminal justice system to community-based mental health services. Justin's mental illness and the minor charges for which he was arrested qualified him for immediate transfer from jail to a crisis unit at Jackson Memorial Hospital, where he received treatment. Once he was stabilized, Justin was given the option of returning to jail or participating in a diversion program. Justin chose the diversion program. He was given shelter in an assisted living facility that was paid for with the monthly Social Security disability checks that staff from the CMHP had helped him secure. As long as Justin complied with the program, he would stay out of jail. Had Justin rejected the opportunity to participate in the diversion program, he would have returned to jail and, if found competent, would have stood trial. In November of 2007, Justin became CMHP's first peer specialist, a job he has held for nearly twelve years. Now, one of eight peer specialists in CMHP, Justin works in Miami's jails, homeless shelters, treatment centers, courts, and streets, helping people with serious mental illness learn to live successfully in the community.

When Steve Leifman first became a judge in 1996, he handled misdemeanor jail diversion cases, the smallest, most minor offenses. Leifman had no idea that he would become gate-keeper to the largest psychiatric facility in Florida. Nor did he have any idea that there was no system of care for people with serious mental illness—in Florida or anywhere else.

One morning, as Leifman was donning his robes, he was approached by the assistant public defender and the assistant state attorney. They said that a couple whose son's case was on the docket that morning asked to talk with him. Leifman agreed. As the well-dressed older couple entered chambers, their distress was visible. The man had dark bags under his eyes; the woman fiddled nervously with her purse. The man said his son was a brilliant, Harvard-educated psychiatrist with late-onset schizophrenia. His wife explained that for years her son had cycled between being homeless and being jailed. This time, their son had been arrested and jailed for stealing a grocery cart. The couple begged Leifman to help their son. The judge promised to do his best.

The young man brought into the courtroom had long, greasy hair. His pants were baggy; his shirt was torn where once there had been a pocket. Yet the man was respectful and well-spoken. He insisted that nothing was wrong with him and promised Leifman that he would get a psychiatric evaluation if the judge would let him out of jail. Leifman looked at the couple. Is it possible that they were overreacting? Confused, Leifman asked the man, "Why would a Harvard-educated psychiatrist be in jail, homeless, and recycling through the system?" Leifman watched as a look of horror grew on the man's face. The man cupped his ears. He shook back and forth. He pointed and screamed at the couple in the back of the courtroom—the woman sobbing, the man trying to comfort her. The young man said the older couple were CIA agents who were trying to kill him and that his real parents had been killed in the Holocaust. He begged Leifman to kick the couple out of the courtroom. He shouted each statement six times.

Judge Leifman did what he had been trained to do when a person acted strangely: he ordered evaluations by three independent psychiatrists. All three evaluators said the man was psychotic and incompetent. All three psychiatrists recommended that the man be involuntarily hospitalized. Nonetheless, at the sentencing hearing, the man's lawyer reminded the judge that a recent ruling by the Florida Supreme Court said that county court judges had no authority to involuntary hospitalize anyone. Leifman knew he had to obey the law. He had to release the man to the street. In doing so, he broke his promise to the man's parents. He put the man and his community at risk. Frustrated, Leifman determined to help change the system so that this never happened again.

Leifman's program, which earned him the 2018 Pardes Humanitarian Prize, began with a grant from the Policy Research Associates that enabled him to convene a group of police chiefs, social service and behavioral health providers, and the state attorney. The group developed a chart of the county's resources, service gaps, and opportunities. As its first priority, the group developed a post-booking diversion program for people arrested for misdemeanors—the program that Justin Volpe eventually would participate in. In 2008, the program expanded to include defendants arrested for less serious, nonviolent felonies. Not surprisingly, the program was popular. Nearly 80 percent of people invited to participate in the program agreed. Over the past decade, the CMHP has facilitated about four thousand diversions. The program has been highly successful. The annual recidivism rate is about 20 percent among participants who committed a misdemeanor, compared with roughly 75 percent among defendants not in the program. People charged with minor felonies have 75 percent fewer jail bookings and jail days after enrollment in the program than had been experienced beforehand, and recidivism rates of people in the program are much lower than those of people not in the program.

Leifman's next challenge was figuring out how to avoid having the police arrest people with mental illnesses in the first place. That meant changing the way Miami-Dade's thirty-six police departments interacted with people having mental illnesses. For this, Leifman looked to the Memphis Crisis Intervention Team (CIT) model, which provides forty hours of training for a select group of police officers. Training includes information on signs and symptoms of mental illness, mental health treatments, co-occurring disorders, legal issues, and de-escalation strategies. The Memphis CIT model was developed by a community task force composed of law enforcement, mental health and addiction professionals, and mental health advocates in 1988 after a Memphis police officer shot and killed a man with a history of mental illness and substance abuse. The model strives to increase safety in encounters between police and people with mental illness and, when appropriate, divert people with mental illness from the criminal justice system to mental health treatment.

In 2003, Leifman's program won a federal grant, allowing him to bring the CIT program to Miami-Dade. Since then, some 4,600 officers have been trained. In five years, officers have responded to 50,000 mental health crisis calls, resulting in 9,000 diversions to crisis units and only 109 arrests. The average daily census in the county jail system dropped from 7,200 to 4,000. One jail was closed, saving the county $12 million per year. Fatal shootings and injuries of people with mental illness by police officers have been dramatically reduced.

Leifman now plans on transforming the former South Florida Evaluation and Treatment Center into a state-of-the-art mental health diversion facility. The 800,000-square-foot, seven-story building once imprisoned inmates who were unfit to stand trial. Now it would be used to nurture people with mental illness. After Leifman convinced Miami-Dade mayor Carlos Gimenez that the facility would save the county $8 million per year, funding of $42.1 million from the county and Jackson Memorial Hospital was secured, and construction has begun. The new facility, scheduled to open in March 2021 but delayed due to the Covid pandemic, will include a crisis stabilization unit, vocational training, and a courtroom. It will have both short- and longer-term housing, creating a safe place where people with serious mental illnesses can live, get treatment, and learn to manage their illnesses and their lives.

One man, Steve Leifman, frustrated that he could not keep his promise to one couple, managed to make changes to an ineffective system that criminalized mental illness. As a result, people like Justin Volpe, once doomed to either languish in jail or roam the streets, can become productive members of the community. Leifman's belief—that there is no such thing as a treatment-resistant person, there are only treatment-resistant programs—helped start a national trend in which mental health courts divert people with mental illnesses from jails/prisons to community-based programs. There are now more than three hundred mental health courts in the United States. Although these diversion programs are effective, their potential is limited by the lack of treatment programs in most American cities.

Homelessness

Just as Penrose's classic study found an inverse relationship between the size of prison and psychiatric hospital populations, so too did a study of eighty-one US cities find that having more psychiatric hospital beds in a city is associated with less homelessness. Although scholars disagree about how to define homelessness, it is clear that homelessness is linked to poverty, food insecurity, and chronic illnesses, including serious mental illness.

According to the annual report from the US Department of Housing and Urban Development (HUD), on a single night in

January 2018, as many as 552,830 people were homeless nationwide, of whom 441,238 were over the age of 18. The prevalence of serious mental illness among homeless people is difficult to identify and hence widely disputed. The HUD data, which found that 111,122 people—25.2 percent of homeless adults—had a serious mental illness, provide a conservative estimate. More likely, given the challenges of finding and gaining cooperation among people with serious mental illness to participate in a study, the proportion of people with serious mental illness is much higher. Still further evidence of the link between mental illness and homelessness comes from research showing that between 4 and 36 percent of people with serious mental illness have experienced homelessness. Among people with serious mental illness, those who are homeless are most likely to be African American men who have a substance use disorder, have a diagnosis of schizophrenia or bipolar disorder, and lack Medicaid coverage. What's more, homeless people with serious mental illnesses are more likely to experience repeated episodes of homelessness, to be homeless for longer periods of time, and to require more health and social services than homeless people who do not have a mental illness.

Homelessness can be devastating for people with serious mental illness. The street drugs, victimization, strained family and friendship ties, and harassment from passersby can make the hallucinations, delusions, and depression of serious mental illness more intense. A study that compared the experiences of 1,533 homeless persons in Los Angeles with and without mental illness found that people with mental illness were more likely to have been victimized (45%) than others (26%). The study also found that homeless people with serious mental illness had poorer physical health and were less likely to have their food needs met than homeless people without serious mental illness. Moreover, the link between homelessness and incarceration is strong, as people who are homeless often turn to illegal activities such as theft, prostitution, and drug sales to survive. Among people with serious mental illness, rates of criminal behavior, contact with the criminal justice system, and victimization are higher for homeless adults than for people who have homes. Additionally, a national study found that recent homelessness was 7.5 to 11.3 times more common among jail inmates than in the general population. These studies highlight the strong connections between mental illness, homelessness, and crime.

Community Programs Can Make a Difference

Like the United States, Canada has hundreds of thousands of people with mental illness who are homeless. Canada's "At Home/Chez Soi" project, funded by Health Canada and carried out by the Mental Health Commission of Canada, is the largest program in the world designed to meet the needs of homeless mentally ill people ever mounted. This program is remarkable, not only for its size and accomplishments but also for how it came to be.

The Backstory

When Atlanta hosted the 1996 Summer Olympics, the city drew criticism for arresting homeless people or offering them one-way tickets out of town. The committee organizing the 2010 Winter Olympics in Vancouver did not want to make this mistake. They committed to addressing their homeless population more humanely. But Canada had a real problem. Vancouver's Downtown Eastside, Canada's most visible geographic concentration of homeless people, was just five blocks from the Olympic venue.

Spurred by housing advocates, local media raised concerns about Olympic-related gentrification of Single Room Occupancy hotels in the Downtown Eastside. Wanting to export

Vancouver's homeless population before the games in a humane manner, Vancouver mayor Sam Sullivan suggested reopening Riverview Psychiatric Hospital in suburban Coquitlam. This was not a popular idea.

Canada's problem was compounded by the release of a United Nation's report on the impact of the Olympics and other mega-events on homeless people. This report resulted in a human rights complaint being filed, which led to a UN special rapporteur being sent to Canada. The rapporteur's findings led the United Nations to release a set of recommendations addressing housing and homelessness in Canada, paying particular attention to Vancouver's situation. In response, the Federation of Canadian Municipalities called for a national plan to end homelessness and deliver affordable housing.

At the same time, Canada's prime minister, Stephen Harper, cared about people with mental illness. Harper had been responsible for the creation of the Mental Health Commission of Canada in 2007. Some say he was motivated by the 1950 disappearance of his grandfather, Harris Harper, a high school principal in Moncton who suffered from depression before jumping off a bridge and drowning. Quickly, the idea of doing something for the homeless on Vancouver's Downtown Eastside expanded into a project targeting the homeless mentally ill.

Of course, Stephen Harper was not working alone. Beginning in 2003, Senator Michael Kirby chaired the Senate Standing Committee on Social Affairs, Science, and Technology. The committee created the Mental Health Commission of Canada; Kirby became the new committee's chair. Politically astute, innovative, well-connected, and gifted with the ability to speak in ways that resonated with decision-makers, Kirby also had firsthand experience with the gaps in Canada's mental health system. He had advocated on behalf of his sister, who had suffered from severe depression. He was perfect for the job.

In January 2008, Prime Minister Harper asked Kirby to help formulate a project for homeless people with mental illness. Kirby understood Canada's problem and knew that the solution had to be a research and demonstration project. The national government could not become a service provider because service delivery is the responsibility of the Canadian provinces. Kirby also knew that to be politically acceptable, a demonstration project could not be run in only one area. Rather, it had to be a nationwide initiative. Moreover, in this case, Kirby knew that if the project were run only in Vancouver, it would appear that the government was pandering to the International Olympics Committee.

Kirby used his skills, resources, and access as an insider—within both the mental health movement and the government—to ascertain the feasibility of the project and build broad-based support among key decision-makers. He recruited Dr. Paula Goering, a researcher with the Centre for Addiction and Mental Health in Toronto, to help formulate the project. He appointed Dr. Jayne Barker, the Mental Health Commission's director of policy and research, to lead the initiative. He named Dr. John Service the Mental Health Commission's chief operating officer, giving him authority to negotiate the funding agreement of the project. Kirby worked quickly and efficiently. In March 2008, just two months after Kirby began working on the project, Canada's federal budget included a commitment to spend $110 million to address the needs of homeless mentally ill people.

At Home / Chez Soi

Meanwhile, a small number of studies conducted in the United States had found that programs that combined housing with support to people with serious mental illness were effective in reducing homelessness and hospitalizations and bettering the quality of life. These programs, known as Housing First, involve providing homeless people with immediate access to subsidized housing and supports. Housing First is guided by the belief that people need basic necessities like food and a place to live before they can work on getting a job or dealing with substance abuse issues. With Housing First programs, there are no preconditions to participation, such as being treated with medications.

Housing First programs targeting people with serious mental illness typically involve a multidisciplinary team, including a psychiatrist and nurse. Support is provided seven days a week, twenty-four hours a day, following a well-defined program model called "Assertive Community Treatment" (ACT). Housing First programs serving a broader population of homeless people typically use intensive case management (ICM), operating seven days a week, twelve hours per day.

Building on the Housing First model, the Canadian demonstration project developed by Kirby and his team was called "At Home/Chez Soi." A randomized controlled trial, it was conducted between 2009 and 2013 in five Canadian cities having different sizes and varied ethnic, racial, and cultural composition: Vancouver, Winnipeg, Toronto, Montreal, and Moncton. Homeless people with mental illness were stratified by level of need and evaluated in order to understand how well the ACT and ICM service delivery models fared when compared with treatment as usual (TAU). People with high needs were randomized into ACT or TAU, while people with moderate needs were randomized into ICM or TAU. The study included 2,148 people, with 1,198 randomized to At Home/Chez Soi (ACT or ICM) and 950 randomized to TAU. People in the At Home/Chez Soi groups were provided with their own apartments as well as rent supplements.

The study found that At Home/Chez Soi was more effective than TAU in helping people exit homelessness and achieve stable housing. Over the course of the two years that people were studied, At Home/Chez Soi participants spent 73 percent of their time in stable housing, compared with TAU participants who spent only 32 percent of their time in stable housing. People in the ACT and ICM groups did equally well. At Home/Chez Soi participants also showed greater improvements in community functioning and quality of life than TAU participants. Moreover, the project showed that At Home/Chez Soi is a sound economic investment. On average, the At Home/Chez Soi intervention cost $22,257 per person per year for the ACT participants and $14,177 per person per year for ICM participants. Further, every $10 invested in At Home/Chez Soi resulted in an average savings of $21.72, as service use shifted from expensive crisis care to less costly community care. These cost savings for communities exist because housed people are less likely to use emergency services, including hospitals, jails, and emergency shelters, than people who are homeless. The program is sustainable and has been widely replicated in the United States. The National Alliance to End Homelessness website has a wealth of information showing how communities can develop Housing First programs and reduce homelessness among people with mental illness.

Victimization of People with Serious Mental Illness

People with serious mental illnesses are more likely to be the victim of a crime than a perpetrator of a crime. A 2008 review of studies in the United States found that, while between 12 and 22 percent of people with mental illness had perpetrated violence within the past eighteen months, 35 percent of people with mental illness had been a victim of a violent crime. People with mental illness who are victimized are younger, more socially active, and more symptomatic than people with mental illness who are not victimized. As is true in the general population, rates of victimization are higher for women than for men. People with serious mental illness are also more likely to be the victim of nonviolent crimes than people without serious mental illness. More specifically, people with serious mental illness were three times more likely to be victims of burglary, theft, and robbery, as well as criminal damage, than people without mental illness.

Sometimes people with serious mental illnesses are victimized by the emergency rooms and hospitals they turn to in times of crisis. Although "patient dumping" is not new—the term was coined in the late 1800s when private hospitals began sending poor patients to public hospitals—a number of high-profile cases have recently come to the public's attention. In 2018, for example, a Las Vegas class action lawsuit found that during the previous five years Rawson-Neal Psychiatric Hospital had bused about 1,500 patients with mental illness out of Nevada. One-third of these patients were sent to California. The hospital failed to organize any type of follow-up care or housing for these people. Once they got off the buses, many became homeless, were arrested, or were rehospitalized.

Patient dumping is heartbreaking and often becomes the subject of news reports. On January 9, 2018, psychotherapist Imamu Baraka was leaving work when he saw and videotaped four security guards walking away from a bus stop with a wheelchair near the University of Maryland Medical Center (UMMC) Midtown Campus. The guards had just abandoned a woman wearing a thin yellow hospital gown and socks. She slouched in her wheelchair, her arms crossed over her chest. She had a gash on her forehead. Several bags of her belongings sat at the bus stop. In the video, the woman moaned, cried, and coughed. Her breath formed white clouds in the cold. Baraka called 911, and rescue workers quickly took the woman back to the hospital that had discharged her just minutes ago. The next day, she was discharged to another Baltimore hospital and then sent to a homeless shelter.

It did not take long for police to identify the woman as 22-year-old Rebecca Hall, who had been diagnosed with Asperger syndrome when she was 4 years old and bipolar disorder with traits of schizoaffective disorder when she was 16. She had taken medication for a few years and had done well. She had lived in a group home where she had her own apartment, had been working toward her GED, and, for a while, had worked a job at Target as a cashier. Things fell apart after Rebecca turned 18. She knew she was an adult, and she asserted her legal right to make decisions on her own. She drank alcohol and smoked marijuana. She stopped taking her medications. Because she had violated the group home's rules, she was kicked out of the program. During the next few months, Rebecca lived with her mother and was hospitalized ten times; her mother called the police three times because Rebecca was out of control. Rebecca left home, and a case manager admitted her to Johns Hopkins Bayview Medical Center. It is not clear how Rebecca ended up at UMMC. Investigation by the Centers for Medicare & Medicaid Services found that the hospital enacted barriers to patients receiving care in the emergency department, failed to discharge a patient in a safe manner from the emergency department, and failed to protect one patient from harassment and potential harm.

Patient dumping violates the federal Emergency Medical Treatment and Active Labor Act (EMTALA). Enacted in 1986, EMTALA seeks to prevent any refusal of care for patients who are unable to pay by imposing requirements on Medicare-participating hospitals and enforcing monetary sanctions against physicians or hospitals that do not comply. Participating hospitals must conduct medical screening examinations and provide necessary stabilizing treatment to any patient seeking emergency medical care in an emergency department.

Hospitals unable to do so may transfer the patient to a facility that can provide those services.

Despite these laws and penalties, hospitals have continued turning patients away. From 1996 to 2000, the watchdog organization Public Citizen confirmed violations by 527 hospitals in forty-six states, the District of Columbia, and Puerto Rico. Of these 527 hospitals, 117 had violated the act more than once, and for-profit hospitals were significantly more likely to do so.

But it is not just hospitals and emergency rooms that victimize people with serious mental illness. The police also play a significant role.

Deborah Danner was one of the 242 people with mental illness killed by police in the United States in 2016.

Deborah had been diagnosed with schizophrenia when she was nearly 30. Her mother, Louise, a nurse at the prison on Rikers Island, sought help for her daughter and arranged for Deborah to have her own apartment in the same Bronx apartment complex where she lived. Deborah blossomed at Manhattan's Fountain House, a community of people with mental illness, where she took art classes, participated in employment programs, and taught a popular acting class for about ten years. Educated at City College and Lehman College, Deborah loved to read; her apartment was filled with books.

But when Louise died in 2006, Deborah became in charge of her own life for the first time since her diagnosis of schizophrenia. She stopped going to Fountain House. She was in and out of psychiatric hospitals. The police responded to at least four 911 calls about disturbances at Danner's apartment. One time, Deborah had barricaded herself inside, forcing authorities to break down the door. Another time she had threatened to jump out a window. After promising Louise that she would always take care of Deborah, her sister Jennifer had been appointed guardian, but Deborah didn't like that idea. Deborah wanted help, but not from Jennifer.

The situation became a crisis on October 18, 2016, when a neighbor of Deborah's called 911. The neighbor told police that 66-year-old Deborah had been diagnosed with paranoid schizophrenia. Deborah was ranting in the apartment hallway and ripping posters off the wall, angry at Jennifer's insistence that she continue as guardian. A team of five police officers and two emergency medical technicians were dispatched. They hoped to persuade Deborah to go to the hospital. The team found five-foot-seven, 233-pound Deborah sitting on her bed, cutting paper.

Accounts of what happened next vary. According to Brittney Mullings, one of the medics dispatched to the apartment, Deborah agreed to put down the scissors, had come out of the bedroom, and had been talking with Mullings. The police had retreated to the living room while Ms. Mullings explained to Deborah why the team had been called. Deborah had stopped screaming, although she remained agitated and talked loudly. While Deborah and Mullings were talking, Sergeant Hugh Barry arrived. Ms. Mullings said that Barry conferred with the other officers, saying nothing to her or to Deborah. Mullings heard one of the officers say, "Are you ready?" Deborah screamed and ran back into her bedroom. She was followed by the pack of officers. Mullings remained in the hallway. A minute later Mullings heard an officer yell "Get down!" Two shots were fired.

Sergeant Barry said that when he arrived, Deborah was sitting on her bed cutting paper with a pair of scissors. Barry said he tried to coax Deborah to the doorway of the bedroom. When Deborah refused to move, Barry said he tried to grab Deborah, but she ran back into the bedroom and pulled a baseball bat from under the bedclothes. Barry said Deborah stood on the bed and "raised the bat like she was stepping onto home plate." Barry said he pulled his gun and told her to drop the bat. Deborah swung the bat at his head. Barry fired twice.

Reports from the other officers differed as well. Officer Camilo Rosario, whom all agreed was the only officer with a clear view of the encounter, said Deborah never swung a bat. Officer Michael Garces, who once reported to Barry, supported Barry's report.

Sergeant Barry, the officers, and Ms. Mullings all said that Barry had been in the apartment only eight minutes before the fatal shots were fired.

Immediately after Deborah's death, Police Commissioner James O'Neill said, "We failed." He placed Sergeant Barry on modified duty, stripped of his badge and gun. New York mayor Bill de Blasio said that Barry had not followed training or protocol for dealing with people with mental illness. Barry had neither used his Taser nor waited for officers specially trained to deal with such situations.

On February 15, 2018, Judge Robert Neary acquitted Sargent Barry of murder, manslaughter, and criminally negligent homicide. On December 13, 2018, New York City agreed to a $2 million settlement with Deborah Danner's family.

Some estimate that the risk of being killed during a police incident in the United States is as high as 16 times greater for people with untreated mental illness than for other people, although rigorously generated data regarding police-involved shootings are lacking.

In 2015, the *Washington Post* assembled a database to track police-involved shootings, revealing that about 25 percent of deaths from police shootings since 2015 have involved people with mental illness. At this rate, having signs of a mental illness is associated with a greater than sevenfold increased risk of death at the hands of a police officer than not having these signs. More in-depth analysis found that being black increased the likelihood of a person with mental illness being killed during interactions with police. Further, like Deborah Danner, people with mental illness were nearly three times more likely to have been at home when they were killed by police than people without mental illness.

In 2012, four years before Deborah Danner's death, she wrote a six-page essay entitled "Living with Schizophrenia" for her adult education class that eerily foreshadowed the final moments of her life. She begins her essay with these words: "Any chronic illness is a curse. Schizophrenia is no different—its only 'saving grace,' if you will, is that as far as I know it's not a fatal disease." In the essay, Danner refers to Eleanor Bumpers, a 260-pound black woman in her late sixties with a history of mental illness who lived alone and was four months behind on her rent. On October 29, 1984, the New York City Housing Authority had called the police because Bumpers screamed through her door at city marshals who had tried to serve an eviction notice. Bumpers had made hostile threats and was considered dangerous. Officers stormed her fourth-floor Bronx apartment. Officer Stephen Sullivan fired twice at Bumpers. The first shot struck Bumpers's hand. The second slammed into her chest and killed her. Danner wrote, "We are all aware of the all too frequent news stories about the mentally ill who come up against law enforcement instead of mental health professionals and end up dead." Danner's essay insisted that we prioritize "teaching law enforcement how to deal with the mentally ill in crisis so as to prevent another Bumpers tragedy," pleading, "there but by the grace of God, go I."

Crisis Intervention Training

Crisis intervention training (CIT) is a term used to describe both a program and a training in law enforcement to help guide interactions between law enforcement and those living with mental illness. CIT is an innovative first-responder program that promotes officer safety and safety of people with mental illness who are in crisis. It is used by many communities, including Miami. Sargent Barry had not participated in a CIT program, an issue raised by reporters and his superiors after he shot and killed Deborah Danners. While research on the effectiveness of CIT is limited, it does appear to lower arrest rates of people with mental illnesses, increase mental health service use, and improve safety outcomes. CIT programs can strengthen communities. Details about starting a CIT program can be found at the CIT International website.

CAHOOTS

In Deborah Danner's case, independent teams of mental health professionals and the police were dispatched to her apartment. Today, when a person in Eugene, Oregon, is in the midst of a nonviolent crisis—when someone is homeless, disoriented, intoxicated, mentally ill, or enmeshed in an escalating dispute—a different response is made. The program, called CAHOOTS (Crisis Assistance Helping Out On The Street), calms people in crisis and directs them to shelters. Developed by social activists in 1989, CAHOOTS provides mobile crisis intervention 24/7 and offers a broad range of services, including crisis counseling, suicide prevention, conflict resolution, substance abuse assistance, first aid, and transportation to services. CAHOOTS is wired into the 911 system and responds to most calls without police. CAHOOTS employees are trained mental health professionals. They dress in black sweatshirts, tones designed to calm people, and they speak in quiet voices. They drive unassuming large white vans stocked with warm clothing, blankets, food, and water. They do not carry weapons, and they do not arrest or detain people. Instead, CAHOOTS transports people to locations where they can receive help.

In 2017, CAHOOTS handled 17 percent of the calls made to Eugene police, freeing up police officers to focus on fighting crime. Moreover, CAHOOTS is fiscally conservative. Salaries for its thirty-nine employees and operating costs run approximately $800,000 a year, a fraction of the Eugene Police Department's $58 million annual budget. Although formal evaluations have yet to be completed, the program is a more humane approach than locking people with mental illness in jail.

Suicide

Suicide is the tenth-leading cause of death in the United States. In 2017, a total of 47,173 people in the United States died by suicide, while an estimated 1,400,000 people attempted suicide. For decades, psychological autopsies—reports based on conversations with a deceased person's family, friends, and acquaintances to determine that person's state of mind at the time of death—found that most people who died by suicide had suffered from mental illnesses, with some figures suggesting that nearly 90 percent of people who kill themselves suffered from a mental illness.

However, recent data from the Centers for Disease Control and Prevention (CDC) suggest that the psychological autopsies may have overestimated the number of people having mental illness. The CDC data suggest that more than half of people who die by suicide did not have a known mental illness. These findings highlight the complex relationship between suicide and serious mental illness and suggest that, although people with serious mental illness are at risk for suicide, mental illness alone does not explain why a person may die by suicide.

Links between psychosis and suicidal thoughts and behaviors are strong. Every year, approximately 30 to 40 percent of people with psychotic disorders think about suicide, 20 to 30 percent make a suicide attempt, and 5 to 10 percent die by suicide. In the general community only 3 percent of people think about suicide, 0.5 percent make a suicide attempt, and 0.013 percent die by suicide. Although women are more likely than men to have suicidal thoughts, the suicide rate among men is four times higher than it is among women.

Among all people diagnosed with major psychological disorders, those with bipolar disorder have the highest risk of suicide: nearly 60 times greater than that of the general population. Approximately 15 to 20 percent of people with bipolar disorder kill themselves, and up to 40 percent make at least one suicide attempt during their lifetime. Risk factors for suicide attempts among people with bipolar disorder include being female, younger age at illness onset, depression during the initial illness episode, current depression, anxiety, substance or alcohol abuse, borderline personality disorder, and having a close blood relative who had died by suicide. Suicide deaths are significantly greater for men and people with first-degree family history of suicide.

People who die by suicide often suffered with depression. Risk factors for suicide death among people with depression include being male, a family history of psychiatric disorder, a previous attempted suicide, feelings of hopelessness and anxiety in the days and weeks prior to death, and drug and alcohol abuse.

Risk factors for suicide attempts among people with schizophrenia include a history of alcohol abuse, family history of psychiatric illness, other physical illnesses, history of depression, family history of suicide, history of drug and tobacco use, being white, and experiencing depressive symptoms. Risk factors for death by suicide in this group include being male, history of attempted suicide, younger age at mental illness onset, higher intelligence, poor adherence to treatment, and feelings of hopelessness.

Two medications—clozapine and lithium—are particularly effective in reducing suicide outcomes among people with serious mental illness. InterSePT, a large, multicenter, international randomized controlled trial that followed 980 patients with schizophrenia and schizoaffective disorder for two years, revealed that clozapine was more effective than olanzapine (a more commonly prescribed atypical antipsychotic) in reducing

suicide attempts. Clozapine is the only medication with a specific US Food and Drug Administration indication for reducing
the risk of recurrent suicidal behavior in patients with schizophrenia or schizoaffective disorder. Although lithium's role in
preventing suicide in patients with serious mental illness is not
as well established as that of clozapine, a significant body of evidence for this claim exists. It is likely that, rather than decreasing suicidal ideation, lithium alleviates suicide by diminishing
impulsivity of people with bipolar disorder and depression.
While no large randomized placebo-controlled study examining the effect of lithium on suicide has been published, several
smaller studies have compared lithium to a variety of other
drugs (antidepressants and anticonvulsant mood stabilizers)
and placebos. A meta-analysis of the data from these trials
showed that rates of mortality were lower in the lithium group
than in the nonlithium groups, providing compelling evidence
for the use of lithium in preventing suicide deaths in patients
with bipolar disorder.

Sometimes people with mental illness kill themselves even
though they have loving, supportive families and access to good
medical care. Collin, the guitar player with bipolar disorder
whom you met in chapter 5, was one of these people.

Collin, who scored a gold record before he was 18, knew he
had a problem. Diagnosed with bipolar disorder at 27, Collin
started using alcohol to calm his depression and anxiety. He
told his mother that the psychotropic medications prescribed
to quell his racing thoughts and spiraling depressions dulled
his creativity. Collin knew he needed help from a program
that would address both his bipolar disorder and his drinking
problem. He did not want an Alcoholics Anonymous program
because it would not address his mental illness. He did not want
an inpatient program because he did not want to take time away
from his music. So, Collin asked his mother, Betty, a nurse, to
research nearby outpatient programs.

Together, Collin and Betty selected an outpatient program about two hours away. The program's marketing materials said they could handle people with both mental illness and alcohol problems. It promised to tailor a program specifically for him and provide as much counseling as he might need.

Collin was frightened. He often thought about killing himself. He had even told his mother about his fear.

The program was primarily outpatient, but during the first three days, when Collin was detoxing from alcohol, he stayed overnight. Although nurses checked on him regularly, they stopped giving him Lamictal, the medication his doctor had prescribed. Without Lamictal, Collin became manic. When Collin told his mother what had happened, Betty said he should come home. Betty called the program director more than once, warning the staff they were losing him and expressing concern about the care. The staff embarrassed Collin, saying, "Your mom's calling all the time. You need to grow up and do this on your own." They told Betty to stop calling. They said they would take care of Collin. But they did not.

On the fourth night, Collin stayed with a friend who lived nearby so he could teach guitar to some kids in a music camp. On the fifth day, Collin went home. He told Betty he was moving out because the counselors told him that he should grow up and recover on his own. Yet he said, "Why can't I feel better? Why can't I stop drinking? I'm so anxious and they won't give me anything for anxiety because they're afraid I'll become addicted to it."

Collin packed his belongings and left, telling Betty not to argue with him. He played gigs with his band all weekend and stayed in hotels or with friends at night. On the seventh day, Collin didn't attend the program, but he did call the program director. He told her he had relapsed with alcohol over the weekend but would be back tomorrow.

Collin never made it. Just eight days after Collin began the program, he killed himself, overdosing on heroin in a motel. He was alone. It was the night before his twenty-ninth birthday.

After Collin died, Betty learned that Collin had seen a counselor only once. The therapist who had promised to call and check up on Collin never did. She said her grandmother had died and that she had forgotten to check on Collin.

Suicide threats and attempts should always be taken seriously. Although we do understand the factors that put a group of people at greater risk for suicide, we cannot predict whether a given individual will attempt self-harm at any point in time. Chapter 3 includes concrete suggestions about what to do when you fear that a family member is likely to harm him- or herself.

Suicide can leave family members grieving for years. In the immediate aftermath of suicide, family survivors are at heightened risk for depression and suicide. Family members bereaved by suicide are at higher risk for cardiovascular disease, hypertension, diabetes, and chronic obstructive pulmonary disease than their peers. Adolescents who experience a family member's death by suicide are more likely than their peers to report marijuana and alcohol use, thoughts of suicide, and suicide attempts. They also experience more emotional distress. Compared with children whose mother or father died of cancer, suicide-bereaved children experience more depressive symptoms, especially those involving negative moods, interpersonal problems, feelings of uselessness, and inability to experience pleasure.

Losing a family member is always difficult, but loss through suicide can be even more traumatic. Some have suggested that families that lose a loved one to suicide experience a grieving process that is qualitatively different from that of people surviving a nonsuicide death. Sometimes, family members feel that they did something to cause the suicide; other times, they feel that they did not do enough to prevent it. Suicide, like mental illness, is laden with stigma; so, not surprisingly, people who lose a loved one to suicide often worry about what and how much to tell people about the death.

Family members coping with a suicide death need more support from other people than family members coping with death from other causes. Ironically, they often get less support. When my mother killed herself, I didn't want to tell anyone. I was sure they would think poorly of my mother or me. I learned years later how wrong I was.

Here are a few things I wish I had told my friends after my mother killed herself:

- Be present. When people avoid family members because they fear saying or doing the wrong thing, survivors feel blamed and isolated. Whatever your doubts, make contact. Survivors will forgive awkward behaviors or clumsy statements as long as support and compassion are evident.

- Avoid hollow reassurance. Listen to the pain and don't try to minimize it. Avoid statements like "Things will get better" or "At least she's not suffering anymore."

- Don't ask for details. Be supportive and listen.

- Share positive memories and stories about the person who died. Don't be afraid to say the person's name.

- Follow the survivor's lead when broaching sensitive topics. Ask the survivor whether he or she wants to talk about what happened. Don't assume that the person's feelings and needs will be the same as yours.

- Ask the survivor what you can do to help. Offer to help with practical things such as running errands or watching over children. Offer to sit quietly or pray with the person.

- Check in with the survivor several times in the weeks and months after the death.
- Be especially sensitive during holidays and anniversaries.

As gut-wrenching as my mother's suicide was for me, the times she attempted suicide but did not kill herself were equally dreadful. Each time my mother tried to kill herself but did not succeed, I worried about whether she would try again. I wanted to help her, but I felt that nothing I did mattered.

Here are some suggestions for what *not to do* after a suicide attempt:

- Do not blame the person. Avoid saying, "You let me / your family down," "I'm disappointed in you," "Why would you do this to your kids?" and "Why would you do this to me?" These statements feed into the person's sense of hopelessness and increase the likelihood of another suicide attempt.
- Do not ignore the situation or pretend that the suicide attempt did not happen.
- Do not hover and monitor every action of the person. No one wants to be smothered, even by a well-meaning family member.
- Do not blame yourself. Remember, it is most likely the symptoms of the person's mental illness that caused the suicide attempt.
- Do not think it will never happen again.

On the other hand, here are some things *to do* after a suicide attempt:

- Come to the person's aid. Be there for them. Talk if they want to talk. Once the person is released from the hospital, make sure they adhere to the follow-up regimen.

Help the person find a doctor and then make and get to appointments. Make sure the person gets prescriptions filled and takes the medications as directed.

- Create a safety plan with the person that they could follow should they once again become distressed or feel suicidal.

- Realize that it will take time for the person to recover. You wouldn't tell a person with cancer or diabetes to "just get over it," so don't say this to a person who attempted suicide.

- Be vigilant for symptoms of depression, mania, or psychosis that may lead to another suicide attempt.

- Take care of yourself. Seek help if you need it.

- Remove or lock up guns and restrict access to lethal means as much as possible. Keep only small quantities of pain relievers such as aspirin, Advil, and Tylenol at home. Remove unused or expired medicines.

- Talk about what happened with trusted friends and/or family members. The support they can give you and the person with mental illness is invaluable.

Destroyed Families and Rippling Grief

Incarceration, homelessness, and death are not the only tragedies associated with mental illness. Untreated mental illnesses can damage not only current parent-child and sibling relationships but also next-generation relationships.

After being gone for seven years, my daughter Sophie called and told me she was pregnant. The baby's father had schizophrenia and did not take medication. Between the two of them, they had one part-time job—Sophie was working in a nursing home laundry.

Shortly after the baby was born, my husband and I traveled to Texas for a visit. Over the next two years, we tried to reestablish our relationship with Sophie. We cooed over our beautiful granddaughter and sent adorable clothes and cuddly stuffed animals. We paid for Sophie's doctor appointments and medications because she said that, now that she had a baby, she had to make sure her bipolar disorder was under control. We embraced the baby's father and helped him find a doctor when he said he wanted treatment to ease his psychotic symptoms. We were hopeful that Sophie was learning to live with her mental illness.

But then both Sophie and the baby's father started using street drugs again. They stopped cleaning. Their apartment was filthy and filled with cockroaches. Hearing loud arguments in the middle of the night, neighbors called the police dozens of times, concerned about the baby's welfare. When I told Sophie that I was worried about her 2-year-old's safety, she dismissed my concerns and refused to talk to me. Frantic, I called Child Protective Services. The baby was removed from Sophie's care and placed with her paternal grandparents, people whom Sophie has told to shun me. My relationship with my daughter Sophie is destroyed. The sole connection I have to my granddaughter is an overworked social worker who says, "I'm sorry, but I'm not allowed to tell you anything about her."

Although conflicted parent-child relationships can lead to heartbreaking rifts between grandparents and grandchildren, when the middle generation suffers mental illness, the stakes are greater and the options fewer. My granddaughter has genes from a mother with bipolar disorder and a father with schizophrenia. Nature is stacked against her. While it is not clear that a structured, drug-free environment could compensate her genetic background, at least it could provide her with a chance for a productive, normal life. Of course, my husband and I could resort to lawyers and the courts for decisions about custody and visits, but that only holds the potential for even more fractured relationships.

Even when parents spend years helping an adult child with mental illness, there are challenges that many people do not expect. My friend Florence's story is a case in point. Here's what she told me one week over lunch.

"Just when I think it can't get any worse, it does," Florence said, holding her fork over her Greek salad.

"What's wrong?" I asked. Florence and I have a lot in common. We're both social scientists, we're both Jewish, and we both have an adult child with a serious mental illness. Florence's son Jacob was diagnosed with schizophrenia nearly thirty years ago, when he was a senior undergraduate student in the physics department at Stanford University. From the onset of his illness, Jacob has refused medications. He saw a psychiatrist on and off for a few years, but then the doctor retired and Jacob rejected the idea of a replacement. Although Jacob eventually completed his bachelor's degree and then got a master's degree in computer science, he has been unemployed most of his life, occasionally working as a lab technician or grocery store bagger. Jacob has always lived with Florence and his father, Yosef, although he insists that they are not his real parents. Jacob is not sure who Yosef and Florence are, but he knows they are people who were made bad by his enemies. On good days, when Florence or Yosef initiates a conversation with Jacob, he responds with a shake of the head or a grunt. On Tuesdays, Jacob refuses to speak at all. Yosef is 84. He has cancer, diabetes, heart disease, and end-stage renal disease. He uses a walker and rarely leaves the house.

Florence said, "I went out to do a few errands yesterday. Jacob was sitting at the kitchen table. Yosef wanted some soup. Using a can opener is difficult for Yosef, so he asked Jacob to help him open the can. Jacob said, 'No.' Yosef struggled with the can opener. It slipped out of his hand and dropped to the floor. When Yosef bent over to pick up the can opener, he lost his balance and fell. He couldn't get up. Jacob watched Yosef fall and he walked out of the room. Yosef cried for help, but Jacob never looked back. I came home and found Yosef on the floor."

"Why wouldn't Jacob help Yosef get up?" I asked.

"Jacob has always had a problem touching people, especially Yosef, so that part doesn't surprise me," Florence said. "What I don't understand is why Jacob didn't call 911. He just left his father lying on the floor."

My heart went out to Florence. I thought about all she and Yosef had done for Jacob over the years—supported him financially, put up with his refusal to communicate with them, and shouldered the embarrassment of watching him walk barefoot through the neighborhood in the winter, wearing threadbare clothes. Although both Florence and Yosef wanted to retire to Israel, they had put their plans on hold because Jacob refused to go with them and they could not bear to leave him behind.

Talking with Florence and wondering what would become of Jacob, I remembered one of the first research projects I had led. Back in 1992, I secured funding from the National Institute of Health to study two groups of older women. One group included 487 mothers of adult children with a developmental disability. The other contained 351 mothers of an adult child with schizophrenia. Although the two groups of women differed in many ways, they shared a never-ending worry about what would happen to their child after they died. However, when I asked the women about plans they had made for their children's future, the most common response was that a well sibling would take care of things. Asking the women about when they had talked with the well sibling and what had been said, I learned that many had casually mentioned the future and secured the well sibling's promise to look after their brother or sister, but few had legal plans in place that would ensure that the child's quality of life would not be compromised.

Planning for the Future: Finances

Relying on a verbal agreement is a very bad idea. While all people need to make sure they have enough money to last the course of their own lifetime, people who have an adult child with serious mental illness must have enough money to last the course of two lifetimes. In his book *When Mental Illness Strikes: Crisis Intervention for the Financial Plan*, Allen Giese, founder of Northstar Financial Planners and the father of an adult son diagnosed with schizophrenia in his late teens, stresses the important role that lifelong financial planning plays.

ABLE Accounts

In addition to government benefits (SSDI, SSI, Medicaid) discussed in chapter 5, ABLE accounts and special needs trusts help ensure that a person with serious mental illness has a quality of life higher than the subsistence level provided by government funding.

ABLE accounts are tax-advantaged savings accounts that were created in 2014 when Congress passed the Stephen Beck Jr. Achieving a Better Life Experience (ABLE) Act. People experiencing the onset of disability before the age of 26 are eligible. Unlike with SSDI, SSI, SNAP, and Medicaid—which require a means test and allow no more than $2,000 to accumulate in savings—families can add up to $15,000 to an ABLE account each year. Funds are controlled by the person with mental illness and can be used to improve health, independence, and quality of life. As such, ABLE accounts can help with housing, transportation, education, employment training and support, assistive technology, personal support services, health care expenses, financial management, and administrative services. As long as the ABLE account does not exceed $100,000, SSDI, SSI, and SNAP benefits are not compromised. Regardless of the size

of an ABLE account, Medicaid eligibility is not affected. However, upon the death of the person with mental illness, the state
may file a claim to all or a portion of the Medicaid funds, so it
is best for people with mental illness to spend the funds on an
ongoing basis and not keep too much money in an ABLE
account.

While the original law stipulated that individuals had to
open an ABLE account in their state of residency, as of 2015
people are free to enroll in any state's program provided that
that program is accepting out-of-state residents. This enables
people to compare different requirements for opening an account, account fees, and investment opportunities and choose
the ABLE account that is best for them. Some states have ABLE
accounts that come with a debit card, making withdrawals easy.

Special Needs Trusts

Special needs trusts are legal instruments that enable a parent,
grandparent, legal guardian, or court order to provide money
for the care of a person with chronic physical or mental illness
in a way that does not jeopardize the person's eligibility for government benefits. These trusts spell out how money should be
used to maintain the person's quality of life. They also protect
the funds from being drained by creditors and from the person
with mental illness making legal or financial mistakes. Because
special needs trusts are legal entities, their provisions remain
in force after the person establishing them dies. However, the
special needs trust should clearly state that Medicaid is entitled
to deduct money remaining in the trust upon the death of the
person with mental illness. Failure to include this statement
may cause the person with mental illness to be deemed ineli-
gible for SSI.

Establishing a trust involves making several important decisions that will determine the future of the person with mental

illness. First, it is critical to hire a lawyer who is an expert in developing special needs trusts. Not every lawyer is able to do this, so shop carefully. It is also a good idea to engage a financial planner in this process.

Next, parents must appoint a trustee who will be in charge of making decisions in the interest of the person with mental illness. The trustee must be responsible and well versed in the provisions of the trust.

Third, parents must determine the succession of trustees. For instance, should the special needs trust be a first-party trust, a third-party trust, or a pooled trust? Will government benefits be protected? How will the trust be funded? Does the trust fund have enough money to last the child's lifetime?

Moving from Rock Bottom to Supported Decisions and Advance Directives

Clearly, waiting for people with serious mental illnesses to hit rock bottom and ask for help is not a good solution—for them, their families, or their communities. Forced treatment, as some suggest, violates basic civil rights and, as such, is not a viable alternative. But what if there were another way? What if there were a way that would enable people to get the help they need in a crisis and maintain their dignity?

Decision-making is central to a person's autonomy, yet throughout history people with serious mental illnesses have been stripped of their decision-making abilities. Asylums removed people's autonomy, responsibility, and self-direction, replacing those with paternalistic care. Guardianships revoke individual rights and transfer authority for making legal, financial, medical, social, and living decisions to another person—a substitute. While these strategies work for some, for the vast majority of people with a serious mental illness they are a miserable failure.

Current law centered on individual rights guides American expectations for how personal decisions should be made. At age 18, people are empowered and encouraged to make decisions on their own, even if they are not able to do so. Individual civil rights dominate. Treatments for mental illnesses, just like treatment for any other illnesses, are voluntary. As a result, people who are unable to make decisions are forced to do so on their own. Families that are willing and able to help are ignored by the medical system and not consulted because that is the law. Under these laws, sick people must reach rock bottom and ask for help before anyone can help them.

But the tide is turning.

In 2006, the United Nations Convention on the Rights of Persons with Disabilities (UNCRPD) passed a mandate that became effective in 2008. The order maintains that people with disabilities, including mental illness, have the right to recognition as persons before the law, that people with disabilities have the right to enjoy legal capacity on an equal basis with other people in all aspects of life, and that appropriate measures must be made to provide persons with disabilities access to the support they may require in exercising their legal capacity. The spirit of this order lies in sharp contrast to guardianship practices or substitute decision-making. It demands a sharp change in how decisions are made.

Supported Decision-Making

A new model called supported decision-making (SDM) is emerging. A law first passed in Canada in 1995 outlined SDM and provides a process that recognizes people with disabilities as persons before the law. This creates a pathway for people with serious mental illness to exercise legal capacity by developing supports that enable autonomous decision-making. This person-centered approach to decision-making enables individuals to exercise legal capacity to the greatest extent possible and changes the central question from "Does a person have the capacity to make a decision?" to "What supports are needed to ensure that this person can best exercise his or her rights?" Since the passages of the Canadian act and the UNCRPD, many countries—including Australia, Germany, Ireland, Scotland, England, Norway, Sweden, Israel, and the United States—have begun to integrate SDM into their legal systems.

While SDM has been embraced by people with developmental disabilities and promoted as a strategy for end-of-life decision-making, its popularity among people with serious mental illness has lagged. This may be because some mental illnesses affect judgment and decision-making, calling into question the capacity of people with serious mental illness to make informed decisions about their care. Depression can make decision-making difficult; schizophrenia can lead to passive acceptance or rigid adherence to a single idea; bipolar disorder, especially during manic episodes, can lower the bar for risk tolerance.

Yet there is also good evidence that people with serious mental illnesses can make competent and prudent treatment decisions. Moreover, the variability of most serious mental illness symptoms means that there are times when thinking is clear enough that competent decisions can be made, especially with support.

SDM offers people with serious mental illness the right to retain their autonomy. With SDM, people with mental illness become the ultimate decision-maker, while enlisting help from family, friends, or other trusted persons who can help clarify the problems and options. In many respects, SDM is like the typical decision-making process used by most adults who consult with trusted partners about important life decisions. SDM recognizes the voice of the person who is ill but does not force them to hit rock bottom before help can be given. What's more, it is a less restrictive strategy than guardianship. This is the model Deborah Danner was hoping for when she consulted a lawyer and said she wanted help. Deborah wanted help, but not from her sister. With SDM, treatment decisions can hinge on a person's ability to function in society, be subject to change, and balance the rights of individuals and society. Unlike guardianships, SDM does not take away anyone's rights. Rather, it protects individual and societal rights.

Unbeknownst to me at the time, my family used an informal SDM model when my husband's grandmother began showing signs of dementia. The model worked very well. When Nana became disoriented at night, forgot to turn off the stove, and kept asking the same questions over and over, we worried. But the next year, it was clear that Nana was more than just a little confused. One afternoon, we took our kids to an amusement park, leaving Nana home alone, at her insistence. When we returned, Nana told us that circus people had jumped the railroad tracks, run around the house sprinkling a white powder, and then collapsed side by side and head to toe in our beds. We realized then that we could no longer leave Nana alone because she could no longer make decisions on her own about her finances, her medical care, or where she should live. However, she could tell us what she wanted, and she could be part of the decision-making process. We had a family meeting that included Nana, my husband, and me. My husband and I told Nana about our concerns and discussed alternatives, and together we made decisions about what to do. Nana lived with us until her care needs became greater than we could accommodate. Then, we helped her move to an assisted living facility and finally to a nursing home. At every step of the way, Nana knew we supported her, and she got the care she wanted in the place where she wanted it. She did not have to roam the streets eating garbage before being able to get help. Nor did she have to be jailed. SDM worked because Nana wanted our help and we were able to have conversations with her when she was able to tell us what she wanted.

Contrast this experience with those of my daughter Sophie, who did not think she needed help. She would not have wanted to be part of such a conversation, especially when she was manic. Refusing help and making decisions on her own because that was what society said she had the right to do, Sophie became homeless, dependent on drugs, and jailed. All my husband and I could do was watch with horror and dismay. I wonder what might have happened had there been better structure and more opportunity to help Sophie make decisions using an SDM model. Maybe Sophie would have been better able to participate in SDM if a social worker had talked with her when she was not in a manic state.

During the past decade, US courts, legislators, policy makers, and national organizations have started paying attention to SDM. The American Bar Association and the National Guardianship Association have endorsed SDM. In 2015, Texas passed a law that made it the first state to mandate that courts must consider SDM agreements as an alternative to guardianship prior to making guardianship appointments. At least ten other states (Delaware, Indiana, Maine, Maryland, Massachusetts, Michigan, New York, North Carolina, Wisconsin, and Virginia) have begun implementing or examining SDM as an alternative to guardianship. Up-to-date information about SDM in each state may be found on the National Resource Center for Supported Decision-Making website.

Emerging evidence from patients and family members indicates that SDM is an acceptable and often superior alternative to substitute decision-making. Creating teams of decision-makers who can participate in SDM seems like a feasible strategy for many people with serious mental illness. However, there is a dearth of information about SDM outcomes, best practices, people who are SDM's optimal candidates, and decisions most likely to be enhanced by SDM. The model is too new for us to know this. We also do not know whether SDM results in better decisions, greater satisfaction with the decision-making process, and increased sense of empowerment among people with mental illness.

Although SDM shows much promise, like guardianships and other forms of substituted decision-making, it holds the potential for abuse. For example, some people worry that SDM may expose people with mental illness to undue influence or coercion from their alleged supporters, thereby effectively disempowering them. However, SDM appears to provide a viable alternative to more restrictive guardianship laws, and there is little doubt that it is better aligned with the goals of ensuring that autonomy, self-determination, and dignity are maintained when people have a serious mental illness.

Advance Directives

In addition to SDM, advance directives can help people with mental illness get the treatment they want. While every state has legislation authorizing some form of advance directive for health care, many of these directives do not provide adequately for the unique problems relating to treatment of serious mental illnesses.

Psychiatric advance directives (PADs), recognized in about half the states (although their orders can be incorporated into health care directives in all states), are legal documents drafted when a person is well enough to consider preferences for future treatment. PADs recognize that people with serious mental illnesses are capable of making important decisions about their treatment most of the time. PADs provide a way for people to express their free will and self-determination by spelling out what they want should they experience a crisis or be unable to make decisions on their own.

There are two types of PADs: *instructional* and *proxy*.

- *Instructional directives* enable a person to indicate medications and treatments they want and those they do not want.
- *Proxy directives* enable the person with mental illness to identify a health care proxy—a lawyer, trusted family member, or friend—who would make decisions for the person with serious mental illness if they were in crisis.

State-by-state information about developing a PAD can be found at the National Resource Center on Psychiatric Advance Directives website.

Once a PAD is established, it is important that it be included in a person's health records so that care managers and health care providers know it exists. If a person with a PAD is determined to lack capacity to make their own treatment decisions, health care providers must follow the treatment instructions in the PAD. However, the health care provider is not required to follow the PAD instructions if they conflict with accepted standards of care or are contrary to needs in an emergency.

Finally, although few people with serious mental illness have a PAD, research finds that people who do establish PADs experience increases in autonomy and are more satisfied with the treatment they receive during a crisis. A review of the effectiveness of PADs found that they can empower patients, minimize coercion, and improve coping strategies, all of which may reduce the frequency of in-patient admissions. Moreover, there is evidence that people who are offered medications that they had requested in advance directives are more likely than people not having advance directives to adhere to these medications, supporting the benefit of patient participation in medication choice.

Of course, PADs, like other medical advance directives, are not perfect. Sometimes, especially in a crisis situation, nobody can find the advance directive paperwork. Unaware that advance directives have been made, family and doctors do what they believe is in the patient's best interest. Other times, the advance directives are not specific enough to guide practice.

PADs and SDM are not magic bullets. Nevertheless, when they are thoughtfully developed and distributed to family and health care providers, they can help people with serious mental illness get the medications and treatments they need without trampling their free will and civil rights. As more people use SDM and develop PADs, the myth of requiring people with serious mental illness to hit rock bottom before they can be helped will fade away and much of the pain and suffering of serious mental illness will be alleviated.

CHAPTER 7

Remarkable Resilience

JOE HAS LIVED with schizophrenia since he was 17 years old. He is now 72. He was last hospitalized for psychosis thirty-two years ago.

Sharon was diagnosed with depression at 51. She is 63 and has not missed a single day of work because of depression since 2007.

Michelle is 61. She was hospitalized seven times over a twenty-three-year period, but for the past eight years Michelle has successfully controlled the symptoms of bipolar disorder with medication and therapy.

Each has lived with a serious mental illness for decades. Today, however, their lives look quite ordinary. Joe is retired. He plays pickup basketball on Wednesday afternoons and fly-fishes whenever he can. In nice weather, he plays golf and rides his bike. Sharon continues to work full-time as a social worker. On weekends, she enjoys strolling through craft festivals, going to the theater, bird watching, and reading a book at the seashore. Michelle dotes on her three grandchildren and pursues crafting, her lifelong passion. When I recently spoke with Michelle, she told me she had spent the weekend teaching forty children how to make candles.

Yet, as we have seen in previous chapters, Joe, Sharon, and Michelle have lived lives that are anything but ordinary. The struggles each has faced and the strength each has shown make them truly resilient and remarkable people.

Scientists have charted the courses of mental illnesses over both short and long periods of time. From their research, we have learned about remission, a period of time during which a person experiences no more than minimal symptoms. We have also learned about recovery and how differently recovery is defined by clinicians and by people with mental illness. Clinicians define "recovery" as the ability to participate actively in society at a given point in time. People with serious mental illness, on the other hand, define recovery as a process by which they learn to live satisfying and fulfilling lives. The next sections examine what we know about remission and recovery and offer strategies for helping people in remission and in recovery.

Remission

In the early twentieth century, pioneering psychiatrist Emil Kraepelin defined dementia praecox—known now as schizophrenia—as a progressive neurodegenerative disease leading to irreversible loss of cognitive functioning. According to Kraepelin, people with schizophrenia were doomed. They would never get better. When people with dementia praecox seemed to improve, Kraepelin and his followers would assert that it was most likely that the illness was misdiagnosed or that the person was experiencing a temporary remission. Nearly one hundred years later, a new conventional wisdom had evolved to explain the "natural course" of schizophrenia. According to this perspective, one-third of people deteriorate, one-third have frequent relapses, and one-third either recover or have occasional relapses with reasonably good functioning between episodes.

More recent studies following people with serious mental illnesses for extended periods of time have revealed an even more optimistic picture. As many as 70 percent of people with schizophrenia who leave psychiatric institutions experience significant periods of symptom reduction, limited hospitalization, and improved functioning. People with bipolar disorder and depression typically experience episodes of distress followed by periods of calm. There are, it seems, more differences than similarities in how serious mental illnesses evolve over time, but it is the unusual person who follows Kraepelin's pathway of doom.

Studies of short-term outcomes of serious mental illness generally focus on remission. Not surprisingly, scientists disagree about how to define remission. In 2003, the Remission in Schizophrenia Working Group convened to develop a consensus definition of remission from schizophrenia. This committee was guided by the goals of a similar group whose work nearly a decade earlier had defined remission from depression. The Schizophrenia Working Group defined remission as "a state in which patients have experienced improvement in core signs and symptoms to the extent that any remaining symptoms are of such low intensity that they no longer interfere significantly with behavior and are below the threshold typically utilized in justifying an initial diagnosis of schizophrenia." Similarly, a group of bipolar disorder experts defined remission as no more than minimal symptoms of both mania and depression for at least one week and sustained remission as experiencing no more than minimal symptoms for between eight and twelve consecutive weeks.

Remission rates over the long term are lower than remission rates over the short term. Research found that, for example, over a two-year period, 58 percent of people diagnosed with depression were in remission; when those same people were followed for six years, remission rates dropped to 17 percent. A national survey of community-dwelling people found that one-third of people who had been diagnosed with major depression, bipolar disorder, manic depression, schizophrenia, or schizoaffective disorder had been in remission for at least the past twelve months.

These findings suggest that, for many people, the symptoms of schizophrenia, depression, and bipolar disorder are episodic. People like Joe, Michelle, and Sharon often live in remission for years. Another national study found that remission rates were related to age. About 25 percent of people between the ages of 20 and 32 experience remission, compared with 58 percent of people age 65 and older. Low rates of remission among younger people are often explained by their reluctance to seek help or inability to find or afford help. Not surprisingly, the higher remission rates that occur with age have been attributed to a patient's growing maturity and willingness to seek and engage in treatment and a natural burning out of psychotic symptoms.

However, when it comes to remission, there is a lot of variability. Joe, for example, experienced a six-year period (from when he was 23 until he was 29) during which he neither took psychotropic medications nor experienced psychotic symptoms. Joe cannot explain the remission he had in his twenties, but the combination of having young children and the fear of experiencing a severe psychotic episode made Joe consciously commit to closely monitoring his symptoms thoughout his thirties. As the primary breadwinner, he knew he could not afford to be sick. By the time Joe was nearly 40, he and his wife Molly had learned to identify the warning signs that his thinking was becoming delusional. These included sleeplessness and loss of appetite. Joe would tell Molly when he had thoughts about being God-like or about being needed to solve international conspiracies. Joe acknowledges and is grateful for the critical role that

Molly has played in keeping him from succumbing to psychosis. Sometimes Molly knew that Joe was in danger of a psychotic episode even before Joe did. When there were indications that his illness was recurring, Joe would increase both the frequency of counseling sessions and the medication dosages. He jokes that doing this was easier than arguing with his wife. Although these strategies often helped prevent the need for hospitalization, there were times when Joe did need to be hospitalized.

Clinical Recovery

The Remission in Schizophrenia Working Group defined not only remission but also recovery. This group contended that to experience recovery, a person must not only be relatively free of disease-related symptoms but also be able to hold a job and engage in social relationships. The group viewed recovery as more demanding and longer-term than remission, and it saw remission as a necessary but insufficient step toward recovery. This perspective has come to be known as "clinical recovery."

Clinical recovery is typically considered to be an outcome, although there is little agreement about where to draw the line between recovered and not recovered. In an effort to advance the state of the science, standardized definitions of recovery have been suggested, but these definitions vary regarding the length of time required, acceptable symptom level, and what it means to function well within the community. Not surprisingly, rates of recovery vary dramatically as a function of how recovery is defined.

The role that medications play for clinical recovery has been debated for years. However, because many definitions of clinical recovery include medication adherence, it is difficult to separate medication use and clinical recovery. Other definitions of recovery, however, do not include medication adherence, providing the opportunity to examine how medications influence recovery.

One of the first long-term studies of the effects of psychotropic medications on remission and recovery among people with schizophrenia and mood disorders was spearheaded by Dr. Martin Harrow. A chess master who played two tournament games against Bobby Fischer, both ending in a draw, Harrow is also the widely cited author of over 250 scientific papers and four books about schizophrenia and bipolar disorders.

Harrow and his colleagues found that clinical recovery is possible for many people with serious mental illnesses who do not continue to take antipsychotic medication. Harrow's study, known as the Chicago Followup Study, recruited 139 young patients (average age 23) with schizophrenia or mood disorders who had been admitted to two psychiatric hospitals in Chicago following an episode of acute psychosis. Because these patients had experienced recent onsets of their illnesses, Harrow's team was able to study how the illnesses unfolded. All patients were treated with psychotropic medications while in the hospital, interviewed extensively, and then reevaluated six times over the next twenty years. As is typically found in studies of people with serious mental illnesses, no uniform treatment plan applied to all the patients that Harrow studied. Over time, some patients stopped taking medication, either on their own or following their doctors' advice, while other patients continued to take medication. At the initial follow-up, two years after the hospitalization, Harrow's team found that there were no significant differences in the severity of psychotic symptoms experienced between people with schizophrenia on antipsychotic medications and those not on these medications.

However, beginning four and a half years after the initial hospitalization and continuing over the next fifteen years, people with schizophrenia who were not on antipsychotic medications experienced significantly fewer psychotic symptoms than those taking antipsychotic medicines. People not taking antipsychotic medications also had fewer rehospitalizations and were more productive in terms of work and social functioning. Although people in Harrow's study with mood disorders had better outcomes than those with schizophrenia, the patterns of the relationships between antipsychotic medication use and indicators of recovery were similar. At each of the six follow-up assessments over the twenty years, significantly more of the unmedicated patients with mood disorders experienced decreases in psychotic symptoms and increases in social and work functioning than those taking antipsychotic medication.

Harrow's team concluded that, while antipsychotic medications were helpful in the short run after the onset of serious mental illness, between 30 and 40 percent of people with schizophrenia did not need to take antipsychotic medications long-term. And it wasn't just Harrow's group that found this. At least seven other studies followed people with schizophrenia for more than seven years in countries such as the United States, the Netherlands, Denmark, England, Finland, and Canada. Unlike short-term studies that consistently find benefits when patients are treated with psychotropic medications for up to three years, many long-term studies find little benefit to continuing psychotropic medications long-term.

However, it would be a mistake to conclude that people with serious mental illnesses should be quick to dump their medications. A 2020 study that followed 62,250 patients with schizophrenia in Finland for twenty years found that mortality rates of people not using antipsychotics were nearly double those of people using any antipsychotic medication, and mortality rates of people using clozapine were especially low. It is also important to know that although longitudinal studies can tell us about how people change over time, findings from longitudinal studies can only be generalized to people who are like those who continue to participate in the research. People who drop out of

studies typically are sicker than those who continue to participate, and because they are sicker, they were probably more
likely to be taking medication before dropping out of the study.
This was true for people in the Chicago Followup Study. Harrow and his team found that people who stopped taking antipsychotic medications for a prolonged period and recovered
were a self-selected group that could be identified as early as
their initial hospitalization. These people were less anxious and
had better neurocognitive skills and resources before their hospitalization than those who continued to take antipsychotic
medications long-term. In sum, because there is much we do
not know about the long-term effects of antipsychotic medications, decisions about medications must be made on a case-
by-case basis with guidance from a skilled clinician.

Over the years, Joe, Sharon, and Michelle have had very different experiences with medications. Many times, Joe tried to
stop taking psychotropic medication, both with and without his
doctor's help. Some attempts were successful; there were even
many years when Joe could go to work and take care of himself
and his family without medication. Eventually, however, Joe
and his doctor found that a low daily dose of Haldol kept his
delusional thinking in check without causing unwanted side effects. Sharon never wanted to try giving up the medications
her doctor prescribed. She feared that the awful depression and
anxiety she had experienced years ago would come crashing
back. And so, for years, Sharon has taken seventy-five milligrams of Effexor each morning. When Michelle was first hospitalized and diagnosed with bipolar disorder, her doctor prescribed lithium. Michelle took the medicine daily for twenty
years. Every three months, she had her blood checked to ensure
that lithium levels were stable. When Michelle was in her early
fifties, blood tests indicated that she had developed kidney disease, a common side effect of lithium. Her doctor changed her
medications, and Michelle now takes ten milligrams of Saphris,

an atypical (second-generation) antipsychotic, and two hundred milligrams of Lamictal, a mood stabilizer. She sees a therapist regularly. Consistent with findings from Harrow's research that people with the mildest forms of mental illness were most able to live without medications, it is likely that Joe, Sharon, and Michelle, who each had very serious psychosis earlier in life, will need to continue taking medication for the rest of their lives. But Joe, Sharon, and Michelle have also experienced clinical recoveries for years.

In sum, serious mental illnesses are often episodic, there is wide variability to their courses, and approximately half of all people with serious mental illness have good long-term outcomes. For many with serious mental illness, the most destructive effects are evident early on, followed by a plateau, and then gradual improvement. Further, a subgroup of people with schizophrenia can discontinue antipsychotic medications after a few years and not experience a relapse. These people tend to be older and have a later onset of illness, shorter duration of untreated psychosis, fewer symptoms, better social functioning, and a history of being maintained on a lower dose of antipsychotics before they stopped taking the medications.

How can an individual with mental illness know whether it is safe to decrease or stop medication? This is one of the greatest challenges for people with serious mental illness. Best practice, however, suggests that working closely with a knowledgeable doctor and monitoring thoughts, feelings, and behavior can help individuals determine what is right for them.

Personal Recovery

Nearly thirty years ago, people with serious mental illnesses began to define recovery on their own terms. They saw recovery not as an outcome as described by clinicians and researchers but as a process. Let's take a look at how one of the most articulate among these people drew strength from her illness and launched a movement that changed the way we think about serious mental illnesses.

Patricia Deegan was the oldest child in a large working-class Irish Catholic family. At 17, the high school senior was a gifted athlete who did just enough academic work to be able to compete on the varsity teams. She dreamt of playing lacrosse for the US Women's Team or maybe joining the Peace Corps because she loved helping people. She applied to college, hoping to become a gym teacher.

One winter afternoon during basketball practice, Pat found it harder and harder to catch the ball. Her depth perception was off. She got hit in the head with passes she usually would catch. Everything looked different. Tables and chairs morphed into frighteningly sharp angles, their utility unclear. She had trouble understanding words. Eventually Pat did not know what people were saying at all. Instead of focusing on words, Pat watched the mechanical ways people moved their mouths. She saw screwdrivers where once she had seen teeth. She did not believe people were whom they said they were. Convinced that people wanted to kill her, she stayed awake for days, ready to defend herself.

Pat's family admitted her to a psychiatric hospital where she was given Haldol. Although Pat graduated from high school, she could not go to college. She was too sick. Pat spent her days sleeping or sitting in a chair in her parents' living room. While her friends went off to college and started new lives, Pat was admitted to the psychiatric hospital for a second time and then a third time.

During her third hospitalization, Pat asked the psychiatrist what was wrong with her. He said, "Miss Deegan, you have a disease called schizophrenia. It is a disease, like diabetes. If you continue to take your medications for the rest of your life and you avoid stress, then you might be able to cope."

Disappointed and angry, Pat left the psychiatrist's office. She did not want to take medication for the rest of her life, and she didn't just want to "cope." She wanted to live. Defiantly, Pat said to herself, "I'll become Dr. Deegan and I'll make the mental health system work the right way." And that is exactly what Pat Deegan did. But it took a long, long time, because Pat's recovery was slow. For months after her third hospitalization, she sat in a chair in her parents' living room, drugged on Haldol, smoking one cigarette after the next. She just wanted to sleep. Every day, Pat's grandmother would come into the living room and ask Pat if she wanted to go food shopping with her. Because her grandmother asked just once a day, Pat said it felt like a real invitation. But each day, Pat said no.

Then, one day, Pat said yes. Although all Pat did that day was push the cart through the grocery store, it was a beginning. Little by little, Pat began talking with friends and taking responsibility for her medications. She got a part-time job. Taking an English composition class at the local community college brought new challenges, as Pat was still very ill. She had to manage her anxiety, quiet the distressing voices she still heard, and ignore thoughts of doom that popped into her mind as she tried to listen to the teacher's lecture. She had to find ways to concentrate so she could do her homework. Over time, Pat discovered strategies that worked for her. She earned a bachelor's degree from Fitchburg State College in 1977. She earned a PhD in clinical psychology from Duquesne University in 1984.

More than thirty years ago, Pat Deegan published a paper defining recovery from serious mental illnesses like schizophrenia, bipolar disorder, and depression. Unlike the clinical definition of recovery, Deegan viewed recovery as accepting and then overcoming the challenges of mental illness. There was more to recovery than being free of disease-related symptoms, holding a job, or engaging in social relationships. Deegan said that people with psychiatric illnesses "need to meet the challenge of the disability and to reestablish a new and valued sense of integrity and purpose within and beyond the limits of the disability; the aspiration is to live, work, and love in a community in which one makes a significant contribution." She acknowledged that, because there are no cures for serious mental illnesses, people do not recover from serious mental illnesses like they recover from acute illnesses. But, she said, people with serious mental illness can enjoy satisfying and fulfilling lives. They can work, they can go to school, they can be parents, and they can have long-term relationships. Hope, willingness to try, and responsible action are key.

As I got to know Joe, Michelle, and Sharon during the course of writing this book, I realized just how true this is. Joe earned a BS in fisheries from the University of Arizona. Before retiring in 2010, Joe worked as a lab technician at PacifiCorp's Naughton Plant for nearly thirty years, where he helped provide affordable electricity to people. He never missed a day of work because of his mental illness. Joe played such an important role at the plant that twice he has been called out of retirement to help out. Sharon continues her career as a social worker and says that she is helped at her job by her personal experiences with depression. She knows what to listen for and when her patients might not be telling the truth. Michelle retired after working in the school cafeteria for years. She remains the anchor of her family, providing support to her husband, children, and grandchildren. Joe and Michelle continue to be in long-term marriages, supported even in their most psychotic states by their spouses, Molly and Tim. Joe, Michelle, and Sharon have all raised children who are productive, healthy adults.

What are their secrets? How have these people been able to live with their mental illness and yet have satisfying, productive lives? I posed these questions to Joe, Michelle, and Sharon. What they told me was poignant and instructive.

Joe said, "I'm not particularly religious. My grandmother, however, was devout. She saw to it that I attended Sunday School every week for nine straight years, never missing once. This taught me to never lose hope. There were times when things seemed very bleak, even hopeless, but I always had an underlying sense that this was only temporary, that things would get better. I just had to keep on keeping on. Maybe for the first time in my life, I am living where I want to live and doing what I want to do." In addition to hope, Joe told me about the importance of the support he has received from his family, friends, and professionals. He knows that without Molly's love, he would have been a very different man. Finally, Joe said, "I am cognizant of my illness every day. I check in with myself every morning and every night and make sure I'm seeing and hearing the same things other people are."

Sharon also is vigilant about sleep, rest, relaxation, and stress. Each morning as she brushes her teeth, she looks in the mirror and asks herself, "Do I feel rested? Is anything bothering me?" She adjusts whenever needed. Sharon remembers too well the beginnings of her illness and does not want to experience ever again the anxiety and depression that made her want to kill herself. She practices yoga and maintains a healthy diet. A few years ago, Sharon was treated for breast cancer. Today, she is healthy physically and mentally.

Michelle told me that she fought her mental illness for the sake of her children. She didn't want them to experience what she had suffered when her father, who also had bipolar disorder, refused to take medications and, instead, drank himself into nightly alcoholic stupors. Michelle said, "I prayed a lot. If my prayers weren't answered, which often they weren't, I realized that God had a bigger plan for me. It taught me patience when I was suffering." Michelle also said that her husband Tim's active involvement in her care—researching options, talking to doctors, helping their children understand her illness—helped make her more resilient.

By the mid-1980s, hoping to gain control over their lives, some people with serious mental illness began referring to themselves as "consumers" rather than "patients." In many respects this mindset change was groundbreaking. Unlike patients, "consumers" have reciprocal relationships with service providers. Unlike patients, consumers have a choice in their treatment. Deegan's work encouraged others with serious mental illness to write about their own recoveries. These narratives describe deeply personal processes of changing attitudes, values, feelings, goals, skills, and roles that stand in clear contrast to the clinical definition of recovery.

From these writings, we see that recovery from serious mental illness is not a uniform process. Rather, it is a process that varies from person to person. Nevertheless, there are some common characteristics. They include connectedness, hope, identity, meaning, and empowerment—together known as CHIME. The CHIME framework has been widely endorsed; many now recognize the importance of personal recovery as distinct from clinical recovery.

Little by little, the consumer-driven movement gained momentum. As it did, interventions designed to address the fundamental principles of recovery were developed. A growing number of programs helped people with serious mental illnesses feel hopeful about their lives, while research documented the improvements that people participating in recovery programs experienced. Today, interventions emphasizing education, self-management skills, and self-determination help promote recovery, hope, and empowerment. Improvement does not appear to be affected by age, gender, or race. Further, because most of the interventions are relatively brief, people can begin to recover in weeks rather than years.

Interventions that include collaborative efforts of mental health professionals and peer providers—people who themselves have serious mental illnesses—also have positive effects, suggesting that partnerships between peers and professionals may be especially effective. Mental health professionals provide information about recovery and goal setting and help people develop new skills. Working alongside professionals, peer specialists provide support and model self-efficacy and agency in everyday settings. They demonstrate coping strategies and reinforce attempts to use new skills outside of treatment settings.

Working in conjunction with a clinician, Michelle facilitates a bipolar support group at St. Mary's Kempf Bipolar Wellness Center. Helping people understand that they are more than their illness, and that despite their illness they can have productive lives, is gratifying to Michelle. Watching people change from being helpless to being hopeful gives Michelle's life meaning.

Few studies have examined whether interventions run exclusively by peers—whether they be mutual support groups, peer support services (support is unidirectional, with one or more peer supporters offering help to other people), or peer mental health service providers (where people who have used mental health services are employed to provide care)—result in lower rates of hospitalization, fewer symptoms, or greater satisfaction with care. As such, it is premature to make conclusions about the value of these interventions. Moreover, there is good evidence that working with peers has benefits to people with serious mental illness, including increasing their willingness and ability to take responsibility for their health care, promoting self-efficacy, and strengthening feelings of empowerment and hope.

Joe volunteers three to four days a week at the Friendly Harbor Community Center, a gathering place founded in 1996 by Chris Hart, Mike Mihalas, and Robin Hill, all of whom have experienced a serious mental illness. At the Friendly Harbor, people with serious mental illness can talk on equal footing with one another. There is no judgment, and the program is free to participants. The program's goal is to restore hope, dignity, and a sense of purpose to people with a mental illness.

In 2013, Michelle became a peer recovery advocate at the PEACE Zone (Peer Empowerment & Advocacy in the Community of Evansville). The PEACE Zone offers peer support for people who suffer mental illnesses. Group discussions provide support and emphasize recovery. People are empowered to become advocates for their own recovery. Additionally, the PEACE Zone has programs that include job readiness, community education and outreach, arts engagement, billiards, music, and physical activity. Several years ago, Michelle took a week's worth of classes and became a certified recovery specialist / community health worker. Michelle provides mentorship to peers and does outreach at four mental health facilities, where she tells her recovery story, provides information about the PEACE Zone, and encourages people to participate in the PEACE Zone. She also does outreach at two local colleges and health fairs.

In addition to his work at Friendly Harbor, Joe is involved in advocacy work and frequently meets with his state representatives in Denver. This past year, Joe lobbied for long-term civil commitment beds at the Colorado Mental Health Institute at Pueblo, the community's 455-bed hospital that provides inpatient care to people with mental illness. Joe has also advocated for: supported housing; Assertive Community Treatment, a team-based treatment model that provides multidisciplinary, flexible treatment and support to people with mental illness 24/7; assisted outpatient treatment, the program used successfully in Miami by Steven Leifman in which a judge orders a qualifying person with symptoms of severe untreated mental illness to adhere to a mental health treatment plan while living in the community; and restoration of the age of consent to 18 from 15 in Colorado. Last year, Joe received Mental Health

America's Phoenix award, given to a person with a serious mental illness who has done exceptional work in the mental health field.

Both Joe and Michelle share their personal stories. The memoir each has written is filled with pain and struggle, but also with hope. Joe and Michelle each participate in Crisis Intervention Team training programs in their communities. A partnership of police officers, mental health professionals, people with mental illness, and advocates, CIT helps people with mental illness access medical treatment as an alternative to putting them in jail. It also promotes police officer safety, as well as safety of people in crisis. The police sergeant in charge of the program told Joe that hearing Joe's story was the most impactful part of the training. Joe and Michelle share their stories at National Alliance on Mental Illness meetings, helping family members understand what people with serious mental illnesses experience. At the invitation of Valerie Baughman, director of Parkview Hospital's Behavioral Health Division, which has sixty-five inpatient beds for people with mental illness or substance abuse, Joe participates in a training program designed to help staff understand what it is like to be hospitalized for mental illness. Not only are staff moved by Joe's personal story, but they also develop greater understanding for their patients as people.

Clinical versus Personal Recovery

Can people with serious mental illness experience personal recovery and not clinical recovery? A recent analysis of thirty-seven studies examined this question and found that the answer is yes. People with mental illness symptoms can have hope, and they can feel empowered. These findings suggest that people with serious mental illnesses can recover despite having psychotic symptoms. That people with serious mental illness can achieve clinical and personal recovery stands in sharp contrast to Kraepelin's pessimistic view of serious mental illnesses. It also raises questions about what the goal of care should be and what it means to function within society.

What People with Serious Mental Illness Can Do to Foster Recovery

Resilience—the ability to handle life's challenges and setbacks—in the face of serious mental illness is not easy, but it is possible. It does, however, require hard work. Here are some ideas for becoming more resilient that I have learned from scientific studies and personal accounts:

- Be mindful of how you feel. Check in with yourself each day. Pick a time that works for you—when you're brushing your teeth or drinking a cup of coffee. Pay attention to how you're feeling.

- Realize that many of the bad things that happen are not your fault. Use your experiences with difficulties in the past to remind you of all that you've overcome. Remind yourself that things that hurt can make you a stronger person.

- Try to maintain control, even during stressful times. Go for a walk or a run. Physical exercise calms people down.

- Get connected. Building strong, positive relationships with family and friends provides support. Join a faith or spiritual community. Offer to volunteer in a community service program.

- Ask someone you admire to tell you about a difficult or a meaningful time in their life.

- Find something that centers you. For some, it is knitting. For others, it may be painting or working with clay. For still others, it may be listening to music or taking a hot shower.

- Make every day count. Do something that makes you happy every day. It doesn't have to be something big. Go for a walk. Listen to music. Do something kind for a stranger. It can be as easy as opening a door, helping someone cross a street, or telling them they have a nice smile.

- Make a list of the things that make you happy. Then, make time each day to do at least one thing on your list. A friend of mine with depression made strips of paper and wrote on each strip one thing she could do at any time that makes her happy (e.g., eat a scoop of ice cream, go for a walk, listen to music). She put the strips of paper in a jar. When she feels overwhelmed, she dips her hand into the jar and does what the paper tells her to do.

- Keep a journal of the things that make you feel grateful or happy.

- Take care of yourself. Make sure you get at least eight hours of sleep each night. Eat a healthy diet. Practice stress management and relaxation techniques such as yoga, meditation, guided imagery, deep breathing, or prayer. Treat yourself to a favorite treat.

- Be practical. Don't ignore problems that come up. Figure out what needs to be done, develop a plan, and act. Don't be afraid to ask friends and family to help you find a doctor or get to an appointment.

- Never lose hope. Focus on positive things. Think about things you can look forward to. It doesn't have to be something big or expensive. Plant some flowers. Buy a ticket to an upcoming concert or sports event. Make plans to visit someone you haven't seen for a while. Do something new—start a hobby; learn a language.

What Families Can Do to Help
a Person in Recovery

While clinical recovery and personal recovery are primarily individual processes, social relationships are integral to both.
Relationships with family and friends—at the heart of most
people's social worlds—are especially important to people with
serious mental illnesses. Families often provide economic support, emotional support, and help with medication compliance.
They can provide important information to the health care
team about the patient's past. Families can help people sustain
meaningful connections, providing identity and hope. The en-
couragement Pat Deegan's grandmother gave Pat with the daily
invitation to join her in a trip to the grocery store launched Pat's
recovery. Over the course of their illnesses, Joe's, Michelle's, and
Sharon's families have supported and nurtured them. Joe and
Michelle both attribute much of their success and recovery to
their spouses. Joe has been married to Molly for forty-four years.
Michelle and Tim have been married for forty-one years. For
Michelle, staying symptom-free has also been motivated by her
love for her children and grandchildren. Sharon attributes the
love and support from her sisters and her daughter to her
recovery.

How can families support a person in recovery?

First, it is important to acknowledge that recovery is a process. Because every person in recovery is different, families
must be aware of the unique concerns of their loved one. For
example, more than anything, Michelle was motivated to help
her children. When her daughter's marriage crumbled and Michelle began planning to drive across several states to help
care for her granddaughter, Michelle's husband, Tim, did not
think that this was a good idea. He worried that the stress of the
trip would reignite the symptoms of Michelle's bipolar disorder.
But Tim supported Michelle's decision. He talked with Michelle

each night, and then, when he was able to take time off work, Tim joined Michelle.

Second, family members must realize that, while they can offer support and encourage the person with mental illness, they cannot make treatment decisions for that person. For example, even though Joe's wife, Molly, wanted him to go to the hospital when his thinking became psychotic, she supported Joe's decision to increase his medications and see his doctor more often. Making this distinction creates a respectful, healing environment within the family.

Third, it is important to remember that a person in recovery continues to struggle with a serious illness. When people with mental illness seem to be acting difficult or making bad decisions intentionally, it is important to give them the benefit of the doubt. Remember, no one wants to experience the hallucinations, delusions, and depression caused by serious mental illnesses.

Finally, it is critical that family members maintain their own mental and physical health. Just as flight attendants remind us to put on our own oxygen masks before attending to others, so too must family members take care of themselves so that they can attend to the needs of others. For example, although Sharon's sister often helped her, there were times when she needed a break, and so she asked other people—her husband, her son, and her daughter—to pitch in.

Here is some advice that may be helpful for families of people in recovery:

- Encourage family cooperation. Assign everyone in the household (including the person with mental illness) roles according to their abilities. For example, if your person in recovery is a good cook, ask him to take responsibility for planning and cooking dinner a couple of times a week.

- Pick your battles. Listen carefully and try to avoid unnecessary arguments. Helping a person stick to a medication plan is important, but fighting about medications is usually counterproductive. Be a partner, not a nag.
- Establish normal routines. Spend time together engaging in activities unconnected to the illness, such as watching a movie or going out for dinner. Learn to live with a mental illness rather than fight it.
- Acknowledge small steps toward recovery. For example, if the person in recovery says she wants to take an art class at the community college but doesn't know how to enroll, tell her that you're proud of her for wanting to take this step and then help her enroll.
- Don't give up. When setbacks occur, as they surely will, try something new.

Family Experiences and Recovery

People with mental illnesses aren't the only ones whose lives are changed when illness strikes. The onset of a serious mental illness can be traumatic to family members who loved the person with mental illness long before the illness made itself known. Over time, as families must bend and adapt to the challenges of serious mental illness, the lives of parents, siblings, spouses, and children are changed. A vast amount of research documents the burden that family members experience when a loved one has a serious mental illness and demonstrates how caregiving burden can lead to physical illnesses and poor quality of life for family members. Parents often provide decades of extended care to their adult son or daughter with serious mental illness, all while the child's debilitating symptoms produce obstacles to his or her ability to work, marry, and function independently. Providing this care can lead to poorer physical and mental health, increased rates of marital disruption, and lower levels of work satisfaction.

For at least a half century, we have known that mental illness in parents is sometimes associated with psychiatric disturbances in their children—effects that last well into the children's middle-age years. Children having a parent with a serious mental illness are more likely to develop psychotic illnesses of their own, have emotional and behavioral problems, and suffer personality disorders, cognitive dysfunction, and feelings of social inadequacy than children whose parents do not have a mental illness. Adult children of parents with schizophrenia often have social adjustment problems affecting their abilities to work and sustain a marriage.

Similarly, siblings of people with serious mental illness have a tendency to be more depressed and experience poorer overall psychological well-being than other people—effects that often are lifelong. One study found that people who grew up with a brother or sister with schizophrenia, bipolar disorder, or depression completed fewer years of education and were less likely to be employed in the early years of midlife than their counterparts who did not have a sibling with mental illness.

A *Modern Love* column by Mark Lukach describes how he was affected by the psychotic break his wife, Giulia, suffered when they were both 27 years old and in their third year of marriage. Giulia had no history of mental illness. What began as mild depression and sleeplessness led Giulia to believe that voices were speaking to her in the night. She also experienced delusions and paranoia.

As her spouse, Mark found that his biggest struggle was keeping his own emotions in check. Mark is not alone. Research finds that spouses of depressed and mentally ill people experience higher levels of anxiety and depression and lower levels of subjective well-being compared with other people.

What can spouses do? Mark made sure Giulia took her medicine. When Giulia said she wanted to die, Mark told her how much he loved her. He held her when she sobbed. He pleaded with her to hang on. As Giulia's spouse, Mark had to learn to manage his own feelings. He was scared and worried, but he did not let Giulia know. Mark learned to compartmentalize his worry and anxiety. He cried when Giulia was not in the room. But Mark also realized that, although Giulia's illness exhausted him, it had also made him feel closer to her.

Families of people who have a relapsing or episodic illness are strained by the transitions between acute illness periods and the ongoing uncertainty about when the next episode might occur. As such, one of the greatest challenges these family members face is adaptation to shifting needs and priorities. What might be important to their loved one with mental illness when he or she is symptomatic often becomes unimportant at other times. Families must learn to shift adeptly from providing care to the person to encouraging autonomy and reciprocity. When Giulia was suicidal, she and Mark washed the dinner dishes together. Mark never wanted to leave her alone. When Giulia was well, they reverted to squabbles that most newlyweds have about household responsibilities.

Families also must learn that support is not one-directional. People with mental illness can provide as well as receive support. For example, as parents age and can no longer drive at night or shop for groceries, their adult children with mental illness may be able to help with these tasks. For many, recovery means assuming intimate family roles, including marriage and parenting. For others, it means reestablishing family relationships that may have deteriorated when the person was unwell. These challenges are difficult, but learning about mental illnesses and how to manage them can help.

Just as people with serious mental illness can experience recovery, so too can family members experience recovery. The first step toward recovery for a family member is to acknowledge the illness and the toll it has taken. Accepting the loss and realizing that the life envisioned may not play out can be a difficult and painful process. Recovery is acknowledging and accepting that attitudes, feelings, and personal relationships have been altered by the family member's mental illness and that, despite the pain, there is hope for the future. Sometimes, as the person with mental illness recovers, so too does the family. This was the case for Mark and Giulia. Other times, even though the person with mental illness does not recover, family members can recover. In my case, I continue to work toward accepting that my daughter Sophie will not become the artist or neuroscientist I had hoped she would be. She will not marry a lawyer, a doctor, or an engineer, as I had hoped she would. She will not have the big fancy wedding I wanted for her. Because Sophie's mental illness has strained our relationship, I will not have the relationship with Sophie's children that many of my friends have with their grandchildren. But my life goes on. I have a strong marriage and a son whom I adore. I have a successful career. I have friends and family whom I love and who love me. While I miss Sophie terribly, I comfort myself knowing that I have done all I can for her, that there is nothing more I can do.

Like patient recovery, family recovery is rarely a linear process. Because family recovery is vulnerable to changes in the person with mental illness, it includes many cycles of despair and hopefulness. Recovery requires a long-term perspective, as it is a process that is often filled with the pain of one stressful event and disappointment after another. Acceptance of the loss is made even more difficult by the cyclical nature of serious mental illnesses. Each time Sophie commits to taking her medicines and seems to be conquering her illness, I support her efforts. I think that maybe this time Sophie will stay on the medications that she needs. Maybe she will go to college. Maybe.

But then the emotional roller coaster crests, gravity takes hold, and down we go. Again. She stops taking her medicine. She goes back to the street drugs. There have been years when I have not even known whether Sophie was alive or dead.

Not surprisingly, each family member recovers at his or her own rate and in his or her own way. A mother's experience is different from a father's experience. A parent's experience differs from a sibling's experience. A younger sibling's experience differs from an older sibling's experience. Because family members recover at different rates, they are likely to be in different phases of recovery at any given time. Communication among family members can help each be aware of where they are in the recovery process so they can be empathic and helpful to one another. Family recovery means dealing with pain yet living a life that includes hope, meaning, intimate connections with others, and goals for the future. NAMI and SARDAA (the Schizophrenia and Related Disorders Alliance of America) offer in-person and online support programs for family members.

What Communities Can Do to Promote Recovery

Just as people with serious mental illness recover within families, so too do they recover within communities. Yet, in most communities in the United States, stigma about mental illnesses, bureaucratic rules and regulations, and the presumption that people will follow predetermined pathways and time frames make recovery difficult, if not impossible. What can communities do to encourage recovery? One strategy can be learned from Geel, Belgium, the oldest therapeutic community in the world. A different approach is modeled by Trieste, Italy, designated by the World Health Organization as the most progressive place on the globe when it comes to caring for people with serious mental illness.

The Role of Community: Geel, Belgium

For seven hundred years, the people of Geel have welcomed strangers with serious mental illnesses into their homes. Geel's tradition hails from the legend of Dymphna, a seventh-century Irish princess who, threatened with rape by her delusional father, King Damon, fled to the forests outside Geel. In a murderous rage, Damon pursued and captured Dymphna. When Dymphna refused to submit to Damon's demands, Damon beheaded Dymphna. Dymphna's resistance to the deranged king made people believe that she could help others fight their "possessions." Pilgrims flocked to Dymphna's tomb to pray for her to intercede and end their suffering. Stories of miraculous cures grew, and the townspeople built a small church honoring her as the influx of pilgrims continued. In 1247, Dymphna was canonized as the patron saint of the mentally ill.

By the fourteenth century, the church in Geel offered a nine-day religious treatment promising to relieve mental illnesses, which were believed to be the result of the devil's work. As stories of wondrous cures continued, the church became such a popular destination that the people of Geel built a larger church—St. Dymphna's Church. In 1480, a small hospice providing shelter to pilgrims was added to the side of the church, providing shelter to people who were required to stay in the church during the nine-day treatment period. Yet the building still overflowed with pilgrims. At the request of the church, citizens of Geel and farmers from the surrounding villages offered housing to pilgrims waiting their turn for treatment. Sometimes, however, families returned home after the religious rituals failed, abandoning their ill relatives in Geel. The people of Geel opened their homes to these pilgrims as well, offering housing and food in exchange for work on the farms. Farmers called the people "guests" or "boarders." In this way, people with mental illness became integrated into the community, rather than secluded from it. Over time, these spontaneous, pragmatic acts evolved into a community tradition of integrated, community residential care.

The tradition begun in Geel survived and developed into the core of Belgium's mental health care system. In the fifteenth century, informal arrangements were made between a villager and either the ill person's family or the church. Over time, authority and supervision of the system moved to the Geel Municipal Council (1838) and then to the Belgian government (1850). Between 1855 and 1938, the Family Care Program in Geel grew from nearly 800 boarders to its height of 3,800 boarders. During and after World War II, the number of people in the Family Care Program declined, falling to 2,600 in 1944. In 1991, Openbaar Psychiatrisch Zorgcentrum (OPZ), the supervising central hospital in Geel, took control of the mental health system in Geel, where the Family Care Program remains an integral part, although the number of boarders has continued to shrink. In 2000, there were 550 boarders, and by 2006, there were 460. In addition to the Family Foster Care program, OPZ has a 285-bed hospital, an outpatient clinic, and mobile health care teams. New patients are evaluated in the hospital and then carefully matched with families.

Today, just as when it began, the mission of the Family Foster Care program is treating people with mental illness as respected family members. Many of Geel's 40,000 residents provide boarders with a safe place to live. The host families integrate the boarders into their households and local community by building on the strengths of each boarder. Some of the boarders provide childcare, while others help with household chores. Boarders become valued members of the household. Respect for people is an essential aspect of the recovery process. As such, foster families usually are not told the boarder's diagnosis. The responsibilities of the foster families and the psychiatric team are clearly defined. Foster families focus on the practical aspects of daily life. The psychiatric team focuses on treatment and helps the families identify strategies to respond to problematic behaviors.

Many host families have two and sometimes three boarders at a time. It is not uncommon for boarders to live with a family for decades. Sometimes when the host becomes too old or dies, the boarder continues to live with the host family's children. Just as their grandparents and parents took in boarders, so too does the current generation. Psychosocial rehabilitation, hospital services, and drug treatment are integrated with family care.

Over the years, some have questioned the wisdom and humanity of Geel's solution. Although the practice of exchanging work on the farms for shelter benefitted most hosts and boarders, there were times when boarders were subjected to abuse. In the fifteenth century, when the townspeople of Geel began welcoming boarders into their homes, Belgian law dictated that if a boarder committed a crime, it was the host family's fault. To avoid stiff fines, some families kept particularly difficult boarders chained or restrained. More recently, social workers have questioned the wisdom of not providing formal training and education about mental illness to the host families and not telling the host families about the diagnoses of their boarders. Further, some physicians have doubted Geel's practice of not medicating all of the boarders.

Yet, in many respects, the Geel model has been successful. Medication compliance is the norm. Many boarders receive long-acting injections of psychotropic medications from the OPZ. In other cases, foster families, instructed by their district nurse, administer medication to their boarders. Although community care for people with serious mental illness began in Geel as a result of an act of violence attributed to King Damon's madness, for the most part Geel's boarders have lived in this peaceful community for centuries. Today, people who have exhibited violent behavior typically are excluded from the Geel program. However, exceptions have been made, and some people who had been violent in other communities have ceased to be violent while living in Geel. If a boarder in Geel's Family Foster Care program becomes agitated or aggressive, the host family will attempt to calm the boarder. Most times they are successful. However, if needed, host families can call the hospital or their district nurse. The OPZ includes physicians, psychologists, social workers, and psychiatrists. Hospitalization is available when needed. Once the person is stabilized, a decision is made about whether the boarder can return to the host family.

I wondered about the Geel model and what lessons we Americans might learn from it. And so, when I was invited to a meeting in Amsterdam in the spring of 2019, my husband and I rented a car and made the two-hour drive to Geel. We found our way to the market square and a café where a waiter who spoke little English helped us order from the Belgian menu. Given the proximity of the café to the OPZ, I knew it was likely that some of the people whom I saw from the café window were boarders. However, I could not tell a boarder from anyone else. Unlike in most American cities, there were no beggars, no disoriented people, and no one sleeping on the sidewalks.

That afternoon we met with Michelle Lambrechts, the social worker on the multidisciplinary team responsible for the Foster Family Care program. She told us that there were only 184 boarders in the program, 60 percent men, 40 percent women. I was surprised to hear that the program had gotten so much smaller than it had been in 2006, and I asked Ms. Lambrechts why that was. She said that the answer is complicated. First, she said, the structure of Geel's families has changed. In Geel, as in the United States, it is common for both husbands and wives to work outside the home. That often means that no one is home to look after the boarders during the day. Second, veteran host families were aging and fewer new families were applying to be hosts. Further, as Geel no longer is the agrarian society it once was, the need for a helping hand on the farm was virtually non-existent. Improved psychotropic medication also has made it less necessary for people with serious mental illness to need supported living, and so fewer people were applying to be boarders. Finally, the program lacks funding. The Belgian government pays 50 euros (approximately $60) per boarder per day to support the practice, with a fraction of that paid to the foster family to cover the boarder's living expenses. Nonetheless, Ms. Lambrechts said that she believes that the Family Foster Care program will continue to be an important part of the way Geel cares for people with mental illness because that is what the people of Geel have always done.

Eager to better understand Geel's Family Foster Care system, I asked Ms. Lambrechts if she would introduce me to one of the host families. I wanted to learn why a family would agree to open its home and provide care to a stranger who is likely depressed or delusional—a person whose behavior could be unpredictable—and I wanted to understand why a family would continue to provide this care for years. Ms. Lambrechts introduced me to Toni Smit.

Toni is 71 years old. She has been married three times and has two grown sons. Toni's paid jobs over the years have varied. She has been a nurse and an orthopedic pedicurist. She worked in sales, where two hundred people once reported to her. Toni, her son, and her husband, Arthur, owned and operated a restaurant. Now retired, Toni teaches cooking classes, reads, gardens, embroiders, and vacations.

But in talking with Toni, it was clear to me that she is most proud of the help she has provided to people during the past several decades. Toni knew she loved helping people when, at age 20, she found joy in helping her fiancé, a psychiatric nurse, plan parties and outings for his mentally ill patients. When her brother-in-law was injured in an accident, Toni helped him. Then, when her son fell sixty-six feet from a scaffold while at work and suffered serious mental and physical injuries, Toni took a five-year absence from work, and she continued to care for him for more than fifteen years. Toni wondered what might have happened to her son if she or another family member had not been able to care for him.

Toni began taking boarders into her home long before she ever heard of Geel and its tradition. When her sister-in-law died and her brother was unable to take care of their 2-year-old daughter, Linda, Toni took Linda in and provided care to her for twenty-four years—until Linda married. Then, Toni and her husband took in two teenaged brothers left homeless after their parents divorced.

Toni first learned about OPZ and the Family Foster Care program twenty-five years ago, when she and Arthur moved to Geel. Toni's neighbors were both host families. When the neighbor's boarder got into trouble and was removed from the program, Toni and Arthur took the young man in and provided a home for him for seven years. Toni and Arthur's second OPZ boarder lived with them for about three years. The boarder was severely depressed, so Toni and Arthur spent many long nights talking with the man, trying to help him. Each night, the man would promise to follow through on suggestions Arthur and Toni made, but the next day he could not even get out of bed. Eventually, the man developed the skills he needed to live on his own, and the OPZ helped him move into his own apartment. Shortly after this man left, the OPZ social worker called Toni and told her they had a 79-year-old man named Dis whom they wanted to place. It has always been difficult for OPZ to place older boarders. Dis lived with Toni and Arthur until he was 91 and needed nursing home care.

About fourteen years ago, while Dis was still living with Toni and Arthur, their current boarder, Luc, moved in. Now 55 years old, Luc is their sole boarder. Toni recalled how nervous Luc had been when they first met. "He was in constant motion. He was constantly playing with his fingers, as though he were checking to make sure they were all still there. He walked around the block several times a day." Prior to living with Arthur and Toni, Luc had lived in an institution. Luc has calmed down, and the nervous behaviors have subsided. Luc fits right into their family. He helps in the yard and in the house. He takes the garbage out. He walks the dog. As Toni and I were talking, Luc came into the room and gave Toni a hug. It was clear how much he enjoys living with Arthur and Toni and how much Toni and Arthur love Luc.

It has not always been easy for Toni and Arthur. Some of their boarders presented daunting challenges. One boarder locked Toni and Arthur out of the bathroom for hours as he furiously washed his hands. Another screamed at night, imagining lions coming out of the walls. Another believed he was in love with Toni. Together, Toni and Arthur came up with strategies that enabled them to manage the odd behaviors while helping their boarders.

Could a program like Geel's work in America? I wondered what it would take for Americans to agree to share their home with a mentally ill stranger. Was there something unique to people who lived in Geel or something about Geel's history that made people so giving and willing to help? I posed the question to Toni. She smiled. "Of course, it could work. Americans are just as capable as people in Geel of caring for other people. There are plenty of good people willing to help others," Toni said. Then, she surprised me and said that she had been born in Salt Lake City, Utah, and had spent the first fifteen years of her life there and in Parchment, Michigan, a small town just two hours from Detroit, where I grew up. "But for a program like this to work in America, Americans would have to figure out how to pay for it. That has been a struggle, even in Geel."

As we were ending our time together, I thought about how kind Toni and Arthur were to have helped so many people by bringing them into their home and treating them like family. With both of them now retired, I wondered how much longer they would want to take in boarders. Before I could ask Toni about their plans, she said, "We haven't told the OPZ yet, but Arthur and I have been talking about taking in another boarder."

The Role of Community: Trieste, Italy

According to the World Health Organization, the "Trieste model" of helping people with serious mental illness is the most progressive in the world. The model puts the person with mental illness—not the disorder—at the center of the health care system. Launched in the 1970s, the model was spearheaded by Franco Basaglia, a charismatic psychiatrist who had directed three psychiatric asylums. Sickened by a morally bankrupt system that had few benefits for the patients, Basaglia abandoned the prevailing belief about keeping people with mental illness secluded from others. Walking the streets of Trieste, a seaport city in northeastern Italy, Basaglia developed the idea that even people with the most serious mental illnesses could live a normal life if their community could learn to accommodate them. Social inclusion, not exclusion, became his goal.

During a time when asylums were closing worldwide, Basaglia became responsible for closing the Trieste asylum and replacing it with a novel community mental health system. Under Basaglia's direction, resources were transferred to a new community system of care. This process culminated in the passage of Law 180 in Italy in 1978, innovative legislation that led to the final closure of all asylums in Italy. Law 180 mandated the creation and public funding of community-based therapeutic alternatives and affordable living arrangements that sought to restore the human, civil, and social rights of people with serious mental illness. Central to the Trieste model were "life projects"—connections between people with mental illness and their care providers that ensure access to housing, jobs, and community interaction—as strategies for fostering the engagement of people with mental illness in community life. Through these life projects, people with mental illness and their care providers plan the unfolding of relationships and resources over the course of the person's entire life, shifting attention from symptoms and bare survival to long-term social integration of the person in the community. Essential to the success of life projects is the availability of resources, including affordable housing, health care services, and employment opportunities.

Today in Trieste, a city of 240,000 people, the model Basaglia envisioned exists. The Department of Mental Health employs 207 mental health workers, including psychiatrists, nurses, psychologists, social workers, rehabilitation specialists, and nursing aides. At the core of Trieste's model is a network of four community mental health centers (CMHCs) operating twenty-four hours a day, seven days a week. Each CMHC is run by a team composed of approximately thirty nurses, two social workers, two psychologists, two rehabilitation specialists, and four to five psychiatrists, serving a catchment area of between 50,000 and 65,000 people. Each CMHC directly responds to the full range of psychiatric needs in its catchment area. Acute situations are managed with a view toward prevention, treatment, and rehabilitation. The CMHCs are located in nonhospital residential facilities, usually a two or three-story house, and include four to eight beds used for those needing inpatient care. The homelike quality of their environment is consistent with staff attitudes that mainly focus on flexibility and reasonable negotiation with users according to their needs. A single multidisciplinary team rotates twenty-four hours a day, covering all functions, from care of people admitted to beds to outpatient and outreach activities. People using the CMHCs are considered "guests" rather than "patients" and can receive visits without restrictions. If a guest chooses to leave, a staff member will follow him or her to ensure that needed help is provided. CMHC guests are encouraged to continue ordinary life activities if they are able. CMHCs provide walk-in services without waiting lists, and they typically meet requests within an hour or two. People in crisis or with acute psychiatric conditions sleep in the CMHC facilities rather than in the hospital. Once a guest's condition improves, care is provided at home or at a community center.

The community centers epitomize the Basaglian philosophy in design, location, and services provided. The Barcola Mental Health Center, for example, is located in an elegant villa surrounded by a manicured garden facing the Adriatic Sea. Its outside walls are painted bright yellow, and a rectangle of rosemary, lavender, and big pink daisies shields the front entrance veranda. Nearby trails lead to the beach or to a pinewoods park. Inside, the first floor has a reception area, office, pharmacy, and large meeting room. The interior of the building is well lit and welcoming, with bright colors, interesting shapes, and a wooden floor.

Supporting the CMHCs is a six-bed psychiatric unit housed within the community's general hospital (used mainly for emergencies at night), a network of group homes, and two day care centers. The CMHCs are also supported by staff from the rehabilitation and residential support service. The center manages forty-five beds in group homes operated by nongovernment organizations. The aim of this service is to encourage people to move toward independent living. Staff help people search for a home. Once one is found, staff introduce the person to their new community and help them integrate into the community by encouraging participation in soccer tournaments, literary and philosophical conversations, bands, and theatrical productions. Another key component of the Trieste model is on-the-job training for staff.

Bascaglia's belief that people with serious mental illness should be fully integrated into the community led the Trieste

Mental Health Department to develop ways to help people manage small businesses and participate in paid employment too. Tax exemptions in Italy are provided for businesses employing people with mental illness. Today, the Tritone Hotel overlooking the sea is managed and operated by people using the services of the Trieste Mental Health Department. Il Posto della Fragole (Strawberry Fields Café) is a busy restaurant managed by users of mental health services. In Trieste, the cafes at the opera house, public radio station, a historic bathhouse, all museums, and public gardens employ people using mental health services.

Resources that once funded institutional care now are used to help people secure housing and jobs and provide subsidies that empower people to live in the community. The allocation of funds by the Trieste Mental Health Department reflects its commitment to providing services in the community. In 2012, 20 percent of the 18 million euros (approximately $21 million) spent by the department were payments to service users in the form of job grants and economic subsidies, as well as payments for group activities, trips, and personalized health care budgets. On average, 180 clients each year receive professional training supported by work grants, and 13 percent of these clients move into nonsubsidized jobs. Additionally, approximately 160 clients each year receive a personal health care budget to cover support services for their "life projects," including housing, work, and relationship building. Only 6 percent of the overall budget was spent on inpatient services, and 6 percent on pharmaceuticals. The remaining funds finance community-based services.

In 2012, Trieste had more than four thousand users of its psychiatric services. Every patient matters. People are not left to fend for themselves. The system is patient based, not bureaucracy driven. People are treated as full-fledged members of the community, with their individual needs identified and addressed. Most crises are handled by the CMHCs. Today, when someone in Trieste has a psychotic episode, a mental health team responds. The police are not involved. Moreover, a team that is familiar to the person in crisis will often spend hours working to diffuse the situation. Readmission rates are low, and involuntary commitments are rare. Neither physical nor chemical restraints are used. None of the clients become homeless because the CMHCs have the capacity to function as shelters until other accommodations can be found. Compliance with antipsychotic medication is high, a situation attributed to the quality of therapeutic relationships. People with mental illness are not in jail. A suicide prevention project has contributed to reducing the suicide rate by half (from 25 to 12 per 1,000,000) over the past twenty years.

The success of the Trieste model is clear. It is especially impressive, standing in sharp contrast to the experience elsewhere in Italy. Although Law 180 applied to all of Italy and it was Basaglia's intention to create a nationwide system of CMHCs, the rest of Italy did not benefit as much as Trieste. Several reasons have been suggested. First, Basaglia's sudden death at age 56 in 1978 left the movement without a leader. What Basaglia had started in Trieste did not have the momentum to progress to the rest of Italy. Second, lacking a national budget to implement the law, each of Italy's twenty-one regions was faced with the challenge of executing the law without the funding needed. And third, care providers throughout much of Italy were uncomfortable providing services outside the institution.

Could the Trieste model work in an American city? Most likely not. In most American cities, the majority of people with serious mental illness depend on the public mental health system. The social safety net is thin, and economic resources are limited. Without adequate housing, health care, and finances, people are doomed to live in poverty. Unlike in Trieste, family members in the United States are often geographically dispersed, limiting their ability to provide help. Drugs are rampant in many American cities, exacerbating problems associated with mental illness. While services for people with serious mental illness exist in many American cities, the public mental health system has not been able to keep pace with the demand. Unlike in Trieste, where services follow patients, in the United States resources generally do not follow patients from the mental hospitals into the community. As such, many formerly hospitalized patients end up without services.

In sum, the combination of a large number of mentally ill people, the lack of affordable housing, the drug epidemic, the thinness of the social safety net, the dearth of affordable housing, and a relatively loose family structure have led to a virtual abandonment of many people with serious mental illness in America. Although many people with mental illness are cared for and supported by state-of-the-art case management programs, many others are treated by overworked staff who can barely manage to control patients' acute and chronic symptoms, much less help people develop life projects, attend to their social needs, or help integrate them into the community. However, the Trieste model is inspiring. It demonstrates what people with mental illness are capable of accomplishing when they are provided with services and not robbed of their economic, social, political, and civil rights.

The Role of Community: The United States

During the past several decades, there have been many attempts to reform the mental health system in the United States. While these reforms have much in common with those of Trieste and Geel, they developed independently and have uniquely American wellsprings. In 1913, Will and Agnes Gould established Gould Farm in the Berkshires of Massachusetts. They welcomed guests experiencing emotional and psychiatric problems to work on their farm and share the joys and challenges of daily life. In 1948, thirty years before Law 180 was passed in Italy, Fountain House, the first Clubhouse model of care, opened in New York. The Clubhouse model centers on supportive vocational services, socialization, member empowerment, and inclusion in the life of the community. Clubhouses offer people living with mental illnesses opportunities for friendship, employment, housing, education, and access to medical and psychiatric services in a single, caring, and safe environment. There are now over three hundred local Clubhouses in more than thirty countries around the world. A directory of Clubhouses can be found on the Clubhouse International website.

Soteria, yet another model that developed in the United States, had great promise to help people with serious mental illness. The story of Soteria is entwined with that of its creator, Loren Mosher, MD. Mosher cared deeply about people with schizophrenia, and research indicates that the program he developed was effective for people newly diagnosed with schizophrenia. However, Soteria suffered from two problems. First, the program encouraged minimal use of medication, which was misinterpreted as eschewing medication, threatening the medical model dominating Mosher's day and leading to Mosher's downfall. Then, when Soteria was launched and operated as an anti-medication program, tragedy followed, virtually ending Soteria in the United States. Let's take a look at Loren Mosher, the program he developed, and what happened.

Before even beginning as a Stanford University undergraduate in 1952, Mosher knew he wanted to become a doctor. In his second year of medical school, Mosher developed "medical school hypochondriasis" and spent a year in psychotherapy, where he experienced firsthand the healing possibilities of a caring, human relationship. He gravitated to psychiatry's humanistic orientation, a strong contrast to the technological, mechanized aspects of other medical specialties, and earned his medical degree at Harvard University.

Mosher's mentor during his psychiatric residency at the Massachusetts Mental Health Center, Elvin Semrad, instructed him not to "treat" or "cure" his patients, but to sit with them and learn about their lives. Mosher came to appreciate people with schizophrenia as people with serious problems. He learned to treat them with dignity and respect and to see things as his patients saw them. Mosher continued his residency at the National Institute of Mental Health, where he studied identical twins, one with schizophrenia and the other without the psychotic disorder, and he learned that genes alone could not explain the onset of schizophrenia. Mosher completed his medical training in 1966 with a year of study at the Tavistock Clinic in London, where he saw firsthand how Kingsley Hall, the small therapeutic community established by R. D. Laing, benefitted people with schizophrenia.

By the end of his residency, Mosher knew both that human relationships could be therapeutic for people with schizophrenia and that hospitals are not good places for people with schizophrenia. After a year on the faculty at Yale University, Mosher knew that his philosophy about how best to help people with schizophrenia differed from that of his supervisors, who believed that antipsychotic drugs were psychiatry's only useful treatment.

In 1968, Mosher returned to the NIMH, where he became the first chief of the Center for Studies of Schizophrenia. There, Mosher designed Soteria, which is the Greek word for "deliverance." The following year, Mosher became the first editor in chief of *Schizophrenia Bulletin*, a position he held for ten years.

Soteria opened for business in 1971, targeted toward patients with newly diagnosed schizophrenia. The program operated in a vintage 1915 twelve-room house in the San Francisco Bay Area that accommodated six patients at a time. There were six paid staff members, including the project director, who acts as friend, counselor, and supervisor to the staff. A quarter-time psychiatrist supervised the staff. Staff were trained not as therapists but as facilitators of patient healing. They were taught to "be with," "put their feet in the other person's shoes," and "stand by attentively"—in other words, to actively engage in empathic relationships with the patients, just like Mosher had been taught in Massachusetts and just like staff at Kingsley Hall interacted with its patients. Staff were responsible for preventing patients from hurting themselves or others. Two of the specially trained nonprofessional staff were on duty at any one time. Volunteers often helped out in the evenings. Staff and patients (to the extent that they were able) shared responsibility for the maintenance of the house, preparation of meals, and cleanup. Organized structure was minimal; meal preparation was planned and tasks assigned at the beginning of each week. Patients and staff ate together each evening and participated in a two-hour meeting each Friday. Patients were encouraged to pursue activities they enjoy, including painting, yoga, and reading.

The first Soteria research study also began in 1971. Patients meeting eligibility criteria were assigned on a consecutively admitted, space-available basis to either Soteria or usual care (the ward of the CMHC). Six-month and one-year outcome data revealed that both groups decreased in levels of psychopathology over time.

Although the study included only seventy-nine people, Soteria patients consistently fared better than the hospitalized patients. They had better overall psychological health at discharge, six months post-discharge, and one year after admission. At both six and twelve months post-discharge, the Soteria patients were more likely to hold a job and more likely to be living independently or with their peers than the hospitalized patients. A second study included one hundred people who were randomly assigned to either Soteria or usual care and followed for two years. Together, these studies found that two years after the experiment Soteria patients were better adjusted, experienced lower levels of psychopathology, and had fewer hospital admissions than patients in the usual care group. More recently, a systematic review of these studies and similar research in Switzerland concluded that Soteria was at least as effective as traditional hospital-based treatment.

Soteria patients, like the Kingsley Hall patients in London, were given neuroleptic drugs when they needed them. In his book *Soteria: Through Madness to Deliverance*, Mosher says, "I neither prescribed nor avoided neuroleptics across the board. When they looked helpful, I suggested them. If they seemed to be working, I continued them under careful scrutiny. And when the benefits—as often—did not seem to outweigh the risks, I avoided them." Antipsychotic medications were ordinarily not used during the first six weeks of treatment, yet there were explicit criteria for their short-term use; 24 percent of Soteria patients received medications during their initial forty-five-day period.

Although Mosher held a lofty position at the NIMH, his reluctance to embrace the philosophy of the day—that psychotropic medications should be the first and only line of defense against serious mental illness—got him in trouble. He lost his job and lost control of Soteria.

Without its primary champion, Soteria lost sight of both its primary target (people with newly diagnosed schizophrenia) and its fundamental principle (to use medication sparingly). In Anchorage, Alaska, for example, Soteria did not attract newly diagnosed patients with schizophrenia but rather people with chronic schizophrenia. Medications were avoided. In 2011, Michael McEvoy, an unmedicated 21-year-old man with schizophrenic delusions, shot and killed 19-year-old Mozelle Nalan, another Soteria patient whom McEvoy thought was a dragon.

Soteria should have had a different future. The program worked. Whether Soteria's downfall was due to a benign misunderstanding or a malevolent rejection is debatable. But

Mosher's Soteria included both a caring environment and medications. Shortly before he died, Mosher made a last attempt to clarify his perspective. He said, "Today, my position is that, since no real alternatives to antipsychotic drugs are currently available, to be totally against them is untenable. Thus, for seriously disturbed people, I occasionally recommend them—as part of collaborative planning with my client—but in the lowest dosage and for the shortest length of time possible."

People with serious mental illness are no longer relegated to the doomed life described by Emil Kraepelin. There are plenty of role models—ordinary people like Joe, Sharon, and Michelle, who have learned to live with schizophrenia, depression, and bipolar disorder and now show others that it is possible to live, work, love, and be loved despite their illness. Medications and therapy can help ease the worst of the symptoms. Families and communities can provide support. Places like Geel and Trieste show what is possible. Living with serious mental illness is by no means easy, but research over the past several decades has identified strategies that can ease the pain and enable people to thrive.

Epilogue

December 2012

"What is the blessing you would like to have?" asked the scribe, entering a letter on the Torah in the small synagogue atop Masada, a rugged natural fortress overlooking Israel's Dead Sea.

He put down his quill and looked at my husband, Josh. I held my breath. Josh is not a religious guy.

The scribe had just told us that there are 304,805 letters in a Torah. If a single letter is missing, the Torah cannot be used in a synagogue.

"Talk about stressful jobs," I'd said.

"I want my new real estate business to be successful," Josh said. "I started the business when I lost my corporate job. So many people in the United States have lost their jobs and I want to help them keep their homes in these difficult times." As Josh spoke about the economic recession and foreclosures, I snapped one picture after the next. Our 16-year-old son Aaron rolled his eyes. My friend Susan jockeyed positions so she could capture the moment on her iPad.

"You have kind thoughts and righteous understanding." The scribe stroked his salt-and-pepper beard and turned back to the Torah scroll. He uttered a blessing and penned a letter for Josh. "You will do well," he proclaimed.

Looking up, the scribe adjusted his glasses. He turned to me and asked, "Do you know why you cannot use the Torah in a synagogue if one letter is missing?"

"Because it would say the wrong thing?" I guessed.

"Yes, but there's a different reason," the scribe said. "Every letter in the Torah represents a general soul which divides into the individual sparks that become each of our souls. The Torah's message is to unite all the people together under God in love and peace. If one letter is missing, it's like one person is missing."

I thought about the missing person in my life.

"I would like to give you a blessing as well. What is your name?" Following Jewish tradition, I said, "Rachel, daughter of Abraham and Zahava."

"You can have any kind of blessing that you would like to have." Picking up his quill, the scribe asked, "What is the blessing you would like to have?"

Tears clouded my eyes. Susan patted my back and handed me a tissue. The scribe looked at me, then at Josh, wondering what had caused such pain. As I wept, Josh explained that our adopted daughter Sophie suffers from serious mental illness and that we hadn't seen her for two years.

The scribe kept his eyes fixed on Josh. He asked our daughter's age, whether she was alone, and how long she had been part of our family. Then he dipped his quill in the black liquid and calmly penned a letter onto the Torah parchment for me. A group of chattering tourists silenced their voices as they entered the room.

The scribe turned back to his desk and wrote a message on a small note card. Handing me the note, he said, "Keep this until your daughter returns. And then, on the day she comes home, give it to her as a gift."

"I will," I promised.

July 2021

I still have the note.

ACKNOWLEDGMENTS

The impetus for this book was a graduate social work student at Columbia University whose name I do not know. She sat in the front row of the auditorium, sipping coffee as I talked about my memoir, *Surrounded by Madness: A Memoir of Mental Illness and Family Secrets*. When I said that my mother, who had suffered from manic depression for nearly a decade, had killed herself when I was a senior in college, she cringed. When I said that it had been years since I'd heard from my adopted daughter, diagnosed with bipolar depression and borderline personality disorder when she was 16, a tear ran down her face. After my talk had ended and the auditorium had emptied, the student approached the lectern. She said that her mother had been hospitalized six times in the past couple years because of depression and that her brother had recently been diagnosed with schizophrenia. Then, she asked me a single question: "What can we do so that people with serious mental illness and their families stop suffering?"

I don't know whether people with serious mental illness and their families will ever stop suffering until there are cures for illnesses such as schizophrenia, bipolar disorder, and depression, but I do know that there are things we can do so people suffer less.

For five years, I sifted through hundreds of published articles about serious mental illness. My goal was to understand what we're doing wrong and to identify evidence-based strategies that can help alleviate suffering. As I read and thought about the issues, I talked about them with my husband. Our lively conversations, most during early morning walks with our dogs, taught me how to think about these complex issues in creative ways. As I drafted each chapter, my husband gave me feedback that sometimes made me frustrated but always made for clearer writing.

I was fortunate to meet E. Fuller Torrey, MD, shortly after I started this project. His willingness to provide historical context and psychiatric perspective helped me better understand the issues. It was rare for one of my e-mails not to be answered within twenty-four hours.

Once again, Laurie Rozakis, PhD, was the perfect editor for me. As I developed each chapter, she painstakingly read my work and told me what she liked and what needed work. She understood that I was writing for a lay audience and helped me find just the right balance of presenting rigorous research and identifying the bottom line. She told me where I needed examples so that readers would stay engaged and where I needed practical advice.

My writing got even stronger when copyeditor Jeremy Horsefield read and edited the book.

Finally, I am indebted to friends who read the manuscript and gave me thoughtful comments about issues I had neglected, matters I hadn't fully developed, and writing that was not clear. Thank you from the bottom of my heart to Nancy Alterman, LSW, Rosemary Blieszner, PhD, Joseph Bowers, Jonathan E. Brill, PhD, Deb Champion, Anne Francisco, Harriet Hartman, PhD, Michelle Krack, Barry Lebowitz, PhD, Sara Qualls, PhD, Thea Singer, PhD, and Sherry Weiss.

NOTES

Chapter 1. Preliminary Points

p. 10, **Still others have claimed that mental illnesses are not real.** Szasz, T. (1961). *The Myth of Mental Illness: Foundations of a Theory of Personal Conduct.* New York: Hoeber-Harper.

p. 10, **Psychoanalytic theory and its treatment.** Garfield, S. R. (1970). The delivery of medical care. *Scientific American, 222 (4)*, 15–23.

p. 10, **The current edition of the American Psychiatric Association's . . .** American Psychiatric Association. (2013). *Diagnostic and Statistical Manual of Mental Disorders.* 5th ed. Arlington, VA: American Psychiatric Association.

p. 11, **47.6 million Americans live with mental illness.** https://www.samhsa .gov/data/sites/default/files/cbhsq-reports/NSDUHNationalFindings Report2018/NSDUHNationalFindingsReport2018.pdf.

p. 11, **"Severe and persistent mental illnesses."** Insel, T. (2013). Director's blog: Getting serious about mental illnesses. NIMH. http://www.nimh.nih .gov/about/director/2013/getting-serious-about-mental-illnesses.shtml.

p. 11, **Brain abnormalities often are visible even before behaviors.** Cole, J., et al. (2011). Hippocampal atrophy in first episode depression: A meta-analysis of magnetic resonance imaging studies. *Journal of Affective Disorders, 134 (1–3)*, 483–87; De Peri, L., et al. (2012). Brain structural abnormalities at the onset of schizophrenia and bipolar disorder: A meta-analysis of controlled magnetic resonance imaging studies. *Current Pharmaceutical Design, 18 (4)*, 486–94.

p. 12, **In 2010 people were more likely to report.** Barry, C. L., et al. (2013). After Newtown—public opinion on gun policy and mental illness. *New England Journal of Medicine, 368 (12)*, 1077–81; Pescosolido, B. A., et al. (2010). "A disease like any other?" A decade of change in public reactions to schizophrenia, depression, and alcohol dependence. *American Journal of Psychiatry, 167*, 1321–30; Phelan, J. C., et al. (2000). Public conceptions of mental illness in 1950 and 1996: What is mental illness and is it to be feared? *Journal of Health and Social Behavior, 41*, 188–207; Schomerus, G., et al. (2012). Evolution of public attitudes about mental illness: A systematic review and meta-analysis. *Acta Psychiatrica Scandinavica, 125 (6)*, 440–52.

p. 12, **Today, more than half of all Americans.** Barry, C. L., et al. (2013). After Newtown—public opinion on gun policy and mental illness. *New England Journal of Medicine, 368 (12)*, 1077–81.

p. 12, **Beliefs that these illnesses are contagious.** Corrigan, P. W. (2012). Where is the evidence supporting public service announcements to eliminate mental illness stigma? *Psychiatry Online, 63*, 79–82; Marsh, J. K., and Shanks, L. L. (2014). Thinking you can catch mental illness: How beliefs about membership attainment and category structure influence interactions with mental health category members. *Memory and Cognition, 42*, 1011–25.

p. 12, **Change in one person's life causes change in the lives of other family members.** Pruchno, R. A., et al. (1984). Life events and interdependent lives: Implications for research and intervention. *Human Development, 27*, 31–41.

p. 13, **11.2 million adults.** NIMH uses this figure, derived from data reported by SAMSHA in 2017 (https://www.nimh.nih.gov/health/statistics /mental-illness.shtml).

p. 13, **1.9 million children.** CDC finds that 1.9 million children are diagnosed with depression (https://www.cdc.gov/childrensmentalhealth/data.html).

p. 13, **For their families, the 20 million people.** The number of family members living in a household with a person with serious mental illness is calculated for 2017 starting with the number of adults with serious mental illness (11.2 million). Subtracting out the estimated 0.1 million people with serious mental illness who are homeless (www .endhomelessness.org/pages/snapshot_of_homelessness) leaves 11.1 million people with serious mental illness living in households. In that year, the average American household size was 2.54 people, yielding 28.19 million adults and children living in a household with a person suffering from a serious mental illness. Subtracting the 11.2 million adults with serious mental illness yields 17 million people who have a front-row view of adult serious mental illness. To this, I add the families of the 1.9 million children with serious mental illness. Assuming an average of 2.54 people per family, there are 4.8 million people living in a household with a mentally ill child. Subtracting the 1.9 million children with mental illness leaves 2.93 million people living in a household with a child who is seriously mentally ill. Together, there are nearly 20 million people living in a household with a person diagnosed with serious mental illness.

p. 16, **In 2012, the annual economic costs.** Bloom, D. E., et al. (2011). *The Global Economic Burden of Non-communicable Diseases.* Geneva, Switzerland: World Economic Forum, 2011; Cloutier, M., et al. (2016). The economic burden of schizophrenia in the United States in 2013. *Journal Clinical Psychiatry, 77 (6),* 764–71; Insel, T. (2015). Director's blog: Mental health awareness month: By the numbers. NIMH. http:// www.nimh.nih.gov/about/director/2015/mental-health-awareness -month-by-the-numbers.shtml; Soni, A. (2009). *The Five Most Costly Conditions, 1996 and 2006: Estimates for the U.S. Civilian Noninstitution- alized Population.* Statistical Brief #248, July 2009. AHRQ, Rockville, MD.

p. 16, **As such, many very sick people.** Druss, B. G., et al. (2011). Understand- ing excess mortality in persons with mental illness: 17-year follow-up of a nationally representative U.S. survey. *Medical Care, 49 (6),* 599–604; Walker, E. R., et al. (2015). Mortality in mental disorders and global disease burden implications: A systematic review and meta-analysis. *JAMA Psychiatry,* Feb. 11.

Chapter 2. Breaking Brains

p. 18, **Joe knew that Satan.** Bowers, J. M. (2013). *Life under a Cloud: The Story of a Schizophrenic.* Spokane, WA: River3 Digital Press. Hoping to learn about the experiences of people with serious mental illness by talking with their family members, I reached out to a Facebook group I had joined. Joe Bowers responded with a note saying that he had been living with schizophrenia for decades and would be happy to talk with me. It took me more than a year to realize that Joe was right: to understand the experiences of people with serious mental illness, I had to talk with them and learn about life on their terms. I read Joe's compelling memoir, talked with him extensively, and communicated with him for more than five years, learning his story and getting all the details right, so that I could not only understand his story but also tell it correctly.

p. 24, **Schizophrenia is not as common.** NIMH. (2015). See http://www.nimh .nih.gov/health/publications/schizophrenia-booklet-12-2015/index.shtml.

p. 24, **Hallucinations are altered sensory experiences.** Cutting, J., and Dunne, F. (1989). Subjective experience of schizophrenia. *Schizophrenia Bulletin, 15,* 217–31.

p. 25, **Most delusions, hallucinations, and movement disorders.** Torrey, E. F. (2013). *Surviving Schizophrenia: A Family Manual.* New York: HarperCollins.

p. 26, **Its association with auditory hallucinations.** Plaze, M., et al. (2011). Where do auditory hallucinations come from? A brain morphometry study of schizophrenia patients with inner or outer space hallucinations. *Schizophrenia Bulletin, 37,* 212–21.

p. 26, **Sharon's illness had a very different beginning.** Although Sharon has been a friend for nearly a decade, it was only when I told her I was writing this book that she told me about her experiences with depression.

p. 35, **A World Health Organization study.** Simon, G. E., et al. (1999). An international study of the relation between somatic symptoms and depression. *New England Journal of Medicine, 341,* 658–59.

p. 35, **The greater the number of physical symptoms.** Kroenke, K., et al. (1994). Physical symptoms in primary care: Predictors of psychiatric disorder and functional impairment. *Archives of Family Medicine, 3,* 774–79.

p. 35, **The more painful the physical symptoms.** Ohayon, M. M., and Schatzberg, A. F. (2003). Using pain to predict depressive morbidity in the general population. *Archives of General Psychiatry, 60,* 39–47.

p. 35, **Approximately 7 percent of people.** American Psychiatric Association. (2013). *Diagnostic and Statistical Manual of Mental Disorders (DSM-5).* Washington, DC: American Psychiatric Publishing.

p. 35, **That was the goal of a team of Canadian scientists.** Wang, J., et al. (2014). A prediction algorithm for first onset of major depression in the general population: Development and validation. *Journal of Epidemiological Community Health, 68,* 418–24.

p. 36, **People who are depressed often consider ending their lives.** Franklin, J. C., et al. (2017). Risk factors for suicidal thoughts and behaviors: A meta-analysis of 50 years of research. *Psychological Bulletin, 143 (2),* 187–232.

p. 36, **The onset of Michelle's illness.** Krack, M. M. (2014). *Michelle May Crack: A Personal Memoir of Bipolar Disorder.* CreateSpace. The positive experience I had learning about Joe's story both from his memoir and from our communications led me to want to have a similar experience with a person diagnosed with bipolar disorder. I read several memoirs. When I found a memoir that presented an honest look at the illness, I contacted the author, inquiring about whether she would be interested in talking with me and sharing her story for this book. I was struck not only by Michelle's story but also by her willingness to answer the many questions I had over a period of nearly five years.

p. 44, **Type I bipolar disorder.** American Psychiatric Association. (2013). *Diagnostic and Statistical Manual of Mental Disorders (DSM-5).* Washington, DC: American Psychiatric Publishing.

p. 44, **Distinguished unipolar depression from bipolar depression.** Mason, B. L., et al. (2016). Historical underpinnings of bipolar disorder diagnostic criteria. *Behavioral Sciences, 6 (3),* 14.

p. 45, **The significant overlap of abnormalities.** Arnone, D., et al. (2009). Magnetic resonance imaging studies in bipolar disorder and schizophrenia: Meta-analysis. *British Journal of Psychiatry, 195 (3),* 194–201; Yuksel, C., et al. (2012). Gray matter volume in schizophrenia and bipolar disorder with psychotic features. *Schizophrenia Research, 138 (2–3)*, 177–82.

p. 46,   **Hypomanic episodes can last for weeks or even months.** American Psychiatric Association. (2013). *Diagnostic and Statistical Manual of Mental Disorders (DSM-5)*. Washington, DC: American Psychiatric Publishing.

p. 46,   **The hypomania of Type II bipolar disorder is less debilitating.** American Psychiatric Association. (2013). *Diagnostic and Statistical Manual of Mental Disorders (DSM-5)*. Washington, DC: American Psychiatric Publishing.

p. 48,   **Contrasting the clinical features and outcomes.** Geoffroy, P. A., et al. (2013). Reconsideration of bipolar disorder as a developmental disorder: Importance of the time of onset. *Journal of Physiology—Paris, 107*, 278–85.

p. 48,   **Children . . . who experience the onset of bipolar disorder very early.** Ortiz, P. L., et al. (2015). Early-onset and very-early-onset bipolar disorder: Distinct or similar clinical conditions? *Bipolar Disorders, 17*, 814–20.

p. 50,   **People exposed to traumatic experiences.** Addington, J., et al. (2013). Early traumatic experiences in those at clinical high risk for psychosis. *Early Intervention in Psychiatry, 7 (3)*, 300–305; Bechdolf, A., et al. (2010). Experience of trauma and conversion to psychosis in an ultra-high-risk (prodromal) group. *Acta Psychiatrica Scandinavica, 121 (5)*, 377–84; Thompson, A. D., et al. (2014). Sexual trauma increases the risk of developing psychosis in an ultra high-risk "prodromal" population. *Schizophrenia Bulletin, 40 (3)*, 697–706.

p. 51,   **The diathesis-stress model best explains the relationship.** Ingram, R. E., and Luxton, D. D. (2005). Vulnerability-stress models. In *Development of Psychopathology: A Vulnerability Stress Perspective*, ed. B. L. Hankin and J. R. Z. Abela, 32–46. Thousand Oaks, CA: Sage; Zubin, J., and Spring, B. (1977). Vulnerability—a new view of schizophrenia. *Journal of Abnormal Psychology, 86 (2)*, 103–26.

p. 51,   **When a person's bucket overflows.** Brabban, A., and Turkington, D. (2002). The search for meaning: Detecting congruence between life events, underlying schema and psychotic symptoms—formulation-driven and schema-focused cognitive behavioral therapy for a neuroleptic-resistant schizophrenic patient with a delusional memory. In *Casebook of Cognitive Therapy for Psychosis*, ed. A. P. Morrison, 59–75. New York: Brunner-Routledge.

p. 59,   **People who have a pet cat.** Torrey, E. F., and Yoklen, R. H. (1995). Could schizophrenia be a viral zoonosis transmitted from house cats? *Schizophrenia Bulletin, 21 (2)*, 167–71; Torrey, E. F., et al. (2015). Is childhood cat ownership a risk factor for schizophrenia later in life? *Schizophrenia Research, 165 (1)*, 1–2; Yuksel, P., et al. (2010). The role of latent toxoplasmosis in the aetiopathogenesis of schizophrenia—the risk factor or an indication of a contact with cat? *Folia Parasitol (Praha), 57 (2)*, 121–28; Palomäki, J., et al. (2019). Cat ownership in childhood and development of schizophrenia. *Schizophrenia Research, 206*, 444–45; Solmi, F., et al. (2017). Curiosity killed the cat: No evidence of an association between cat ownership and psychotic symptoms at ages 13 and 18 years in a UK general population cohort. *Psychological Medicine, 47 (9)*, 1659–67.

p. 59, **Torrey and his team found that exposure to a pet dog.** Yolken, R., et al. (2019). Exposure to household pet cats and dogs in childhood and risk of subsequent diagnosis of schizophrenia or bipolar disorder. *Plos One, 14 (12)*, e0225320.

p. 59, **Children born of mothers who had inflammation.** Allswede, D. M., et al. (2020). Cytokine concentrations throughout pregnancy and risk for psychosis in adult offspring: A longitudinal case-control study. *Lancet Psychiatry, 7 (3)*, 254–61.

p. 59, **Most likely serious mental illnesses are the product.** Mas, S., et al. (2020). Examining gene-environment interactions using aggregate scores in a first-episode psychosis cohort. *Schizophrenia Bulletin, 46 (4)*, 1019–25.

p. 60, **The National Alliance for Mental Illness has free programs.** See https://www.nami.org/Find-Support/NAMI-Programs/NAMI-Ending-the-Silence.

p. 61, **The National Comorbidity Study-Adolescent Supplement.** Merikangas, K. R., et al. (2010). Lifetime prevalence of mental disorders in U.S. adolescents: Results from the National Comorbidity Study-Adolescent Supplement (NCS-A). *Journal of American Academy of Child and Adolescent Psychiatry, 49 (10)*, 980–89.

Chapter 3. Crisis Care

p. 64, **On November 18, 2013, a man.** https://www.therecorderonline.com /articles/he-could-do-anything-and-do-it-well/; https://www .washingtonpost.com/national/a-fathers-scars-for-deeds-every-day -brings-questions/2014/11/01/2217a604-593c-11e4-8264-deed989ae9a2 _story.html?utm_term=.c973b40c2b56.

p. 66, **In colonial America.** Grob, G. N. (1994). *The Mad among Us: A History of the Care of America's Mentally Ill.* New York: Free Press.

p. 67, **Between 1752 and 1754, 18 of the 117 people.** Grob, G. N. (1994). *The Mad among Us: A History of the Care of America's Mentally Ill.* New York: Free Press.

p. 67, **A farmer had burned down his barn.** Torrey, E. F., and Miller, J. (2002). *The Invisible Plague: The Rise of Mental Illness from 1750 to the Present.* New Brunswick, NJ: Rutgers University Press.

p. 67, **Patients with mental illness did not stay long.** Grob, G. N. (1994). *The Mad among Us: A History of the Care of America's Mentally Ill.* New York: Free Press.

p. 67,   **Pennsylvania Hospital.** Torrey, E. F., and Miller, J. (2002). *The Invisible Plague: The Rise of Mental Illness from 1750 to the Present.* New Brunswick, NJ: Rutgers University Press.

p. 69,   **McLean, for example, admitted sixty-one patients.** Grob, G. N. (1994). *The Mad among Us: A History of the Care of America's Mentally Ill.* New York: Free Press.

p. 69,   **Of the 666 patients discharged.** Grob, G. N. (1994). *The Mad among Us: A History of the Care of America's Mentally Ill.* New York: Free Press.

p. 70,   **Worcester State Hospital could not meet the demands.** Torrey, E. F., and Miller, J. (2002). *The Invisible Plague: The Rise of Mental Illness from 1750 to the Present.* New Brunswick, NJ: Rutgers University Press.

p. 70,   **In the first year of its existence.** Torrey, E. F., and Miller, J. (2002). *The Invisible Plague: The Rise of Mental Illness from 1750 to the Present.* New Brunswick, NJ: Rutgers University Press.

p. 70,   **In 1841, 39-year-old Dorothea Dix.** Gollaher, D. (1995). *Voice for the Mad.* New York: Free Press.

p. 71,   **People were chained, naked, beaten with rods.** Torrey, E. F., and Miller, J. (2002). *The Invisible Plague: The Rise of Mental Illness from 1750 to the Present.* New Brunswick, NJ: Rutgers University Press.

p. 71,   **As many people with mental illness in jails.** Torrey, E. F., and Miller, J. (2002). *The Invisible Plague: The Rise of Mental Illness from 1750 to the Present.* New Brunswick, NJ: Rutgers University Press.

p. 71,   **By 1846 . . . the facility had deteriorated.** Torrey, E. F., and Miller, J. (2002). *The Invisible Plague: The Rise of Mental Illness from 1750 to the Present.* New Brunswick, NJ: Rutgers University Press.

p. 72,   **More than one new state asylum.** Torrey, E. F., and Miller, J. (2002). *The Invisible Plague: The Rise of Mental Illness from 1750 to the Present.* New Brunswick, NJ: Rutgers University Press.

p. 72,   **The first state hospitals.** Payne, C. (2009). *Asylum: Inside the Closed World of State Mental Hospitals.* Cambridge, MA: MIT Press.

p. 73,   **Dix was responsible for founding.** Grob, G. N. (1994). *The Mad among Us: A History of the Care of America's Mentally Ill.* New York: Free Press.

p. 73,   **As long as asylums remained small.** Grob, G. N. (1994). *The Mad among Us: A History of the Care of America's Mentally Ill.* New York: Free Press.

p. 73,   **By 1860, there were forty-one asylums.** Torrey, E. F., and Miller, J. (2002). *The Invisible Plague: The Rise of Mental Illness from 1750 to the Present.* New Brunswick, NJ: Rutgers University Press.

p. 74,   **The population of people with mental illness living in poorhouses.** Grob, G. N. (1994). *The Mad among Us: A History of the Care of America's Mentally Ill.* New York: Free Press.

p. 75, **These articles became the source.** See https://digital.library.upenn.edu /women/bly/madhouse/madhouse.html.

p. 76, **In his memoir, Beers.** Beers, C. (1908). *A Mind That Found Itself.* New York: Longmans, Green (quote on 46).

p. 77, **In his autobiography.** Beers, C. (1908). *A Mind That Found Itself.* New York: Longmans, Green (quote on 37).

p. 77, **He walked its beautiful grounds.** Beers, C. (1908). *A Mind That Found Itself.* New York: Longmans, Green (quote on 38).

p. 77, **Convinced that he had found.** Beers, C. (1908). *A Mind That Found Itself.* New York: Longmans, Green (quote on 45).

p. 78, **"The pendulum had swung too far."** Beers, C. (1908). *A Mind That Found Itself.* New York: Longmans, Green (quote on 48).

p. 80, **Despite all the brutality.** Beers, C. (1908). *A Mind That Found Itself.* New York: Longmans, Green (quote on 106).

p. 80, **Some asylums, immense to begin with.** Sacks, O. (2009). The lost virtues of the asylum. *New York Review*, 50–52.

p. 80, **By the mid-twentieth century.** Torrey, E. F., et al. (2012). *No Room at the Inn: Trends and Consequences of Closing Public Psychiatric Hospitals.* Treatment Advocacy Center.

p. 81, **Mental illness could be transformed.** Sacks, O. (2009). The lost virtues of the asylum. *New York Review*, 50–52.

p. 83, **From the smoking room.** https://web.archive.org/web/20151004024419 /http://history.tomrue.net/mpc/1874-1974_Centennial_Chronicle_of _Middletown_State_Hospital.pdf.

p. 90, **In 1955, when state hospital beds were the dominant option.** Torrey, E. F., et al. (2012). *No Room at the Inn: Trends and Consequences of Closing Public Psychiatric Hospitals.* Treatment Advocacy Center.

p. 90, **General hospitals.** Pinals, D. A., and Fuller, D. A. (2017). *Beyond Beds: The Vital Role of a Full Continuum of Psychiatric Care.* Treatment Advocacy Center.

p. 91, **There are an estimated 800,000 emergency room visits.** Pinals, D. A., and Fuller, D. A. (2017). *Beyond Beds: The Vital Role of a Full Continuum of Psychiatric Care.* Treatment Advocacy Center.

p. 91, **Arica Nesper and her colleagues.** Nesper, A., et al. (2015). Effect of decreasing county mental health services on the emergency department. *Annals of Emergency Medicine, 67 (4)*, 525–30.

p. 92, **The antipsychotic medications.** Sacks, O. (2009). The lost virtues of the asylum. *New York Review*, 50–52.

p. 94, **The average length of hospital stays.** Pinals, D. A., and Fuller, D. A. (2017). *Beyond Beds: The Vital Role of a Full Continuum of Psychiatric Care.* Treatment Advocacy Center.

p. 97,   **The model is cost-effective.** Murphy, S., et al. (2012). Crisis intervention for people with severe mental illnesses. *Cochrane Database Systematic Review, 5*, CD001087. doi:10.1002/14651858.CD001087.pub4.

p. 97,   **Rates of hospitalization were relatively low.** Kane, J. M., et al. (2016). Comprehensive versus usual community care for first-episode psychosis: 2-year outcomes from the NIMH RAISE Early Treatment Program. *American Journal of Psychiatry, 173*, 362–72.

p. 99,   **Scholars from King's College in London.** Dazzi, T., et al. (2014). Does asking about suicide and related behaviors induce suicidal ideation? What is the evidence? *Psychological Medicine, 44*, 3361–63.

Chapter 4. New Normal

p. 108,   **Yet few psychiatrists are available.** https://www.thenationalcouncil .org/wp-content/uploads/2017/03/Psychiatric-Shortage_National -Council-.pdf.

p. 108,   **Finding a psychiatrist and a therapist.** https://www.thenationalcouncil .org/wp-content/uploads/2017/03/Psychiatric-Shortage_National-Council -.pdf.

p. 108,   **Between 2003 and 2013, the average number of psychiatrists.** Bishop, T. F., et al. (2016). Population of U.S. practicing psychiatrists declined, 2003–2013, which may help explain poor access to mental health care. *Health Affairs, 35 (7)*, 1271–77.

p. 108,   **A 2018 report by Merritt Hawkins.** https://www.merritthawkins.com /uploadedFiles/MerrittHawkins/Content/News_and_Insights/Thought _Leadership/mhawhitepaperpsychiatry2018.pdf.

p. 109,   **There are only 8,300 child and adolescent psychiatrists.** https://www .aacap.org/aacap/resources_for_primary_care/Workforce_Issues.aspx.

p. 109,   **In New Jersey . . . there are sixteen child and adolescent psychiatrists.** https://www.aacap.org/aacap/Advocacy/Federal_and_State _Initiatives/Workforce_Maps/Home.aspx.

p. 109,   **Nearly 60 percent of practicing psychiatrists.** https://www .merritthawkins.com/uploadedFiles/MerrittHawkins/Content/News_and _Insights/Thought_Leadership/mhawhitepaperpsychiatry2018.pdf.

p. 110,   **While diversity in the workforce increases.** https://bhw.hrsa.gov/sites /default/files/bhw/health-workforce-analysis/research/projections /behavioral-health2013-2025.pdf.

p. 110,   **The likelihood of securing an appointment.** Williams, M. O., et al. (2017). Challenges for insured patients in accessing behavioral health care. *Annals of Family Medicine, 15 (4)*, 363–65.

p. 110,   **Another study in which researchers posed as parents.** Steinman, K. J., et al. (2015). How long do adolescents wait for psychiatry appointments? *Community Mental Health, 51*, 782–89.

p. 110, **Between 2005 and 2010, the percentage of psychiatrists.** Bishop, T. F., et al. (2014). Acceptance of insurance by psychiatrists and the implications for access to mental health care. *JAMA Psychiatry, 71 (2)*, 176–81.

p. 110, **A 2017 report from the National Council Medical Director Institute.** https://www.thenationalcouncil.org/wp-content/uploads/2017/03/Psychiatric-Shortage_National-Council-.pdf.

p. 116, **According to Irish lore.** https://www.irishtimes.com/news/health/recovering-well-1.556572.

p. 116, **Results from dozens of water samples.** http://westkerry.com/blog/?page_id=271.

p. 116, **Consistent with more than seventy years of scientific evidence.** Baldessarini, R. J., et al. (2006). Decreased risk of suicides and attempts during long-term lithium treatment: A meta-analytic review. *Bipolar Disorder, 8*, 625–39; Cipriani, A., et al. (2005). Lithium in the prevention of suicidal behavior and all-cause mortality in patients with mood disorders: A systematic review of randomized trials. *American Journal of Psychiatry, 162*, 1805–19; Goodwin, F. K., et al. (2003). Suicide risk in bipolar disorder during treatment with lithium and divalproex. *JAMA, 290*, 1467–73.

p. 117, **Treatments used for serious mental illness.** Czobor, P., et al. (2015). Treatment adherence in schizophrenia: A patient-level meta-analysis of combined CATIE and EUFEST studies. *European Neuropsychopharmacology, 25 (8)*, 1158–66; Furukawa, T. A., et al. (2015). Initial severity of schizophrenia and efficacy of antipsychotics: Participant-level meta-analysis of 6 placebo-controlled studies. *JAMA Psychiatry, 72 (1)*, 14–21; Orfanos, S., et al. (2015). Are group psychotherapeutic treatments effective for patients with schizophrenia? A systematic review and meta-analysis. *Psychotherapy and Psychosomatics, 84 (4)*, 241–49.

p. 117, **Experimenting with a surgical anesthetic.** Shorter, E. (1997). *A History of Psychiatry: From the Era of the Asylum to the Age of Prozac.* New York: John Wiley; Swazey, J. P. (1974). *Chlorpromazine in Psychiatry: A Study of Therapeutic Innovation.* Cambridge, MA: MIT Press.

p. 117, **Patients did not lose consciousness.** Shen, W. W. (1999). A history of antipsychotic drug development. *Comprehensive Psychiatry, 40 (6)*, 407–14.

p. 118, **The hospital released him.** Swazey, J. P. (1974). *Chlorpromazine in Psychiatry: A Study of Therapeutic Innovation.* Cambridge, MA: MIT Press.

p. 119, **By 1964, some 50 million people.** Zincavage, R. (2014). Drugs and deinstitutionalization. In *Cultural Sociology of Mental Illness: An A to Z Guide*, ed. A. Scull. New York: Sage.

p. 119, **Not only did Thorazine revolutionize.** Overholser, W. (1956). Has chlorpromazine inaugurated a new era in mental hospitals? *Journal of Clinical and Experimental Psychopathology, 17*, 197–201.

p. 120, **"They initiate relationships with other people."** Brown, W. A., and
Rosdolsky, M. (2015). The clinical discovery of imipramine. *American
Journal of Psychiatry, 172 (5)*, 426–29 (quote on 427).

p. 121, **While it is plausible that drugs.** Carlat, D. (2010). *Unhinged: The
Trouble with Psychiatry—a Doctor's Revelations about a Profession in
Crisis.* New York: Free Press; Kirsch, I. (2011). *The Emperor's New Drugs:
Exploding the Antidepressant Myth.* New York: Basic Books.

p. 121, **"All psychotropic drugs cause perturbations."** Hyman, S., and Nestler,
E. (1996). Initiation and adaptation: A paradigm for understanding
psychotropic drug action. *American Journal of Psychiatry 153*, 151–61
(quote on 153).

p. 121, **His best-selling book.** Whitaker, R. (2010). *Anatomy of an Epidemic:
Magic Bullets, Psychiatric Drugs, and the Astonishing Rise of Mental
Illness in America.* New York: Broadway Books.

p. 122, **Clozapine (marketed as Clozaril).** Crilly, J. (2007). The history of
clozapine and its emergence in the U.S. market: A review and analysis.
History of Psychiatry, 18 (1), 39–60.

p. 122, **While clozapine is the only medication licensed.** Farooq, S., and
Taylor, M. (2011). Clozapine. *Br J Psychiatry, 198 (4)*, 247–49; Leucht, S.,
et al. (2009). Second-generation versus first-generation antipsychotic
drugs for schizophrenia: A meta-analysis. *Lancet, 373*, 31–41; Lewis, S. W.,
et al. (2006). Randomized controlled trial of effect of prescription of
clozapine versus other second-generation antipsychotic drugs in
resistant schizophrenia. *Schizophrenia Bulletin, 32*, 715–23; McEvoy, J. P.,
et al. (2006). Effectiveness of clozapine versus olanzapine, quetiapine,
and risperidone in patients with chronic schizophrenia who did not
respond to prior atypical antipsychotic treatment. *Am J Psychiatry, 63*,
600–610.

p. 122, **Although long-acting injectable (LAI) medications for treating
schizophrenia were first introduced.** Johnson, D. A. (2009). Historical
perspective on antipsychotic long-acting injections. *Br J Psychiatry
Suppl, 52*, S7–12.

p. 123, **Today, five second-generation LAIs.** Citrome, L. (2017). Long-acting
injectable antipsychotics update: Lengthening the dosing interval and
expanding the diagnostic indications. *Expert Rev Neurother, 17 (10)*,
1029–43.

p. 123, **Consistent evidence indicates that.** Fang, S.-C., et al. (2020). The
effectiveness of long-acting injectable antipsychotics versus oral
antipsychotics in the maintenance treatment of outpatients with chronic
schizophrenia. *Hum Psychopharmacol, 35 (3)*, e2729; Park, S.-C., et al.
(2018). Comparative efficacy and safety of long-acting injectable and oral
second-generation antipsychotics for the treatment of schizophrenia: A

systematic review and meta-analysis. *Clinical Psychopharmacology and Neuroscience: The Official Scientific Journal of the Korean College of Neuropsychopharmacology, 16 (4)*, 361–75.

p. 123, **Lower rates of psychiatric services utilization and hospitalization.** Fang, S.-C., et al. (2020). The effectiveness of long-acting injectable antipsychotics versus oral antipsychotics in the maintenance treatment of outpatients with chronic schizophrenia. *Hum Psychopharmacol, 35 (3)*, e2729; Kim, H. O., et al. (2020). Real-world effectiveness of long-acting injections for reducing recurrent hospitalizations in patients with schizophrenia. *Ann Gen Psychiatry 19*, https://doi.org/10.1186/s12991 -019-0254-2; Kishimoto, T., et al. (2018). Effectiveness of long-acting injectable vs oral antipsychotics in patients with schizophrenia: A meta-analysis of prospective and retrospective cohort studies. *Schizophrenia Bulletin, 44 (3)*, 603–19; Park, S.-C., et al. (2018). Comparative efficacy and safety of long-acting injectable and oral second-generation antipsychotics for the treatment of schizophrenia: A systematic review and meta-analysis. *Clinical Psychopharmacology and Neuroscience: The Official Scientific Journal of the Korean College of Neuropsychopharmacology, 16 (4)*, 361–75.

p. 123, **Better psychosocial functioning.** Olagunji, A. T., et al. (2019). Long-acting atypical antipsychotics in schizophrenia: A systematic review and meta-analyses of effects on functional outcome. *Australian and New Zealand Journal of Psychiatry*, https://doi.org/10.1177 /0004867419837358.

p. 123, **Although they also have higher rates of extrapyramidal syndrome.** Park, S.-C., et al. (2018). Comparative efficacy and safety of long-acting injectable and oral second-generation antipsychotics for the treatment of schizophrenia: A systematic review and meta-analysis. *Clinical Psychopharmacology and Neuroscience: The Official Scientific Journal of the Korean College of Neuropsychopharmacology, 16 (4)*, 361–75.

p. 124, **Emerging evidence suggests that LAI antipsychotic medications.** Pacchiarotti, I., et al. (2019). Long-acting injectable antipsychotics (LAIs) for maintenance treatment of bipolar and schizoaffective disorders: A systematic review. *Eur Neuropsychopharmacol, 29 (4)*, 457–70.

p. 124, **For preventing relapse in patients with rapid cycling bipolar disorder.** Kishi, T., et al. (2016). Long-acting injectable antipsychotics for prevention of relapse in bipolar disorder: A systematic review and meta-analysis of randomized controlled trials. *International Journal of Neuropsychopharmacology, 19 (9)*, pyw038, https://doi.org/10.1093/ijnp/pyw038.

p. 124, **Side effects.** Boyce, P., et al. (2018). Long-acting injectable antipsychotics as maintenance treatments for bipolar disorder—a critical review of the evidence. *Bipolar Disord, 20 Suppl 2*, 25–36.

p. 125, **Although many people fear even trying ECT.** Dukakis, K., and Tye, L. (2006). *Shock: The Healing Power of Electroconvulsive Therapy.* New York: Avery.

p. 126, **For others, like writer Jonathan Cott.** Cott, J. (2005). *On the Sea of Memory: A Journey from Forgetting to Remembering.* New York: Random House.

p. 127, **Much to the scientists' surprise.** Lieberman, J. A., et al. (2005). Effectiveness of antipsychotic drugs in patients with chronic schizophrenia. *New England Journal of Medicine, 353,* 1209–23.

p. 127, **Treatment of schizophrenia . . . is more effective than nontreatment.** Kreyenbuhl, J., et al. (2009). The Schizophrenia Patient Outcomes Research Team (PORT): Updated treatment recommendations 2009. *Schizophrenia Bulletin, 36 (1),* 94–103; Leucht, S., et al. (2013). Comparative efficacy and tolerability of 15 antipsychotic drugs in schizophrenia: A multiple-treatments meta-analysis. *Lancet, 382,* 951–62.

p. 127, **A 2012 analysis of sixty-five studies.** Leucht, S., et al. (2012). Antipsychotic drugs versus placebo for relapse prevention in schizophrenia: A systematic review and meta-analysis. *Lancet, 379,* 2063–71.

p. 128, **Regarding antidepressants.** Gartiehner, G., et al. (2011). https://www.ncbi.nlm.nih.gov/books/NBK83442/.

p. 130, **This "switching" of mood.** Offidani, E., et al. (2013). Excessive mood elevation and behavioral activation with antidepressant treatment of juvenile depressive and anxiety disorders: Systematic review. *Psychotherapy and Psychosomatics, 82,* 132–41.

p. 130, **An analysis that combined results from nearly 100,000 patients.** Baldessarini, R. J., et al. (2013). Antidepressant-associated mood-switching and transition from unipolar major depression to bipolar disorder: A review. *Journal of Affective Disorders, 148,* 129–35.

p. 130, **Switching rates were 4.3 times greater.** Baldessarini, R. J., et al. (2013). Antidepressant-associated mood-switching and transition from unipolar major depression to bipolar disorder: A review. *Journal of Affective Disorders, 148,* 129–35.

p. 131, **The longer a person goes untreated.** Penttila, M., et al. (2014). Duration of untreated psychosis as predictor of long-term outcome in schizophrenia: Systematic review and meta-analysis. *British Journal of Psychiatry, 205 (2),* 88–94.

p. 131, **Earlier treatment of first-episode psychosis.** Ito, S., et al. (2015). Differential impacts of duration of untreated psychosis (DUP) on cognitive function in first-episode schizophrenia according to mode of onset. *European Psychiatry: The Journal of the Association of European Psychiatrists, 30 (8),* 995–1001. Challis, S., et al. (2013). Systematic meta-analysis of the risk factors for deliberate self-harm before and after treatment for first-episode psychosis. *Acta Psychiatrica Scandinavica, 127 (6)*, 442–54.

p. 131, **It also decreases schizophrenia's negative symptoms.** Boonstra, N., et al. (2012). Duration of untreated psychosis and negative symptoms: A systematic review and meta-analysis of individual patient data. *Schizophrenia Research, 142 (1–3)*, 12–19.

p. 131, **People experiencing first-episode psychosis.** Nasrallah, H. A. (2017). For first-episode psychosis, psychiatrists should behave like cardiologists. *Current Psychiatry*, August 4–7.

p. 131, **The importance of aggressively treating first-episode psychosis.** Emsley, R., et al. (2008). Remission in patients with first-episode schizophrenia receiving assured antipsychotic medication: A study with risperidone long-acting injection. *International Clinical Psychopharmacology, 23 (6)*, 325–31; Gardner, K. N., and Nasrallah, H. A. (2015). Managing first-episode psychosis: Rationale and evidence for nonstandard first-line treatments for schizophrenia. *Current Psychiatry, 14 (7)*, 33, 38–45, e3; Subotnik, K. L., et al. (2015). Long-acting injectable risperidone for relapse prevention and control of breakthrough symptoms after a recent first episode of schizophrenia. A randomized clinical trial. *JAMA Psychiatry, 72 (8)*, 822–29.

p. 131, **Reasons for nonuse of LAIs.** Heres, S., et al. (2011). Psychiatrists' attitude to antipsychotic depot treatment in patients with first-episode schizophrenia. *European Psychiatry, 26*, 297–301; Iyer, S., et al. (2013). A qualitative study of experiences with and perceptions regarding long-acting injectable antipsychotics: Part II—physician perspectives. *Canadian Journal of Psychiatry, 58 (supp 1)*, 23S–29S; Robinson, D. G., et al. (2020). Focused ethnographic examination of barriers to use of long-acting injectable antipsychotics. *Psychiatric Services, 71 (4)*, 337–42; Samalin, L., et al. (2013). Clinicians' attitudes toward the use of long-acting injectable antipsychotics. *J Nerv Ment Dis, 201*, 553–59; Correll, C. U., et al. (2016). The use of long-acting injectable antipsychotics in schizophrenia: Evaluating the evidence. *J Clin Psychiatry, 77 (supp 3)*, 1–24; Jager, M., and Rossler, W. (2010). Attitudes towards long-acting depot antipsychotics: A survey of patients, relatives and psychiatrists. *Psychiatry Res, 175*, 58–62; Pilon, D., et al. (2017). Treatment patterns, health care resource utilization, and spending in Medicaid beneficiaries initiating second-generation long-acting injectable agents versus oral atypical antipsychotics. *Clin Ther., 39*, 1972–85.

p. 131, **Yet there is good evidence among patients.** Waddell, L., and Taylor, M. (2009). Attitudes of patients and mental health staff to antipsychotic long-acting injections: Systematic review. *Br. J. Psychiatry Suppl, 52*, S43–S50.

p. 131, **Approximately one-quarter of people who develop a schizophrenia-like psychosis.** Hegarty, J. D., et al. (1994). One hundred years of schizophrenia: A meta-analysis of the outcome literature. *American Journal of Psychiatry, 151 (10),* 1409–16; Stalker, H. (1939). The prognosis in schizophrenia. Based on a follow-up study of 129 cases treated by ordinary methods. *Journal of Mental Science, 85,* 122–40; Stephens, J. H. (1978). Long-term psychosis and follow-up in schizophrenia. *Schizophrenia Bulletin, 4 (1),* 25–47.

p. 133, **Finally, Fuller Torrey's book.** Torrey, E. F. (2019). *Surviving Schizophrenia: A Family Manual.* 7th ed. New York: Harper Perennial.

p. 134, **Erving Goffman . . . used the term "stigma."** Goffman, E. (1963). *Stigma: Notes on the Management of Spoiled Identity.* Upper Saddle River, NJ: Prentice Hall.

p. 134, **Knowing a few sociological terms.** Hinshaw, S. P. (2005). The stigmatization of mental illness in children and parents: Developmental issues, family concerns, and research needs. *Journal of Child Psychology and Psychiatry, 46 (7),* 714–34.

p. 135, **To understand mental illness stigma.** Woodward, J. L. (1951). Changing ideas on mental illness and its treatment. *American Sociological Review, 16 (4),* 443–54.

p. 136, **Rather, they feared that the person with mental illness.** Star, S. (1955). The public's ideas about mental illness. Paper presented at the annual meeting of the National Association for Mental Health, Indianapolis, IN (quote on 7).

p. 136, **Perceptions that people with mental illness are physically violent.** Phelan, J. D., et al. (2000). Public conceptions of mental illness in 1950 and 1996: What is mental illness and is it to be feared? *Journal of Health and Social Behavior, 41 (2),* 188–207.

p. 136, **On July 17, 1990, President George H. W. Bush.** http://www.loc.gov/loc/brain/proclaim.html.

p. 137, **A clever analysis of magazine articles.** Clarke, J., and Gawley, A. (2009). The triumph of pharmaceuticals: The portrayal of depression from 1980 to 2005. *Adm Policy Mental Health, 36,* 91–101.

p. 137, **Nationwide studies conducted in 1996 and 2006.** Pescosolido, B. A., et al. (2010). "A disease like any other"? A decade of change in public reactions to schizophrenia, depression, and alcohol dependence. *American Journal of Psychiatry, 167 (11),* 1321–30.

p. 138, **Across sixteen countries in Europe.** Pescosolido, B. A., et al. (2013). The "backbone" of stigma: Identifying the global core of public prejudice associated with mental illness. *American Journal of Public Health, 103 (5),* 853–60.

p. 138, **Nevertheless, even as public beliefs.** Schomerus, G., et al. (2012). Evolution of public attitudes about mental illness: A systematic review and meta-analysis. *Acta Psychiatrica Scandinavica, 125,* 440–52.

p. 138, **The 1999 US surgeon general's report.** US Department of Health and Human Services. (1999). *Mental Health: A Report of the Surgeon General.* Bethesda, USDHHS (quote on 454).

p. 139, **A nationwide study comparing stigma in 1996 and 2006.** Pescosolido, B. A., et al. (2010). "A disease like any other"? A decade of change in public reactions to schizophrenia, depression, and alcohol dependence. *American Journal of Psychiatry, 167 (11),* 1321–30.

p. 139, **In 2006, 53 percent of people said.** Pescosolido, B. A., et al. (2010). "A disease like any other"? A decade of change in public reactions to schizophrenia, depression, and alcohol dependence. *American Journal of Psychiatry, 167 (11),* 1321–30.

p. 140, **More than one-third of respondents were unwilling.** Pescosolido, B. A., et al. (2013). The "backbone" of stigma: Identifying the global core of public prejudice associated with mental illness. *American Journal of Public Health, 103 (5),* 853–60.

p. 140, **The international data.** Pescosolido, B. A., et al. (2013). The "backbone" of stigma: Identifying the global core of public prejudice associated with mental illness. *American Journal of Public Health, 103 (5),* 853–60.

p. 140, **However, biogenetic explanations increase beliefs.** Kvaale, E. P., et al. (2013). Biogenetic explanations and stigma: A meta-analytic review of associations among laypeople. *Social Science and Medicine, 96,* 95–103; Read, J., et al. (2006). Prejudice and schizophrenia: A review of the "mental illness is an illness like any other" approach. *Acta Psychiatrica Scandinavia, 114,* 303–18; Schomerus, G., et al. (2012). Evolution of public attitudes about mental illness: A systematic review and meta-analysis. *Acta Psychiatrica Scandinavica, 125,* 440–52.

p. 140, **American children . . . endorse stigmatizing beliefs.** Parcesepe, A. M., and Cobassa, L. J. (2013). Public stigma of mental illness in the United States: A systematic literature review. *Adm Policy Mental Health, 40 (5),* 1–21. Walker, J. S., et al. (2008). Children's stigmatization of childhood depression and ADHD: Magnitude and demographic variation in a national sample. *Journal of the American Academy of Child and Adolescent Psychiatry, 47(8),* 912–20.

p. 140, **A systematic review of studies of stigma.** Larkings, J. S., and Brown, P. M. (2018). Do biogenetic causal beliefs reduce mental illness stigma in people with mental illness and in mental health professionals? A systematic review. *International Journal of Mental Health Nursing, 27,* 928–41.

p. 144, **In 1963, Erving Goffman.** Goffman, E. (1963). *Stigma: Notes on the Management of Spoiled Identity.* Upper Saddle River, NJ: Prentice Hall.

p. 144, **One of the first studies about courtesy stigma.** Yarrow, M., et al. (1955). The social meaning of mental illness. *Journal of Social Issues, 11,* 33–48.

p. 144, **Between 25 and 50 percent of family members.** Angermeyer, M. C., et al. (2003). Courtesy stigma—a focus group study of relatives of schizophrenia patients. *Social Psychiatry and Psychiatric Epidemiology, 38,* 593–602; Phelan, J. C., et al. (1998). Psychiatric illness and family stigma. *Schizophrenia Bulletin, 24,* 115–26; Thompson, E. H., and Doll, W. (1982). The burden of families coping with the mentally ill: An invisible crisis. *Family Relations, 31,* 379–88; Wahl, O. F., and Harman, C. R. (1989). Family views of stigma. *Schizophrenia Bulletin, 15,* 131–39.

p. 145, **Nearly half of parents and spouses.** Phelan, J. C., et al. (1998). Psychiatric illness and family stigma. *Schizophrenia Bulletin, 24,* 115–26.

p. 145, **Shame is forty times more prevalent.** Ohaeri, J. U., and Fido, A. A. (2001). The opinion of caregivers on aspects of schizophrenia and major affective disorders in a Nigerian setting. *Social Psychiatry and Psychiatric Epidemiology, 36,* 493–99.

p. 145, **Stephen Hinshaw, an eminent scholar.** Hinshaw, S. P. (2005). The stigmatization of mental illness in children and parents: Developmental issues, family concerns, and research needs. *Journal of Child Psychology and Psychiatry, 46 (7),* 714–34 (quote on 720).

p. 145, **Between 20 and 30 percent of family members.** Oestmann, M., and Kjellin, L. (2002). Stigma by association: Psychological factors in relatives of people with mental illness. *British Journal of Psychiatry, 181,* 494–98; Struening, E. L., et al. (2001). Stigma as a barrier to recovery: The extent to which caregivers believe most people devalue consumers and their families. *Psychiatric Services, 52,* 1633–38; Wahl, O. F., and Harman, C. R. (1989). Family views of stigma. *Schizophrenia Bulletin, 15,* 131–39.

p. 145, **More than 70 percent of people disagreed.** Struening, E. L., et al. (2001). Stigma as a barrier to recovery: The extent to which caregivers believe most people devalue consumers and their families. *Psychiatric Services, 52,* 1633–38.

p. 145, **Incompetent parenting skills are blamed.** Phelan, J. C. (2002). Genetic biases of mental illness—a cure for stigma? *Trends in Neurosciences, 25,* 430–31; Phelan, J. C., et al. (2002). Genes and stigma: The connection between perceived genetic etiology and attitudes and beliefs about mental illness. *Psychiatric Rehabilitation Skills, 6,* 159–85.

p. 145, **The public believes that a parent's mental illness.** Corrigan, P. W., and Miller, F. E. (2004). Shame, blame, and contamination: A review of the impact of mental illness stigma on family members. *Journal of Mental Health, 13 (6)*, 537–48.

p. 145, **The genetic attributions of mental illness.** Phelan, J. C. (2005). Geneticization of deviant behavior and consequences for stigma: The case of mental illness. *Journal of Health and Social Behavior, 46*, 307–22.

p. 146, **An analysis of more than sixty studies.** Morgan, A. J., et al. (2018). Interventions to reduce stigma towards people with severe mental illness: Systematic review and meta-analysis. *Journal of Psychiatric Research, 103*, 120–33.

p. 146, **However, contact, especially face-to-face.** Corrigan, P. W., et al. (2012). Challenging the public stigma of mental illness: A meta-analysis of outcome studies. *Psychiatric Services, 63 (10)*, 963–73.

p. 146, **A study . . . integrated a mental health module.** Milin, R., et al. (2016). Impact of a mental health curriculum on knowledge and stigma among high school students: A randomized controlled trial. *Journal of the American Academy of Child and Adolescent Psychiatry, 55 (5)*, 383–91.

p. 146, **Some have suggested that stigma continues.** Pescosolido, B. A., et al. (2010). "A disease like any other"? A decade of change in public reactions to schizophrenia, depression, and alcohol dependence. *American Journal of Psychiatry, 167 (11)*, 1321–30.

p. 147, **Public attitudes were more positive.** McGinty, E. E., et al. (2015). Portraying mental illness and drug addiction as treatable health conditions: Effects of a randomized experiment on stigma and discrimination. *Social Science and Medicine, 126*, 73–895.

p. 147, **Most existing interventions are short-term.** Corrigan, P. W., et al. (2013). The California Schedule of key ingredients for contact-based antistigma programs. *Psychiatric Rehabilitation Journal, 36 (3)*, 173–79.

p. 147, **Much of the progress gained by the LGBT community.** Herek, G. M., and Capitanio, J. P. (1996). "Some of my best friends": Intergroup contact, concealable stigma, and heterosexuals' attitudes toward gay men and lesbians. *Personality and Social Psychology Bulletin, 22*, 412–24.

p. 147, **This same strategy may be productive.** Corrigan, P. W., and Matthews, A. K. (2003). Stigma and disclosure: Implications for coming out of the closet. *Journal of Mental Health, 12 (3)*, 235–48; Corrigan, P. W., et al. (2001). Three strategies for changing attributions about severe mental illness. *Schizophrenia Bulletin, 27*, 187–95; Pettigrew, T. F., and Tropp, L. R. (2006). A meta-analytic test of intergroup contact theory. *Journal of Personality and Social Psychology, 90*, 751–83.

p. 148, **For Dr. Corrigan, stigma is personal.** Corrigan, P. W. (2015). What's there to be proud of? In *Coming Out Proud to Erase the Stigma of Mental*

Illness: Stories and Essays of Solidarity, ed. P. W. Corrigan, J. E. Larson, and P. W. Michaels. Collierville, TN: Instant; Corrigan, P. W. (2018). The disabling effects of mental illness on my education. *Psychiatric Services, 69 (8)*, 847–48.

p. 148, **Although he had been diagnosed.** Corrigan, P. W. (2015). What's there to be proud of? In *Coming Out Proud to Erase the Stigma of Mental Illness: Stories and Essays of Solidarity*, ed. P. W. Corrigan, J. E. Larson, and P. W. Michaels. Collierville, TN: Instant.

p. 148, **Dr. Corrigan's understanding of the literature.** Corrigan, P. W., et al. (2012). Challenging the public stigma of mental illness: A meta-analysis of outcome studies. *Psychiatric Services, 63 (10)*, 963–73.

p. 149, **Dr. Corrigan began to share his personal experiences.** Corrigan, P. W. (2015). What's there to be proud of? In *Coming Out Proud to Erase the Stigma of Mental Illness: Stories and Essays of Solidarity*, ed. P. W. Corrigan, J. E. Larson, and P. W. Michaels. Collierville, TN: Instant.

p. 149, **Corrigan's program, called "Honest, Open, Proud."** http://comingoutproudprogram.org/index.php.

p. 149, **Here are some of the benefits identified by Dr. Corrigan.** http://comingoutproudprogram.org/images/Honest_Open_Proud_COP_ManualBooster_FINAL_updated_2.1.2017-min.pdf.

p. 150, **Disclosing mental illness to a potential employer.** Rusch, N., et al. (2018). Attitudes toward disclosing a mental health problem and reemployment: A longitudinal study. *Journal of Nervous and Mental Disease, 206 (5)*, 383–85; Hipes, C., et al. (2016). The stigma of mental illness in the labor market. *Social Science Research, 56*, 16–25.

p. 153, **She felt free to come forward.** https://www.nami.org/Blogs/NAMI-Blog/October-2018/What-Happens-When-Celebrities-Speak-Out.

p. 154, **A study of female students.** Ferrari, A. (2016). Using celebrities in abnormal psychology as teaching tools to decrease stigma and increase help seeking. *Teaching of Psychology, 43 (4)*, 329–33.

Chapter 5. Ongoing Obstacles

p. 155, **These extraordinary accomplishments.** Saks, E. R. (2007). *The Center Cannot Hold: My Journey through Madness*. New York: Hyperion.

p. 155, **Saks blurted, "What year is this?"** Saks, E. R. (2007). *The Center Cannot Hold: My Journey through Madness*. New York: Hyperion (quote on 191).

p. 156, **She said, "They passed me up."** Saks, E. R. (2007). *The Center Cannot Hold: My Journey through Madness*. New York: Hyperion (quote on 199).

p. 156, **She said, "I think I want to get off my medication."** Saks, E. R. (2007). *The Center Cannot Hold: My Journey through Madness*. New York: Hyperion (quote on 202).

p. 157, **She felt like she was "going to melt."** Saks, E. R. (2007). *The Center Cannot Hold: My Journey through Madness.* New York: Hyperion (quote on 203).

p. 157, **Saks's conviction that "the people in the sky poison me."** Saks, E. R. (2007). *The Center Cannot Hold: My Journey through Madness.* New York: Hyperion (quote on 204).

p. 157, **Saks explains, "In spite of my history."** Saks, E. R. (2007). *The Center Cannot Hold: My Journey through Madness.* New York: Hyperion (quote on 244).

p. 157, **She continues, "My brain was the instrument."** Saks, E. R. (2007). *The Center Cannot Hold: My Journey through Madness.* New York: Hyperion (quote on 245).

p. 158, **She says, "If I'd had a broken leg."** Saks, E. R. (2007). *The Center Cannot Hold: My Journey through Madness.* New York: Hyperion (quote on 282).

p. 158, **About half of people with a serious mental illness.** Garcia, S., et al. (2016). Adherence to antipsychotic medication in bipolar disorder and schizophrenic patients: A systematic review. *J Clin Psychopharmacol, 36 (4),* 355–71; Kessler, R. C., et al. (2001). The prevalence and correlates of untreated serious mental illness. *Health Serv Res, 36 (6 Pt 1),* 987–1007; Mojtabai, R., et al. (2009). Unmet need for mental health care in schizophrenia: An overview of literature and new data from a first-admission study. *Schizophrenia Bulletin, 35 (4),* 679–95; SAMSHA. (2018). *Key Substance Use and Mental Health Indicators in the United States: Results from the 2017 National Survey on Drug Use and Health.* https://www.samhsa.gov/data/sites/default/files/cbhsq-reports /NSDUHFFR2017/NSDUHFFR2017.htm; Vanelli, M., et al. (2001). Refill patterns of atypical and conventional antipsychotic medications at a national retail pharmacy chain. *Psychiatr Serv, 52 (9),* 1248–50.

p. 158, **The National Survey on Drug Use and Health . . . provides important information.** SAMSHA. (2018). *Key Substance Use and Mental Health Indicators in the United States: Results from the 2017 National Survey on Drug and Health.* https://www.samhsa.gov/data/sites/default/files /cbhsq-reports/NSDUHFFR2017/NSDUHFFR2017.htm.

p. 160, **A report from the Centers for Disease Control.** Weissman, J. F., et al. (2015). Serious psychological distress among adults: United States, 2009–2013. *NCHS Data Brief* (203), 1–8.

p. 160, **For decades, studies have shown that whether SES is measured.** Dohrenwend, B. P. (1980). *Mental Health in the United States: Epidemiological Estimates.* New York: Praeger; Faris, R. E. L., and Dunham, W. W. (1939). *Mental Disorders in Urban Areas.* Chicago: University of Chicago Press; Hollingshead, A. B., and Redlich, F. C. (1958). *Social Class and Mental Illness.* New York: Wiley; Hudson, C. G. (1988). Socioeconomic status and mental illness: Implications of the research for policy and practice. *Journal of Sociology and Social Welfare, 15 (1)*, 27–54.

p. 160, **While we still don't understand.** Hudson, C. G. (2005). Socioeconomic status and mental illness: Tests of the social causation and selection hypotheses. *American Journal of Orthopsychiatry, 75 (1)*, 3–18.

p. 160, **These problems are even greater for racial and ethnic minority members.** Maura, J., and Weisman de Mamani, A. (2017). Mental health disparities, treatment engagement, and attrition among racial/ethnic minorities with severe mental illness: A review. *J Clin Psychol Med Settings, 24 (3–4)*, 187–210.

p. 160, **Nearly 60 percent of mental health care.** SAMSHA. (2014). *Projections of National Expenditures for Treatment of Mental and Substance Use Disorders, 2010–2020.*

p. 160, **Medicaid is the single largest payer.** CBHSQ. (2017). *2016 National Survey on Drug Use and Health: Detailed Tables.*

p. 160, **The Medicaid website provides comprehensive information.** https://www.medicaid.gov/state-overviews/index.html.

p. 161, **Information about applying for SSI.** https://www.ssa.gov/pubs/EN-05-11000.pdf.

p. 161, **Eleven categories of mental illness.** https://www.disability-benefits-help.org/disabling-conditions/mental-disorders.

p. 162, **The Benefit Eligibility Screening Tool.** https://ssabest.benefits.gov/.

p. 162, **Many people who are eligible for SSI and SSDI never apply.** Dennis, D., et al. (2011). Helping adults who are homeless gain disability benefits: The SSI/SSDI Outreach, Access, and Recovery (SOAR) program. *Psychiatr Serv, 62 (11)*, 1373–76.

p. 162, **Not only do most people not know about these benefits.** Dennis, D., et al. (2011). Helping adults who are homeless gain disability benefits: The SSI/SSDI Outreach, Access, and Recovery (SOAR) program. *Psychiatr Serv, 62 (11)*, 1373–76.

p. 162, **Since the Substance Abuse and Mental Health Services Administration established.** Dennis, D., et al. (2011). Helping adults who are homeless gain disability benefits: The SSI/SSDI Outreach, Access, and Recovery (SOAR) program. *Psychiatr Serv, 62 (11)*, 1373–76; Lowder, E. M., et al. (2017). SSI/SSDI Outreach, Access, and Recovery (SOAR): Disability application outcomes among homeless adults. *Psychiatr Serv, 68 (11)*, 1189–92.

p. 162, **Information about SOAR by state.** https://soarworks.prainc.com/directory.

p. 163, **A complete list of mandatory and optional benefits.** https://www.medicaid.gov/medicaid/benefits/list-of-benefits/index.html.

p. 163, **Compared with people who are uninsured.** Fry, C. E., and Sommers, B. D. (2018). Effect of Medicaid expansion on health insurance coverage and access to care among adults with depression. *Psychiatr Serv*, doi:10.1176/appi.ps.201800181; Walker, E. R., et al. (2015). Insurance status, use of mental health services, and unmet need for mental health care in the United States. *Psychiatr Serv, 66 (6)*, 578–84; Wen, H., et al. (2015). Effect of Medicaid expansions on health insurance coverage and access to care among low-income adults with behavioral health conditions. *Health Serv Res, 50 (6)*, 1787–1809.

p. 163, **The overall shortage of doctors.** Bishop, T. F., et al. (2014). Acceptance of insurance by psychiatrists and the implications for access to mental health care. *JAMA Psychiatry, 71 (2)*, 176–81.

p. 163, **The ACA changed Medicaid.** SAMSHA. (2014). *Projections of National Expenditures for Treatment of Mental and Substance Use Disorders, 2010–2020.*

p. 164, **According to US Census data.** Smith, J. C., and Medalia, C. (2015). *Health Insurance Coverage in the United States: 2014.*

p. 165, **That number fell to 13.1 percent in 2016.** Barnett, J. C., and Berchick, E. R. (2017). *Health Insurance Coverage in the United States: 2016.*

p. 165, **Being insured . . . increased the number of young adults.** Kozloff, N., and Sommers, B. D. (2017). Insurance coverage and health outcomes in young adults with mental illness following the Affordable Care Act Dependent Coverage Expansion. *J Clin Psychiatry, 78 (7)*, e821–e827.

p. 165, **The ACA has improved the lives.** Thomas, K. C., et al. (2018). Impact of ACA health reforms for people with mental health conditions. *Psychiatr Serv, 69 (2)*, 231–34.

p. 165, **Yet a recent comprehensive report.** Melek, S. P., et al. (2017). *Addiction and Mental Health vs. Physical Health: Analyzing Disparities in Network Use and Provider Reimbursement Rates.*

p. 165, **A study in Denver found.** Williams, M. O., et al. (2017). Challenges for insured patients in accessing behavioral health care. *Annals of Family Medicine, 15 (4)*, 363–65.

p. 165, **Studies in other regions.** Haeder, S. F., et al. (2016). Secret shoppers find access to providers and network accuracy lacking for those in marketplace and commercial plans. *Health Aff (Millwood), 35 (7)*, 1160–66.

p. 165, **The ACA extended Medicaid coverage.** https://www.kff.org/uninsured/fact-sheet/key-facts-about-the-uninsured-population/.

p. 165, **A 2019 study by the US Bureau of Labor Statistics.** https://www.bls.gov/news.release/pdf/ebs2.pdf.

p. 166, **Lack of health insurance puts people.** Hadley, J. (2007). Insurance coverage, medical care use, and short-term health changes following an unintentional injury or the onset of a chronic condition. *Jama, 297 (10)*, 1073–84; McMorrow, S., et al. (2014). Determinants of receipt of recommended preventive services: Implications for the Affordable Care Act. *Am J Public Health, 104 (12),* 2392–99.

p. 166, **They are more likely to be hospitalized.** Castaneda, M. A., and Saygili, M. (2016). The health conditions and the health care consumption of the uninsured. *Health Economics Review, 6 (1),* 55–55; Christopher, A. S., et al. (2016). Access to care and chronic disease outcomes among Medicaid-insured persons versus the uninsured. *Am J Public Health, 106 (1),* 63–69.

p. 166, **Uninsured people face unaffordable medical bills.** Dusetzina, S. B., et al. (2015). For uninsured cancer patients, outpatient charges can be costly, putting treatments out of reach. *Health Aff (Millwood), 34 (4),* 584–91; Xu, T., et al. (2017). Variation in emergency department vs internal medicine excess charges in the United States. *JAMA Intern Med, 177 (8),* 1139–45.

p. 170, **The National Survey on Drug Use and Health revealed that . . . 32.2 percent.** SAMSHA. (2018). *Key Substance Use and Mental Health Indicators in the United States: Results from the 2017 National Survey on Drug Use and Health.* https://www.samhsa.gov/data/sites/default/files /cbhsq-reports/NSDUHFFR2017/NSDUHFFR2017.htm.

p. 171, **In many states, Medicaid already reimburses telehealth.** http://www .securetelehealth.com/medicaid-reimbursement.html.

p. 172, **There were significant decreases in hospital admissions.** Pratt, S. I., et al. (2015). Automated telehealth for managing psychiatric instability in people with serious mental illness. *J Ment Health, 24 (5),* 261–65.

p. 172, **A review of forty-six telepsychiatry studies.** Naslund, J. A., et al. (2015). Emerging mHealth and eHealth interventions for serious mental illness: A review of the literature. *J Ment Health, 24 (5),* 321–32.

p. 172, **The Center for Collegiate Mental Health's 2019 report.** https://ccmh .psu.edu/files/2020/01/2019-CCMH-Annual-Report.pdf.

p. 173, **The rule of thumb.** https://iacsinc.org/staff-to-student-ratios/.

p. 173, **The Jed Foundation.** https://www.jedfoundation.org/.

p. 173, **In 2002, Alison Malmon.** https://www.activeminds.org/.

p. 174, **She says, "I didn't want them to worry."** Saks, E. R. (2007). *The Center Cannot Hold: My Journey through Madness.* New York: Hyperion (quote on 74).

p. 174, **Like Saks, many people with a serious mental illness.** SAMSHA. (2018). *Key Substance Use and Mental Health Indicators in the United States: Results from the 2017 National Survey on Drug Use and Health.* https://www.samhsa.gov/data/sites/default/files/cbhsq-reports /NSDUHFFR2017/NSDUHFFR2017.htm.

p. 174, **A systematic review of 144 studies.** Clement, S., et al. (2015). What is the impact of mental health-related stigma on help-seeking? A systematic review of quantitative and qualitative studies. *Psychol Med, 45 (1),* 11–27.

p. 174, **She adds, "Nevertheless, there were whole parts of myself."** Saks, E. R. (2007). *The Center Cannot Hold: My Journey through Madness.* New York: Hyperion (quote on 95).

p. 175, **Elyn wanted Steve as a lifelong friend.** Saks, E. R. (2007). *The Center Cannot Hold: My Journey through Madness.* New York: Hyperion (quote on 195).

p. 177, **In the 2001 movie *A Beautiful Mind*.** *A Beautiful Mind.* Screenplay by Akiva Goldsman, 2002, Newmarket Press.

p. 179, **People with anosognosia.** Buckley, P. F., et al. (2007). Lack of insight in schizophrenia: Impact on treatment adherence. *CNS Drugs, 21 (2),* 129–41; Elowe, J., and Conus, P. (2017). Much ado about everything: A literature review of insight in first episode psychosis and schizophrenia. *Eur Psychiatry, 39,* 73–79.

p. 180, **Some scholars have suggested that lack of insight.** Comparelli, A., et al. (2013). Relationships between psychopathological variables and insight in psychosis risk syndrome and first-episode and multiepisode schizophrenia. *J Nerv Ment Dis, 201 (3),* 229–33; Ghaemi, S. N., and Rosenquist, K. J. (2004). Is insight in mania state-dependent? A meta-analysis. *J Nerv Ment Dis, 192 (11),* 771–75.

p. 180, **Between 27 and 57 percent of people.** Amador, X., et al. (1994). Awareness of illness in schizophrenia and schizoaffective and mood disorders. *Archives of General Psychiatry, 51,* 826–36.

p. 180, **Lack of awareness is less of a problem.** Amador, X., et al. (1994). Awareness of illness in schizophrenia and schizoaffective and mood disorders. *Archives of General Psychiatry, 51,* 826–36.

p. 180, **People with schizophrenia and those with bipolar disorder.** Pini, S., et al. (2001). Insight into illness in schizophrenia, schizoaffective disorder, and mood disorders with psychotic features. *Am J Psychiatry, 158 (1),* 122–25.

p. 180, **Not surprisingly, insight is greater.** Varga, M., et al. (2006). Insight, symptoms and neurocognition in bipolar I patients. *J Affect Disord, 91 (1),* 1–9.

p. 180, **Moreover, insight is more impaired.** Peralta, V., and Cuesta, M. J. (1998). Lack of insight in mood disorders. *J Affect Disord, 49 (1),* 55–58.

p. 180, **Lack of insight . . . results from physical damage.** Williams, A. R., et al. (2015). Assessing and improving clinical insight among patients "in denial." *JAMA Psychiatry, 72 (4),* 303–4.

p. 180, **People with poorer insight have lower gray matter volumes.** Berge, D., et al. (2011). Gray matter volume deficits and correlation with insight and negative symptoms in first-psychotic-episode subjects. *Acta Psychiatr Scand, 123 (6),* 431–39; Morgan, K. D., et al. (2010). Insight, grey matter and cognitive function in first-onset psychosis. *Br J Psychiatry, 197 (2),* 141–48;

Buchy, L., et al. (2018). A longitudinal study of cognitive insight and cortical thickness in first-episode psychosis. *Schizophr Res, 193*, 251–60; McEvoy, J. P., et al. (2006). Insight in first-episode psychosis. *Psychol Med, 36 (10)*, 1385–93; Shad, M. U., et al. (2004). Insight and prefrontal cortex in first-episode schizophrenia. *Neuroimage, 22 (3)*, 1315–20.

p. 181, **In a mental illness like schizophrenia, nonadherence.** Buckley, P. F., et al. (2007). Lack of insight in schizophrenia: Impact on treatment adherence. *CNS Drugs, 21 (2)*, 129–41.

p. 181, **Surprisingly, while there is strong evidence.** Buckley, P. F., et al. (2007). Lack of insight in schizophrenia: Impact on treatment adherence. *CNS Drugs, 21 (2)*, 129–41.

p. 181, **Psychosocial interventions.** Macpherson, R., et al. (1996). A controlled study of education about drug treatment in schizophrenia. *Br J Psychiatry, 168 (6)*, 709–17; Rossotto, E., et al. (2004). Rehab rounds: Enhancing treatment adherence among persons with schizophrenia by teaching community reintegration skills. *Psychiatr Serv, 55 (1)*, 26–27.

p. 182, **She says, "None of it's been real, John."** *A Beautiful Mind*. Screenplay by Akiva Goldsman, 2002, Newmarket Press (79–80).

p. 182, **Nash responded, "Because the ideas I had."** Nasar, S. (1998). *A Beautiful Mind*. New York: Simon & Schuster (quote on 11).

p. 183, **Nearly twenty years later, Xavier.** Amador, X. F. (2000). *I Am Not Sick. I Don't Need Help!* New York: Vida.

p. 183, **To be creative, ideas.** Kaufman, S. B., and Paul, E. S. (2014). Creativity and schizophrenia spectrum disorders across the arts and sciences. *Frontiers in Psychology, 5*, 1145–45.

p. 184, **Plato suggested that poets.** Jamison, K. R. (1993). *Touched with Fire: Manic-Depressive Illness and the Artistic Temperament*. New York: Simon & Schuster.

p. 184, **It cannot simply be a matter of chance that among geniuses.** Lange-Eichbaum, W. (1931). *The Problem of Genius*. Trans. E. C. Paul. London: Kegan Paul.

p. 184, **A study that compared people attending the Iowa Writers Workshop.** Andreasen, N. C. (1987). Creativity and mental illness: Prevalence rates in writers and their first-degree relatives. *Am J Psychiatry, 144 (10)*, 1288–92.

p. 185, **Another study compared award-winning artists.** Jamison, K. R. (1989). Mood disorders and patterns of creativity in British writers and artists. *Psychiatry, 52 (2)*, 125–34.

p. 185, **In her book.** Jamison, K. R. (1993). *Touched with Fire: Manic-Depressive Illness and the Artistic Temperament*. New York: Simon & Schuster.

p. 185, **More recently, Jamison examined.** Jamison, K. R. (2017). *Setting the River on Fire: A Study of Genius, Mania, and Character*. New York: Penguin Random House.

p. 185, **An analysis based on more than thirty studies.** Taylor, C. L. (2017). Creativity and mood disorder: A systematic review and meta-analysis. *Perspect Psychol Sci, 12 (6)*, 1040–76.

p. 185, **Some studies find that people with mental illness.** Taylor, C. L. (2017). Creativity and mood disorder: A systematic review and meta-analysis. *Perspect Psychol Sci, 12 (6)*, 1040–76.

p. 186, **An exception was people with bipolar disorder.** Kyaga, S., et al. (2013). Mental illness, suicide and creativity: 40-year prospective total population study. *J Psychiatr Res, 47 (1)*, 83–90.

p. 186, **Research consistently finds that creativity.** Taylor, C. L. (2017). Creativity and mood disorder: A systematic review and meta-analysis. *Perspect Psychol Sci, 12 (6)*, 1040–76.

p. 186, **The authors of four major textbooks.** Kaufman, J. C. (2014). *Creativity and Mental Illness.* Cambridge: Cambridge University Press; Runco, M. A. (2007). *Creativity: Theories and Themes: Research, Development, and Practice.* Burlington, MA: Elsevier; Sawyer, R. K. (2012). *Explaining Creativity: The Science of Human Innovation.* New York: Oxford University Press; Weisberg, R. W. (2006). *Creativity: Understanding Innovation in Problem Solving, Science, Invention and the Arts.* Hoboken, NJ: Wiley.

p. 186, **Some scholars suggest that the question.** Silvia, P. J., and Kaurman, J. C. (2010). Creativity and mental illness. In *Cambridge Handbook of Creativity*, ed. J. C. Kaufman and R. J. Sternberg, 381–94. New York: Cambridge University Press.

p. 186, **Others find that when there are connections.** Richards, R., et al. (1988). Creativity in manic-depressives, cyclothymes, their normal relatives, and control subjects. *J Abnorm Psychol, 97 (3)*, 281–88.

p. 186, **Relatives of people with bipolar disorder.** Kyaga, S., et al. (2011). Creativity and mental disorder: Family study of 300,000 people with severe mental disorder. *Br J Psychiatry, 199 (5)*, 373–79; Simeonova, D. I., et al. (2005). Creativity in familial bipolar disorder. *J Psychiatr Res, 39 (6)*, 623–31.

p. 186, **Either there is a hereditary connection.** Power, R. A., et al. (2015). Polygenic risk scores for schizophrenia and bipolar disorder predict creativity. *Nat Neurosci, 18 (7)*, 953–55.

p. 186, **Based on results from neuroimaging.** Carson, S. H. (2011). Creativity and psychopathology: A shared vulnerability model. *Can J Psychiatry, 56 (3)*, 144–53; Kaufman, S. B., and Paul, E. S. (2014). Creativity and schizophrenia spectrum disorders across the arts and sciences. *Frontiers in Psychology, 5*, 1145–45.

p. 186, **Others propose a "mad-genius paradox."** Simonton, D. K. (2014). The mad-genius paradox: Can creative people be more mentally healthy but highly creative people more mentally ill? *Perspect Psychol Sci, 9 (5)*, 470–80.

p. 186, **Particularly gifted people.** Kinney, D. K., and Richards, R. (2014). Creativity as "compensatory advantage": Bipolar and schizophrenic liability, the inverted-U hypothesis, and practical implications. In *Creativity and Mental Illness*, ed. J. C. Kaufman, 295–317. Cambridge: Cambridge University Press.

p. 187, **"When I was crazy, that's all I was."** Wagner-Martin, L. (1987). *Sylvia Plath: A Biography*. New York: Simon & Schuster (quote on 112).

p. 187, **Although the scientific evidence indicates.** Schou, M. (1979). Artistic productivity and lithium prophylaxis in manic-depressive illness. *Br J Psychiatry, 135*, 97–103.

p. 188, **John Nash, for example.** Nasar, S. (1998). *A Beautiful Mind*. New York: Simon & Schuster.

p. 188, **His depression relapsed.** Max, D. T. (2012). *Every Love Story Is a Ghost Story: A Life of David Foster Wallace*. New York: Penguin.

p. 188, **"It was a brilliant cure."** https://www.healthyplace.com/depression /articles/famous-shock-therapy-patients.

p. 188, **"It was like a magic wand."** https://people.com/archive/goodbye -darkness-vol-38-no-5/.

p. 188, **Finally, a collection of essays.** Berlin, R. M. (2008). *Poets on Prozac: Mental Illness, Treatment, and the Creative Process*. Baltimore: Johns Hopkins University Press.

p. 189, **She says, "I can still make."** Berlin, R. M. (2008). *Poets on Prozac: Mental Illness, Treatment, and the Creative Process*. Baltimore: Johns Hopkins University Press (quote on 176).

p. 189, **Romantic notions of the "suffering artist."** Rothenberg, A. (2001). Bipolar illness, creativity, and treatment. *Psychiatr Q, 72 (2)*, 131–47; Verhaeghen, P., et al. (2005). Why we sing the blues: The relation between self-reflective rumination, mood, and creativity. *Emotion, 5 (2)*, 226–32.

p. 189, **When creative people suffer.** Murray, G., and Johnson, S. L. (2010). The clinical significance of creativity in bipolar disorder. *Clin Psychol Rev, 30 (6)*, 721–32; Rothenberg, A. (2001). Bipolar illness, creativity, and treatment. *Psychiatr Q, 72 (2)*, 131–47.

p. 189, **Some medications seem to have less impact.** Flaherty, A. W. (2011). Brain illness and creativity: Mechanisms and treatment risks. *Canadian Journal of Psychiatry, 56 (3)*, 132–43.

p. 190, **Weight gain is common.** Velligan, D. I., et al. (2009). The expert consensus guideline series: Adherence problems in patients with serious and persistent mental illness. *J Clin Psychiatry, 70 (supp 4)*, 1–46.

p. 191, **Collin's decision to use alcohol.** CBHSQ. (2015). *Behavioral Health Trends in the United States: Results from the 2014 National Survey on Drug Use and Health* (HHS Publication no. SMA 15-4927).

p. 191, **Relative to the general population.** Hartz, S. M., et al. (2014). Comorbidity of severe psychotic disorders with measures of substance use. *JAMA Psychiatry, 71 (3)*, 248–54.

p. 191, **Adolescents with a past-year major depressive episode.** CBHSQ. (2015). *Behavioral Health Trends in the United States: Results from the 2014 National Survey on Drug Use and Health* (HHS Publication no. SMA 15-4927).

p. 191, **People with serious mental illnesses who use and abuse alcohol.** Czobor, P., et al. (2015). Treatment adherence in schizophrenia: A patient-level meta-analysis of combined CATIE and EUFEST studies. *European Neuropsychopharmacology: The Journal of the European College of Neuropsychopharmacology, 25 (8)*, 1158–66; Gonzalez-Pinto, A., et al. (2006). Suicidal risk in bipolar I disorder patients and adherence to long-term lithium treatment. *Bipolar Disord, 8 (5 Pt 2)*, 618–24; van Nimwegen-Campailla, L., et al. (2010). Effect of early dysphoric response and cannabis use on discontinuation of olanzapine or risperidone in patients with early psychosis. *Pharmacopsychiatry, 43 (7)*, 281; Verdoux, H., et al. (2000). Medication adherence in psychosis: Predictors and impact on outcome. A 2-year follow-up of first-admitted subjects. *Acta Psychiatr Scand, 102 (3)*, 203–10.

Chapter 6. Senseless Suffering

p. 199, **The myth persists.** Meynen, G. (2010). Free will and mental disorder: Exploring the relationship. *Theoretical Medicine and Bioethics, 31 (6)*, 429–43.

p. 199, **Allowing, even requiring, individuals to make decisions.** Gillon, R. (2015). Defending the four principles approach as a good basis for good medical practice and therefore for good medical ethics. *J Med Ethics, 41 (1)*, 111–16.

p. 200, **Andrew Goldstein rose early.** News reports about Andrew Goldstein and Kendra Webdale: http://www.nbcnews.com/id/16713078/ns/dateline_nbc /t/deadly-encounter/#.XQJs_IhKhPY; https://www.nytimes.com/1999/01 /05/nyregion/new-york-nightmare-kills-a-dreamer.html; http://nymag .com/intelligencer/2018/09/andrew-goldstein-release-kendras-law.html; https://www.nytimes.com/2018/09/11/nyregion/kendras-law-andrew -goldstein-subway-murder.html; https://www.wamc.org/post/story -behind-kendra-s-law; https://www.nytimes.com/1999/01/11/nyregion /subway-killing-casts-light-on-suspect-s-mental-torment.html; https:// www.nytimes.com/1999/05/23/magazine/bedlam-on-the-streets.html.

p. 200, **The link between mental illness and violence is complex.** Swanson, J. W., et al. (2015). Mental illness and reduction of gun violence and suicide: Bringing epidemiologic research to policy. *Annals of Epidemiology, 25 (5)*, 366–76.

p. 200, **Nearly half of Americans.** Barry, C. L., et al. (2013). After Newtown–
public opinion on gun policy and mental illness. *New England Journal of
Medicine, 368 (12)*, 1077–81.

p. 200, **In 1990, the first large study.** Swanson, J. W., et al. (1990). Violence and
psychiatric disorder in the community: Evidence from the Epidemiologic Catchment Area surveys. *Hosp Community Psychiatry, 41 (7)*,
761–70.

p. 201, **A more recent survey reported similar patterns.** Van Dorn, R., et al.
(2012). Mental disorder and violence: Is there a relationship beyond
substance use? *Soc Psychiatry Psychiatr Epidemiol, 47 (3)*, 487–503.

p. 201, **However, once we account for the effects of poverty.** Swanson, J. W.,
et al. (2002). The social-environmental context of violent behavior in
persons treated for severe mental illness. *American Journal of Public
Health, 92 (9)*, 1523–31.

p. 201, **Psychiatric symptoms, especially delusions.** Elbogen, E. B., et al.
(2006). Treatment engagement and violence risk in mental disorders. *Br
J Psychiatry, 189*, 354–60; Swanson, J. W., et al. (2008). Comparison of
antipsychotic medication effects on reducing violence in people with
schizophrenia. *Br J Psychiatry, 193 (1)*, 37–43; Witt, K., et al. (2013). Risk
factors for violence in psychosis: Systematic review and meta-regression
analysis of 110 studies. *PLoS One, 8 (2)*, e55942.

p. 201, **The complex relationship between violence and psychosis.** Swanson,
J. W., et al. (2006). A national study of violent behavior in persons with
schizophrenia. *Arch Gen Psychiatry, 63 (5)*, 490–99.

p. 201, **The violent behavior of this group.** Swanson, J. W., et al. (2008). Alternative pathways to violence in persons with schizophrenia: The role of
childhood antisocial behavior problems. *Law Hum Behav, 32 (3)*, 228–40.

p. 202, **People with delusional thinking.** Swanson, J. W., et al. (2006). A
national study of violent behavior in persons with schizophrenia. *Arch
Gen Psychiatry, 63 (5)*, 490–99.

p. 202, **People who knew the shooters.** Silver, J., et al. (2018). *A Study of the
Pre-attack Behaviors of Active Shooters in the United States between
2000–2013.*

p. 202, **Paranoia, hallucinations, delusions.** https://www.secretservice.gov
/forms/USSS_NTAC-Mass_Attacks_in_Public_Spaces-2017.pdf.

p. 203, **In comparison, about 16 percent of homicides.** Torrey, E. F. (2012). *The
Insanity Offense: How America's Failure to Treat the Seriously Mentally Ill
Endangers Its Citizens.* New York: W. W. Norton.

p. 207, **Kendra's Law establishes a procedure.** https://www.omh.ny.gov
/omhweb/kendra_web/ksummary.htm.

p. 208, **A 2005 report by the New York State Office of Mental Health.** https://
www.omh.ny.gov/omhweb/kendra_web/finalreport/aotfinal2005.pdf.

p. 209, **These findings led New York to reauthorize Kendra's Law.** https://
www.omh.ny.gov/omhweb/kendra_web/finalreport/resources.htm.

p. 209, **An independent evaluation of Kendra's Law.** Swartz, M. S., et al. (2009).
New York State Assisted Outpatient Treatment Program Evaluation.
https://www.omh.ny.gov/omhweb/resources/publications/aot_program
_evaluation/report.pdf.

p. 209, **In a follow-up study examining the cost of AOT.** Swanson, J. W., et al.
(2013). The cost of assisted outpatient treatment: Can it save states
money? *Am J Psychiatry, 170 (12),* 1423–32.

p. 210, **Today, forty-seven states.** Cripps, S. N., and Swartz, M. S. (2018).
Update on assisted outpatient treatment. *Curr Psychiatry Rep, 20 (12),*
112.

p. 210, **Even within New York.** Robbins, P. C., et al. (2010). Regional differences
in New York's assisted outpatient treatment program. *Psychiatric
Services, 61 (10),* 970–75.

p. 210, **Mentally ill people still push strangers.** http://nymag.com
/intelligencer/2018/09/andrew-goldstein-release-kendras-law.html.

p. 210, **Given this, it is not surprising that the benefits.** Cripps, S. N., and
Swartz, M. S. (2018). Update on assisted outpatient treatment. *Curr
Psychiatry Rep, 20 (12),* 112.

p. 211, **When the prison population is large.** Penrose, L. S. (1939). Mental
disease and crime: Outline of a comparative study of European statistics.
British Journal of Medical Psychology, 18 (1), 1–15.

p. 211, **More than 40 percent of people with a serious mental illness have
been in jail.** https://www.treatmentadvocacycenter.org/storage
/documents/final_jails_v_hospitals_study.pdf; Kim, K., et al. (2015). *The
Processing and Treatment of Mentally Ill Persons in the Criminal Justice
System: A Scan of Practice and Background Analysis.*

p. 218, **A Yale Law School report found.** https://law.yale.edu/system/files
/documents/pdf/asca-liman_administrative_segregation_report_sep_2
_2015.pdf.

p. 218, **Suicide by hanging.** Metzner, J. L., and Fellner, J. (2010). Solitary
confinement and mental illness in U.S. prisons: A challenge for medical
ethics. *Journal of the American Academy of Psychiatry and the Law
Online, 38 (1),* 104.

p. 219, **A medical witness said, "The history of his past life."** Low, P. W., et al.
(1986). *The Trial of John W. Hinckley, Jr.: A Case Study in the Insanity
Defense.* New York: Foundation Press (quote on 10).

p. 219, **"Every man is to be presumed to be sane."** Low, P. W., et al. (1986). *The
Trial of John W. Hinckley, Jr.: A Case Study in the Insanity Defense.* New
York: Foundation Press (quote on 11).

p. 219, **On average, fewer than 1 defendant in 100.** Melton, G., et al. (2017). *Psychological Evaluations for the Courts: A Handbook for Mental Health Professionals and Lawyers.* New York: Guilford.

p. 219, **To be released from the hospital.** Low, P. W., et al. (1986). *The Trial of John W. Hinckley, Jr.: A Case Study in the Insanity Defense.* New York: Foundation Press.

p. 220, **"My actions of March 30, 1981."** https://www.nytimes.com/1982/07/09/us/hinckley-hails-historical-shooting-to-win-love.html.

p. 221, **Instead, the Supreme Court said that competence means.** https://supreme.justia.com/cases/federal/us/362/402/.

p. 222, **He must, for example, understand.** https://juvenilecompetency.virginia.edu/legal-precedents/dusky-v-united-states.

p. 223, **In April of 2007, 23-year-old Justin Volpe.** News reports about Justin Volpe and Steve Leifman: https://www.governing.com/topics/public-justice-safety/gov-miami-mental-health-jail.html; https://www.bridgemi.com/michigan-health-watch/after-surviving-mental-illness-he-works-keep-others-him-out-jail; https://www.youtube.com/watch?v=UFbyI6I0Mlk.

p. 225, **People charged with minor felonies.** Iglehart, J. K. (2016). Decriminalizing mental illness—the Miami model. *New England Journal of Medicine, 374 (18)*, 1701–3.

p. 226, **Training includes information on signs and symptoms.** Watson, A. C., et al. (2012). The Crisis Intervention Team model of police response to mental health crises: A primer for mental health practitioners. *Best Practices in Mental Health, 8 (2)*, 71–71.

p. 226, **Fatal shootings and injuries.** Iglehart, J. K. (2016). Decriminalizing mental illness—the Miami model. *New England Journal of Medicine, 374 (18)*, 1701–3.

p. 227, **There are now more than three hundred mental health courts.** https://csgjusticecenter.org/mental-health-court-project/.

p. 227, **Just as Penrose's classic study.** Markowitz, F. E. (2006). Psychiatric hospital capacity, homelessness, and crime and arrest rates. *Criminology, 44 (1)*, 45–72.

p. 227, **Although scholars disagree about how to define homelessness.** Lee, B. A., et al. (2010). The new homelessness revisited. *Annual Review of Sociology, 36 (1)*, 501–21.

p. 227, **According to the annual report from the US Department of Housing and Urban Development.** https://files.hudexchange.info/resources/documents/2018-AHAR-Part-1.pdf.

p. 228, **The HUD data.** https://files.hudexchange.info/reports/published/CoC_PopSub_NatlTerrDC_2018.pdf.

p. 228, **Still further evidence of the link.** Kuno, E., et al. (2000). Homelessness among persons with serious mental illness in an enhanced community-based mental health system. *Psychiatr Serv, 51 (8)*, 1012–16.

p. 228, **Among people with serious mental illness, those who are homeless.** Folsom, D. P., et al. (2005). Prevalence and risk factors for homelessness and utilization of mental health services among 10,340 patients with serious mental illness in a large public mental health system. *Am J Psychiatry, 162 (2)*, 370–76.

p. 228, **What's more, homeless people with serious mental illnesses.** Kuhn, R., and Culhane, D. P. (1998). Applying cluster analysis to test a typology of homelessness by pattern of shelter utilization: Results from the analysis of administrative data. *Am J Community Psychol, 26 (2)*, 207–32.

p. 228, **The study also found that homeless people.** Sullivan, G., et al. (2000). Quality of life of homeless persons with mental illness: Results from the course-of-homelessness study. *Psychiatr Serv, 51 (9)*, 1135–41.

p. 229, **Among people with serious mental illness, rates of criminal behavior.** Roy, L., et al. (2014). Criminal behavior and victimization among homeless individuals with severe mental illness: A systematic review. *Psychiatr Serv, 65 (6)*, 739–50.

p. 229, **A national study found that recent homelessness.** Greenberg, G. A., and Rosenheck, R. A. (2008). Jail incarceration, homelessness, and mental health: A national study. *Psychiatr Serv, 59 (2)*, 170–77.

p. 229, **When Atlanta hosted the 1996 Summer Olympics.** Burbank, M. J., et al. (2001). *Olympic Dreams: The Impact of Mega-events on Local Politics.* Boulder, CO: Lynne Reiner.

p. 230, **This was not a popular idea.** https://archive.macleans.ca/article/2007/6/18/reinventing-the-asylum.

p. 230, **In response, the Federation of Canadian Municipalities.** Macnaughton, E., et al. (2013). Bringing politics and evidence together: Policy entrepreneurship and the conception of the At Home / Chez Soi Housing First Initiative for addressing homelessness and mental illness in Canada. *Soc Sci Med, 82*, 100–107.

p. 230, **Some say he was motivated by the 1950 disappearance.** https://www.theglobeandmail.com/opinion/a-family-tragedy-that-stephen-harper-has-not-forgotten/article787903/.

p. 231, **A small number of studies conducted in the United States.** Nelson, G., et al. (2007). A review of the literature on the effectiveness of housing and support, assertive community treatment, and intensive case management interventions for persons with mental illness who have been homeless. *Am J Orthopsychiatry, 77 (3)*, 350–61.

p. 232, **Housing First programs serving a broader population.** Goering, P. N., et al. (2011). The At Home / Chez Soi trial protocol: A pragmatic, multi-site, randomised controlled trial of a Housing First intervention for homeless individuals with mental illness in five Canadian cities. *BMJ Open, 1 (2)*, e000323.

p. 232, **The study found that At Home/Chez Soi was more effective.** Goering, P., et al. (2014). *National At Home/Chez Soi Final Report.* https://www .mentalhealthcommission.ca/sites/default/files/mhcc_at_home_report _national_cross-site_eng_2_0.pdf.

p. 233, **Further, every $10 invested in At Home/Chez Soi.** https://www .mentalhealthcommission.ca/sites/default/files/mhcc_at_home_report _national_cross-site_eng_2_0.pdf.

p. 233, **The program is sustainable.** Nelson, G., et al. (2016). *The At Home/Chez Soi Project: Cross-Site Report on the Sustainability of Housing and Support Programs Implemented.* https://www.mentalhealthcommission.ca/sites /default/files/2016-11/at_home_sustainability_crosssite_report_eng.pdf.

p. 233, **The National Alliance to End Homelessness website.** https:// endhomelessness.org/.

p. 233, **A 2008 review of studies in the United States.** Choe, J. Y., et al. (2008). Perpetration of violence, violent victimization, and severe mental illness: Balancing public health concerns. *Psychiatr Serv, 59 (2)*, 153–64.

p. 233, **People with mental illness who are victimized.** Swartz, M. S., and Bhattacharya, S. (2017). Victimization of persons with severe mental illness: A pressing global health problem. *World Psychiatry: Official Journal of the World Psychiatric Association (WPA), 16 (1)*, 26–27.

p. 234, **Rates of victimization are higher for women.** Latalova, K., et al. (2014). Violent victimization of adult patients with severe mental illness: A systematic review. *Neuropsychiatr Dis Treat, 10*, 1925–39; Tsai, A. C., et al. (2015). Violent victimization, mental health, and service utilization outcomes in a cohort of homeless and unstably housed women living with or at risk of becoming infected with HIV. *Am J Epidemiol, 181 (10)*, 817–26.

p. 234, **People with serious mental illness were three times more likely.** Khalifeh, H., et al. (2015). Violent and non-violent crime against adults with severe mental illness. *British Journal of Psychiatry, 206 (4)*, 275–82.

p. 234, **Once they got off the buses.** https://www.beckershospitalreview.com /legal-regulatory-issues/mental-health-patients-win-patient-dumping -suit-against-nevada-psych-hospital.html.

p. 235, **It did not take long for police to identify the woman as 22-year-old Rebecca Hall.** News reports about Rebecca Hall: https://www.npr.org /sections/thetwo-way/2018/01/24/580347464/federal-investigation -launched-after-baltimore-patient-left-at-a-bus-stop-in-a-g; https://www .baltimoresun.com/health/bs-hs-patient-dumping-press-conference -20180118-story.html; https://www.washingtonpost.com/local/she-was -tossed-from-a-hospital-on-a-cold-night-wearing-only-a-gown-the-viral

-video-followed-years-of-struggles/2018/04/12/a768f3c2-061c-11e8
-a602-3b8549a2d1ac_story.html?utm_term=.210dd8e7831a; https://
www.washingtonpost.com/local/she-was-tossed-from-a-hospital-on-a
-cold-night-wearing-only-a-gown-the-viral-video-followed-years-of
-struggles/2018/04/12/a768f3c2-061c-11e8-a602-3b8549a2d1ac_story
.html?utm_term=.928eede2c5a7.

p. 236, **Hospitals unable to do so may transfer.** Kahntroff, J., and Watson, R.
(2009). Refusal of emergency care and patient dumping. *Health Law, 11
(1)*, 49–53.

p. 236, **From 1996 to 2000, the watchdog organization Public Citizen.** Black,
K., and Wolfe, S. M. (2001). *Questionable Hospitals: 527 Hospitals That
Violate the Emergency Medical Treatment and Labor Act: A Detailed Look
at "Patient Dumping."* https://www.citizen.org/wp-content/uploads
/qhcompletereport.pdf.

p. 236, **Deborah Danner was one of the 242 people.** News reports about
Deborah Danner: https://www.nbcnews.com/news/us-news/troubled
-bronx-woman-deborah-danner-was-battling-own-family-when
-n670826; https://www.nytimes.com/2018/02/01/nyregion/barry-bronx
-shooting-trial.html; https://www.nytimes.com/2018/01/29/nyregion
/sergeant-murder-trial-danner.html; https://www.nbcnewyork.com
/news/local/NYPD-Officer-Hugh-Barry-Trial-Testimony-Deborah
-Danner-Shooting-Death-Baseball-Bat-472966703.html; https://www
.wsj.com/articles/fellow-officer-muddies-prosecutions-case-in-new-york
-sergeants-murder-trial-1517617873; https://www.nytimes.com/2016
/10/21/opinion/the-death-of-deborah-danner.html; https://assets
.documentcloud.org/documents/3146953/Living-With-Schizophrenia
-by-Deborah-Danner.pdf; https://www.washingtonpost.com/graphics
/national/police-shootings-2016/?noredirect=on.

p. 238, **Some estimate that the risk of being killed.** Fuller, D. A., et al. (2015).
*Overlooked in the Undercounted: The Role of Mental Illness in Fatal Law
Enforcement Encounters.* https://www.treatmentadvocacycenter.org/storage
/documents/overlooked-in-the-undercounted.pdf; Lane-McKinley, K., et al.
(2018). The Deborah Danner story: Officer-involved deaths of people living
with mental illness. *Acad Psychiatry, 42 (4)*, 443–50.

p. 238, **At this rate, having signs of a mental illness.** Saleh, A. Z., et al.
(2018). Deaths of people with mental illness during interactions with
law enforcement. *International Journal of Law and Psychiatry, 58*,
110–16.

p. 238, **People with mental illness were nearly three times more likely to
have been at home.** Saleh, A. Z., et al. (2018). Deaths of people with
mental illness during interactions with law enforcement. *International
Journal of Law and Psychiatry, 58*, 110–16.

p. 239, **In 2012, four years before Deborah Danner's death.** https://assets
.documentcloud.org/documents/3146953/Living-With-Schizophrenia
-by-Deborah-Danner.pdf.

p. 240, **While research on the effectiveness of CIT is limited.** Steadman, H. J.,
et al. (2000). Comparing outcomes of major models of police responses
to mental health emergencies. *Psychiatr Serv, 51 (5)*, 645–49; Broner, N.,
et al. (2004). Effects of diversion on adults with co-occurring mental
illness and substance use: Outcomes from a national multi-site study.
Behav Sci Law, 22 (4), 519–41; Dupont, R., and Cochran, S. (2000). Police
response to mental health emergencies—barriers to change. *Journal of
the American Academy of Psychiatry and the Law, 28 (3)*, 338–44.

p. 240, **Details about starting a CIT program.** http://www.citinternational.org
/Learn-About-CIT.

p. 240, **CAHOOTS provides mobile crisis intervention.** https://whitebirdclinic
.org/cahoots/.

p. 241, **Although formal evaluations have yet to be completed.** https://www
.wsj.com/articles/when-mental-health-experts-not-police-are-the-first
-responders-1543071600.

p. 241, **In 2017, a total of 47,173 people in the United States died by suicide.**
https://afsp.org/about-suicide/suicide-statistics/.

p. 241, **For decades, psychological autopsies.** Brådvik, L. (2018). Suicide risk
and mental disorders. *International Journal of Environmental Research
and Public Health, 15 (9)*, 2028.

p. 241, **Recent data from the Centers for Disease Control and Prevention.**
https://www.cdc.gov/vitalsigns/pdf/vs-0618-suicide-H.pdf.

p. 241, **Every year, approximately 30 to 40 percent.** Huang, X., et al. (2018).
Psychosis as a risk factor for suicidal thoughts and behaviors: A
meta-analysis of longitudinal studies. *Psychol Med, 48 (5)*, 765–76.

p. 241, **In the general community only 3 percent.** Kochanek, K. D., et al. (2016).
Deaths: Final data for 2014. *Natl Vital Stat Rep, 65 (4)*, 1–122.

p. 241, **Although women are more likely.** https://www.cdc.gov/violence
prevention/pdf/suicide-datasheet-a.pdf.

p. 242, **Approximately 15 to 20 percent of people with bipolar disorder.**
Simon, G. E., et al. (2007). Risk of suicide attempt and suicide death in
patients treated for bipolar disorder. *Bipolar Disord, 9 (5)*, 526–30.

p. 242, **Suicide deaths are significantly greater for men.** Schaffer, A., et al.
(2014). International Society for Bipolar Disorders Task Force on Suicide:
Meta-analyses and meta-regression of correlates of suicide attempts and
suicide deaths in bipolar disorder. *Bipolar Disord, 17*, 1–16.

p. 242, **Risk factors for suicide death.** Hawton, K., et al. (2013). Risk factors for
suicide in individuals with depression: A systematic review. *J Affect
Disord, 147 (1–3)*, 17–28.

p. 242, **Risk factors for suicide attempts.** Cassidy, R. M., et al. (2018). Risk factors for suicidality in patients with schizophrenia: A systematic review, meta-analysis, and meta-regression of 96 studies. *Schizophr Bull, 44 (4)*, 787–97.

p. 242, **Risk factors for death by suicide.** Cassidy, R. M., et al. (2018). Risk factors for suicidality in patients with schizophrenia: A systematic review, meta-analysis, and meta-regression of 96 studies. *Schizophr Bull, 44 (4)*, 787–97.

p. 242, **Two medications—clozapine and lithium.** Griffiths, J. J., et al. (2014). Existing and novel biological therapeutics in suicide prevention. *Am J Prev Med, 47 (3 supp 2)*, S195–S203.

p. 242, **InterSePt, a large, multicenter, international randomized controlled trial.** Meltzer, H. Y., et al. (2003). Clozapine treatment for suicidality in schizophrenia: International Suicide Prevention Trial (InterSePT). *Arch Gen Psychiatry, 60 (1)*, 82–91.

p. 243, **It is likely that, rather than decreasing suicidal ideation.** Lauterbach, E., et al. (2008). Adjunctive lithium treatment in the prevention of suicidal behaviour in depressive disorders: A randomised, placebo-controlled, 1-year trial. *Acta Psychiatr Scand, 118 (6)*, 469–79; Oquendo, M. A., et al. (2011). Treatment of suicide attempters with bipolar disorder: A randomized clinical trial comparing lithium and valproate in the prevention of suicidal behavior. *Am J Psychiatry, 168 (10)*, 1050–56.

p. 243, **A meta-analysis of the data from these trials.** Cipriani, A., et al. (2013). Lithium in the prevention of suicide in mood disorders: Updated systematic review and meta-analysis. *BMJ, 346*, f3646.

p. 245, **In the immediate aftermath of suicide.** Bolton, J. M., et al. (2013). Parents bereaved by offspring suicide: A population-based longitudinal case-control study. *JAMA Psychiatry, 70 (2)*, 158–67; Brent, D., et al. (2009). The incidence and course of depression in bereaved youth 21 months after the loss of a parent to suicide, accident, or sudden natural death. *Am J Psychiatry, 166 (7)*, 786–94; Pitman, A., et al. (2014). Effects of suicide bereavement on mental health and suicide risk. *Lancet Psychiatry, 1 (1)*, 86–94; Pitman, A. L., et al. (2016). Bereavement by suicide as a risk factor for suicide attempt: A cross-sectional national UK-wide study of 3432 young bereaved adults. *BMJ Open, 6 (1)*, e009948; Rostila, M., et al. (2013). Suicide following the death of a sibling: A nationwide follow-up study from Sweden. *BMJ Open, 3 (4)*.

p. 245, **Family members bereaved by suicide are at increased risk.** Spillane, A., et al. (2017). Physical and psychosomatic health outcomes in people bereaved by suicide compared to people bereaved by other modes of death: A systematic review. *BMC Public Health, 17 (1)*, 939.

p. 245, **They also experience more emotional distress.** Cerel, J., and Roberts, T. A. (2005). Suicidal behavior in the family and adolescent risk behavior. *J Adolesc Health, 36 (4)*, 352.e359-16.

p. 245, **Compared with children whose mother or father died of cancer.** Pfeffer, C. R., et al. (2000). Child survivors of parental death from cancer or suicide: Depressive and behavioral outcomes. *Psychooncology, 9 (1)*, 1–10.

p. 245, **Some have suggested that families that lose a loved one.** Maple, M., et al. (2014). Uncovering and identifying the missing voices in suicide bereavement. *Suicidology Online, 5*, 1–12.

p. 246, **Suicide, like mental illness, is laden with stigma.** Pitman, A. L., et al. (2016). Bereavement by suicide as a risk factor for suicide attempt: A cross-sectional national UK-wide study of 3432 young bereaved adults. *BMJ Open, 6 (1)*, e009948.

p. 251, **Asking the women about when they had talked.** Pruchno, R. A., et al. (1996). Aging women and their children with chronic disabilities: Perceptions of sibling involvement and effects on well-being. *Family Relations, 45*, 318–26.

p. 252, **In his book.** Giese, A. (2018). *When Mental Illness Strikes: Crisis Intervention for the Financial Plan.* Austin, TX: Lioncret.

p. 252, **ABLE accounts are tax-advantaged savings accounts.** http://ablenrc .org/about/what-are-able-accounts.

p. 255, **In 2006, the United Nations Convention on the Rights of Persons with Disabilities.** https://www.un.org/development/desa/disabilities /convention-on-the-rights-of-persons-with-disabilities/article-12-equal -recognition-before-the-law.html.

p. 256, **Depression can make decision-making difficult.** Velligan, D. I., et al. (2016). What patients with severe mental illness transitioning from hospital to community have to say about care and shared decision-making. *Issues in Mental Health Nursing, 37 (6)*, 400–405.

p. 256, **People with serious mental illnesses can make competent and prudent treatment decisions.** Carpenter, W. T., et al. (2000). Decisional capacity for informed consent in schizophrenia research. *Arch Gen Psychiatry, 57 (6)*, 533–38; Corrigan, P. W., et al. (2012). From adherence to self-determination: Evolution of a treatment paradigm for people with serious mental illnesses. *Psychiatr Serv, 63 (2)*, 169–73; Hamann, J., et al. (2006). Shared decision making for in-patients with schizophrenia. *Acta Psychiatr Scand, 114 (4)*, 265–73.

p. 256, **With SDM, people with mental illness.** Jeste, D. V., et al. (2018). Supported decision making in serious mental illness. *Psychiatry, 81 (1)*, 28–40.

p. 258, **US courts, legislators, policy makers, and national organizations.** Jeste, D. V., et al. (2018). Supported decision making in serious mental illness. *Psychiatry, 81 (1)*, 28–40.

p. 258, **In 2015, Texas passed a law.** Van Puymbrouck, L. (2017). *Supported Decision Making in the United States: A White Paper by CQL.*

p. 258, **Up-to-date information about SDM in each state.** http://supported decisionmaking.org/states.

p. 258, **Emerging evidence from patients and family.** Kokanovic, R., et al. (2018). Supported decision-making from the perspectives of mental health service users, family members supporting them and mental health practitioners. *Aust N Z J Psychiatry, 52 (9),* 826–33.

p. 259, **Some people worry that SDM may expose.** Kohn, N. A., et al. (2013). Supported decision making: A viable alternative to guardianship? *Penn State Law Review, 117,* 1111–57.

p. 260, **State-by-state information.** https://www.nrc-pad.org/.

p. 260, **Although few people with serious mental illness have a PAD.** Nicaise, P., et al. (2013). Psychiatric Advance Directives as a complex and multistage intervention: A realist systematic review. *Health Soc Care Community, 21 (1),* 1–14; Elbogen, E. B., et al. (2007). Effectively implementing psychiatric advance directives to promote self-determination of treatment among people with mental illness. *Psychol Public Policy Law, 13 (4).*

p. 260, **A review of the effectiveness of PADs.** Khazaal, Y., et al. (2014). Psychiatric advance directives, a possible way to overcome coercion and promote empowerment. *Frontiers in Public Health, 2 (37).*

p. 260, **There is evidence that people who are offered medications.** Wilder, C. M., et al. (2010). Medication preferences and adherence among individuals with severe mental illness and psychiatric advance directives. *Psychiatr Serv, 61 (4),* 380–85.

Chapter 7. Remarkable Resilience

p. 263, **Pioneering psychiatrist Emil Kraepelin defined dementia praecox.** Ebert, A., and Bär, K.-J. (2010). Emil Kraepelin: A pioneer of scientific understanding of psychiatry and psychopharmacology. *Indian Journal of Psychiatry, 52 (2),* 191–92.

p. 263, **According to this perspective, one-third of people deteriorate.** Liberman, R. P., et al. (2002). Operational criteria and factors related to recovery from schizophrenia. *International Review of Psychiatry, 14 (4),* 256–72.

p. 264, **As many as 70 percent of people with schizophrenia.** Bellack, A. S. (2006). Scientific and consumer models of recovery in schizophrenia: Concordance, contrasts, and implications. *Schizophr Bull, 32 (3),* 432–42.

p. 264, **People with bipolar disorder and depression typically experience.** Goldberg, J. F., et al. (2005). Long-term remission and recovery in bipolar disorder: A review. *Curr Psychiatry Rep, 7 (6),* 456–61; Verduijn, J., et al.

(2017). Reconsidering the prognosis of major depressive disorder across diagnostic boundaries: Full recovery is the exception rather than the rule. *BMC Med, 15 (1)*, 215.

p. 264, **In 2003, the Remission in Schizophrenia Working Group.** Andreasen, N. C., et al. (2005). Remission in schizophrenia: Proposed criteria and rationale for consensus. *Am J Psychiatry, 162 (3)*, 441–49.

p. 264, **This committee was guided by the goals of a similar group.** Frank, E., et al. (1991). Conceptualization and rationale for consensus definitions of terms in major depressive disorder. Remission, recovery, relapse, and recurrence. *Arch Gen Psychiatry, 48 (9)*, 851–55.

p. 264, **The Schizophrenia Working Group defined remission.** Andreasen, N. C., et al. (2005). Remission in schizophrenia: Proposed criteria and rationale for consensus. *Am J Psychiatry, 162 (3)*, 441–49 (quote on 442).

p. 264, **A group of bipolar disorder experts defined remission.** Hirschfeld, R. M., et al. (2007). Defining the clinical course of bipolar disorder: Response, remission, relapse, recurrence, and roughening. *Psychopharmacol Bull, 40 (3)*, 7–14.

p. 264, **Over a two-year period, 58 percent of people diagnosed with depression.** Verduijn, J., et al. (2017). Reconsidering the prognosis of major depressive disorder across diagnostic boundaries: Full recovery is the exception rather than the rule. *BMC Med, 15 (1)*, 215.

p. 265, **A national survey of community-dwelling people.** Salzer, M. S., et al. (2018). National estimates of recovery-remission from serious mental illness. *Psychiatr Serv, 69 (5)*, 523–28.

p. 265, **About 25 percent of people between the ages of 20 and 32.** Salzer, M. S., et al. (2018). National estimates of recovery-remission from serious mental illness. *Psychiatr Serv, 69 (5)*, 523–28.

p. 266, **This group contended that to experience recovery.** Andreasen, N. C., et al. (2005). Remission in schizophrenia: Proposed criteria and rationale for consensus. *Am J Psychiatry, 162 (3)*, 441–49.

p. 266, **Clinical recovery is typically considered to be an outcome.** Harrow, M., et al. (2012). Do all schizophrenia patients need antipsychotic treatment continuously throughout their lifetime? A 20-year longitudinal study. *Psychol Med, 42 (10)*, 2145–55; Torgalsbøen, A.-K., and Rund, B. (2009). Lessons learned from three studies of recovery from schizophrenia. *International Review of Psychiatry, 14*.

p. 266, **In an effort to advance the state of the science.** Liberman, R. P., et al. (2002). Operational criteria and factors related to recovery from schizophrenia. *International Review of Psychiatry, 14 (4)*, 256–72; Nasrallah, H. A., et al. (2005). Defining and measuring clinical effectiveness in the treatment of schizophrenia. *Psychiatr Serv, 56 (3)*, 273–82.

p. 266, **Not surprisingly, rates of recovery vary.** Hegarty, J. D., et al. (1994). One hundred years of schizophrenia: A meta-analysis of the outcome literature. *Am J Psychiatry, 151 (10)*, 1409–16; Jaaskelainen, E., et al. (2013). A systematic review and meta-analysis of recovery in schizophrenia. *Schizophr Bull, 39 (6)*, 1296–1306; Menezes, N. M., et al. (2006). A systematic review of longitudinal outcome studies of first-episode psychosis. *Psychol Med, 36 (10)*, 1349–62.

p. 266, **Because many definitions of clinical recovery include medication adherence.** Nasrallah, H. A., et al. (2005). Defining and measuring clinical effectiveness in the treatment of schizophrenia. *Psychiatr Serv, 56 (3)*, 273–82.

p. 266, **Other definitions of recovery.** Harrow, M., et al. (2005). Do patients with schizophrenia ever show periods of recovery? A 15-year multi-follow-up study. *Schizophr Bull, 31 (3)*, 723–34.

p. 268, **At each of the six follow-up assessments.** Harrow, M., et al. (2012). Do all schizophrenia patients need antipsychotic treatment continuously throughout their lifetime? A 20-year longitudinal study. *Psychol Med, 42 (10)*, 2145–55; Harrow, M., et al. (2017). A 20-year multi-followup longitudinal study assessing whether antipsychotic medications contribute to work functioning in schizophrenia. *Psychiatry Res, 256*, 267–74.

p. 268, **Harrow's team concluded.** Harrow, M., et al. (2012). Do all schizophrenia patients need antipsychotic treatment continuously throughout their lifetime? A 20-year longitudinal study. *Psychol Med, 42 (10)*, 2145–55; Harrow, M., et al. (2017). A 20-year multi-followup longitudinal study assessing whether antipsychotic medications contribute to work functioning in schizophrenia. *Psychiatry Res, 256*, 267–74.

p. 268, **At least seven other studies.** Bland, R. C. P., J.H. (1978). Prognosis in schizophrenia. Prognostic predictors and outcome. *Archives of General Psychiatry, 35*, 72–77; Harrison, G., et al. (2001). Recovery from psychotic illness: A 15- and 25-year international follow-up study. *British Journal of Psychiatry, 178 (6)*, 506–17; Kotov, R., et al. (2017). Declining clinical course of psychotic disorders over the two decades following first hospitalization: Evidence from the Suffolk County Mental Health Project. *Am J Psychiatry, 174 (11)*, 1064–74; Moilanen, J., et al. (2013). Characteristics of subjects with schizophrenia spectrum disorder with and without antipsychotic medication—a 10-year follow-up of the Northern Finland 1966 Birth Cohort study. *Eur Psychiatry, 28 (1)*, 53–58; Morgan, C., et al. (2014). Reappraising the long-term course and outcome of psychotic disorders: The AESOP-10 study. *Psychol Med, 44 (13)*, 2713–26; Wils, R. S., et al. (2017). Antipsychotic medication and remission of psychotic symptoms 10 years after a first-episode psychosis. *Schizophr Res, 182*, 42–48; Wunderink, L., et al. (2013). Recovery in remitted first-episode psychosis at 7 years of follow-up of an early dose reduction/discontinuation or maintenance treatment strategy: Long-term follow-up of a 2-year randomized clinical trial. *JAMA Psychiatry, 70 (9)*, 913–20.

p. 268, **Unlike short-term studies that consistently find benefits.** Leucht, S., et al. (2012). Antipsychotic drugs versus placebo for relapse prevention in schizophrenia: A systematic review and meta-analysis. *Lancet, 379 (9831)*, 2063–71.

p. 268, **A 2020 study that followed 62,250 patients.** Taipale, H., et al. (2020). 20-year follow-up study of physical morbidity and mortality in relationship to antipsychotic treatment in a nationwide cohort of 62,250 patients with schizophrenia (FIN20). *World Psychiatry, 19 (1)*, 61–68.

p. 269, **Harrow and his team.** Harrow, M., et al. (2012). Do all schizophrenia patients need antipsychotic treatment continuously throughout their lifetime? A 20-year longitudinal study. *Psychol Med, 42 (10)*, 2145–55.

p. 270, **In sum, serious mental illnesses are often episodic.** Bellack, A. S. (2006). Scientific and consumer models of recovery in schizophrenia: Concordance, contrasts, and implications. *Schizophr Bull, 32 (3)*, 432–42.

p. 270, **These people tend to be older.** Tani, H., et al. (2018). Clinical characteristics of patients with schizophrenia who successfully discontinued antipsychotics: A literature review. *J Clin Psychopharmacol, 38 (6)*, 582–89.

p. 271, **Patricia Deegan was the oldest child.** Deegan, P. E. (1997). Recovery and empowerment for people with psychiatric disabilities. *Soc Work Health Care, 25 (3)*, 11–24.

p. 271, **He said, "Miss Deegan, you have a disease called schizophrenia."** Deegan, P. E. (1997). Recovery and empowerment for people with psychiatric disabilities. *Soc Work Health Care, 25 (3)*, 11–24 (quote on 16).

p. 272, **Pat said to herself, "I'll become Dr. Deegan."** Deegan, P. E. (2002). Recovery as a self-directed process of healing and transformation. *Occupational Therapy in Mental Health, 17 (3–4)*, 5–21 (quote on 11).

p. 272, **More than thirty years ago, Pat Deegan published a paper.** Deegan, P. E. (1988). Recovery: The lived experience of rehabilitation. *Psychosocial Rehabilitation Journal, 11 (4)*, 11–19.

p. 272, **She said that people with psychiatric illnesses "need to meet the challenge."** Deegan, P. E. (1988). Recovery: The lived experience of rehabilitation. *Psychosocial Rehabilitation Journal, 11 (4)*, 11–19 (quote on 11).

p. 275, **Deegan's work encouraged others.** Anonymous. (1989). How I've managed chronic mental illness. *Schizophrenia Bulletin, 15 (4)*, 635–40; Leete, E. (1989). How I perceive and manage my illness. *Schizophrenia Bulletin, 15 (2)*, 197–200; Mead, S., and Copeland, M. E. (2000). What recovery means to us: Consumers' perspectives. *Community Ment Health J, 36 (3)*, 315–28; Unzicker, R. (1989). On my own: A personal journey through madness and re-emergence. *Psychosocial Rehabilitation Journal, 13 (1)*, 71–77.

p. 275, **Rather, it is a process that varies.** Lysaker, P. H., et al. (2010). Recovery and wellness amidst schizophrenia: Definitions, evidence, and the implications for clinical practice. *J Am Psychiatr Nurses Assoc, 16 (1)*, 36–42.

p. 275, **Connectedness, hope, identity, meaning, and empowerment.** Leamy, M., et al. (2011). Conceptual framework for personal recovery in mental health: Systematic review and narrative synthesis. *Br J Psychiatry, 199 (6)*, 445–52.

p. 275, **The CHIME framework.** Van Weeghel, J., et al. (2019). Conceptualizations, assessments, and implications of personal recovery in mental illness: A scoping review of systematic reviews and meta-analyses. *Psychiatr Rehabil J, 42 (2)*, 169–81.

p. 275, **A growing number of programs helped people.** Thomas, E. C., et al. (2018). Person-oriented recovery of individuals with serious mental illnesses: A review and meta-analysis of longitudinal findings. *Psychiatr Serv, 69 (3)*, 259–67.

p. 276, **Interventions that include collaborative efforts.** Barbic, S., et al. (2009). A randomized controlled trial of the effectiveness of a modified recovery workbook program: Preliminary findings. *Psychiatr Serv, 60 (4)*, 491–97.

p. 276, **They demonstrate coping strategies.** King, A. J., and Simmons, M. B. (2018). A systematic review of the attributes and outcomes of peer work and guidelines for reporting studies of peer interventions. *Psychiatr Serv, 69 (9)*, 961–77.

p. 278, **A recent analysis of thirty-seven studies.** Van Eck, R. M., et al. (2018). The relationship between clinical and personal recovery in patients with schizophrenia spectrum disorders: A systematic review and meta-analysis. *Schizophr Bull, 44 (3)*, 631–42.

p. 281, **Families often provide economic support.** Clark, R. E. (2001). Family support and substance use outcomes for persons with mental illness and substance use disorders. *Schizophr Bull, 27 (1)*, 93–101; Cohen, A. N., et al. (2013). Preferences for family involvement in care among consumers with serious mental illness. *Psychiatr Serv, 64 (3)*, 257–63; Gerson, L. D., and Rose, L. E. (2012). Needs of persons with serious mental illness following discharge from inpatient treatment: Patient and family views. *Arch Psychiatr Nurs, 26 (4)*, 261–71.

p. 281, **They can provide important information to the health care team.** Wilkinson, C., and McAndrew, S. (2008). "I'm not an outsider, I'm his mother!" A phenomenological enquiry into carer experiences of exclusion from acute psychiatric settings. *Int J Ment Health Nurs, 17 (6)*, 392–401.

p. 283, **Over time, as families must bend and adapt.** Hatfield, A. B., and Lefley, H. P. (1987). *Families of the Mentally Ill: Coping and Adaption*. New York: Guilford.

p. 283, **A vast amount of research documents the burden.** Dore, G., and Romans, S. E. (2001). Impact of bipolar affective disorder on family and partners. *J Affect Disord, 67 (1–3)*, 147–58; Ogilvie, A. D., et al. (2005). The burden on informal caregivers of people with bipolar disorder. *Bipolar Disord, 7 Suppl 1*, 25–32; Smith, L., et al. (2014). Mental and physical illness in caregivers: Results from an English national survey sample. *Br J Psychiatry, 205 (3)*, 197–203.

p. 283, **Parents often provide decades of extended care.** Judd, L. L., et al. (2002). The long-term natural history of the weekly symptomatic status of bipolar I disorder. *Arch Gen Psychiatry, 59 (6)*, 530–37; Mueser, K. T., and McGurk, S. R. (2004). Schizophrenia. *Lancet, 363 (9426)*, 2063–72.

p. 283, **Providing this care can lead to poorer physical and mental health.** Aschbrenner, K. A., et al. (2009). Parenting an adult child with bipolar disorder in later life. *J Nerv Ment Dis, 197 (5)*, 298–304.

p. 284, **Mental illness in parents is associated with psychiatric disturbances.** Mednick, S. A. (1966). A longitudinal study of children with a high risk for schizophrenia. *Ment Hyg, 50 (4)*, 522–35; Perlick, D. A., et al. (2007). Prevalence and correlates of burden among caregivers of patients with bipolar disorder enrolled in the Systematic Treatment Enhancement Program for Bipolar Disorder. *Bipolar Disord, 9 (3)*, 262–73; Rutter, M. (1966). *Children of Sick Parents: An Environmental and Psychiatric Study*. Oxford: Oxford University Press; Rutter, M., and Quinton, D. (1984). Parental psychiatric disorder: Effects on children. *Psychol Med, 14 (4)*, 853–80; Weissman, M. M., et al. (2016). Offspring of depressed parents: 30 years later. *Am J Psychiatry, 173 (10)*, 1024–32; Weissman, M. M., et al. (2006). Offspring of depressed parents: 20 years later. *Am J Psychiatry, 163 (6)*, 1001–8; Williams, O. B., and Corrigan, P. W. (1992). The differential effects of parental alcoholism and mental illness on their adult children. *J Clin Psychol, 48 (3)*, 406–14.

p. 284, **Children having a parent with a serious mental illness.** Goodman, S. H. (1984). Children of disturbed parents: The interface between research and intervention. *Am J Community Psychol, 12 (6)*, 663–87; Parnas, J., et al. (1993). Lifetime DSM-III-R diagnostic outcomes in the offspring of schizophrenic mothers. Results from the Copenhagen High-Risk Study. *Arch Gen Psychiatry, 50 (9)*, 707–14; Rutter, M., and Quinton, D. (1984). Parental psychiatric disorder: Effects on children. *Psychol Med, 14 (4)*, 853–80.

p. 284, **Adult children of parents with schizophrenia.** Terzian, A. C., et al. (2007). A cross-sectional study to investigate current social adjustment of offspring of patients with schizophrenia. *Eur Arch Psychiatry Clin Neurosci, 257 (4)*, 230–36.

p. 284, **Similarly, siblings of people with serious mental illness.** Farmer, A., et al. (2003). A sib-pair study of the Temperament and Character Inventory scales in major depression. *Arch Gen Psychiatry, 60 (5)*, 490–96; Masi, G., et al. (2003). Temperament in adolescents with anxiety and depressive disorders and in their families. *Child Psychiatry Hum Dev, 33 (3)*, 245–59; Taylor, J. L., et al. (2008). Siblings of adults with mild intellectual deficits or mental illness: Differential life course outcomes. *J Fam Psychol, 22 (6)*, 905–14.

p. 284, **People who grew up with a brother or sister with schizophrenia.** Wolfe, B., et al. (2014). Ripple effects of developmental disabilities and mental illness on nondisabled adult siblings. *Soc Sci Med, 108*, 1–9.

p. 284, **A *Modern Love* column by Mark Lukach.** https://www.nytimes.com/2011/11/27/fashion/out-of-the-darkness-modern-love.html.

p. 284, **Research finds that spouses of depressed.** Idstad, M., et al. (2010). Mental disorder and caregiver burden in spouses: The Nord-Trondelag health study. *BMC Public Health, 10*, 516; Wittmund, B., et al. (2002). Depressive disorders in spouses of mentally ill patients. *Soc Psychiatry Psychiatr Epidemiol, 37 (4)*, 177–82.

p. 285, **What might be important to their loved one.** Reupert, A., et al. (2015). Place of family in recovery models for those with a mental illness. *Int J Ment Health Nurs, 24 (6)*, 495–506.

p. 285, **These challenges are difficult.** Sin, J., et al. (2017). Effectiveness of psychoeducational interventions for family carers of people with psychosis: A systematic review and meta-analysis. *Clin Psychol Rev, 56*, 13–24.

p. 286, **The first step toward recovery for a family member.** Spaniol, L. (2010). The pain and the possibility: The family recovery process. *Community Ment Health J, 46 (5)*, 482–85.

p. 287, **Not surprisingly, each family member recovers.** Spaniol, L., and Nelson, A. (2015). Family recovery. *Community Ment Health J, 51 (7)*, 761–67.

p. 287, **NAMI and the Schizophrenia and Related Disorders Alliance of America offer.** https://www.nami.org/Find-Support/NAMI-Programs; https://sardaa.org/about-sardaa/.

p. 287, **In most communities in the United States, stigma about mental illnesses.** Van Bilsen, H. P. J. G. (2016). Lessons to be learned from the oldest community psychiatric service in the world: Geel in Belgium. *BJPsych Bulletin, 40 (4)*, 207–11.

p. 288, **In 1247, Dymphna was canonized.** Goldstein, J. L., and Godemont, M. M. (2003). The legend and lessons of Geel, Belgium: A 1500-year-old legend, a 21st-century model. *Community Ment Health J, 39 (5)*, 441–58.

p. 289, **Over time, these spontaneous, pragmatic acts evolved.** Roosens, E. (1979). *Mental Patients in Town Life: Geel—Europe's First Therapeutic Community.* London: Sage.

p. 289, **In 1991, Openbaar Psychiatrisch Zorgcentrum.** Goldstein, J. L., and Godemont, M. M. (2003). The legend and lessons of Geel, Belgium: A 1500-year-old legend, a 21st-century model. *Community Ment Health J, 39 (5)*, 441–58.

p. 289, **In 2000, there were 550 boarders.** Roosen, E., and Van de Walle, L. (2007). *Geel Revisited: After Centuries of Mental Rehabilitation.* Antwerp: E. Roosens, L. Van de Walle & Garant.

p. 290, **To avoid stiff fines, some families.** Jay, M. (2016). *This Way Madness Lies: The Asylum and Beyond.* London: Thames & Hudson.

p. 290, **Some physicians have doubted Geel's practice.** Goldstein, J. L., and Godemont, M. M. (2003). The legend and lessons of Geel, Belgium: A 1500-year-old legend, a 21st-century model. *Community Ment Health J, 39 (5)*, 441–58.

p. 290, **Although community care for people with serious mental illness began.** Goldstein, J. L., and Godemont, M. M. (2003). The legend and lessons of Geel, Belgium: A 1500-year-old legend, a 21st-century model. *Community Ment Health J, 39 (5)*, 441–58.

p. 295, **The "Trieste model" of helping people with serious mental illness.** Portacolone, E., et al. (2015). A tale of two cities: The exploration of the Trieste Public Psychiatry Model in San Francisco. *Cult Med Psychiatry, 39 (4)*, 680–97.

p. 295, **Launched in the 1970s, the model was spearheaded.** Foot, J. (2014). Franco Basaglia and the radical psychiatry movement in Italy, 1961–78. *Critical and Radical Social Work, 2 (2)*, 235–49.

p. 296, **Essential to the success of life projects.** Portacolone, E., et al. (2015). A tale of two cities: The exploration of the Trieste Public Psychiatry Model in San Francisco. *Cult Med Psychiatry, 39 (4)*, 680–97.

p. 296, **Today in Trieste . . . the model Basaglia envisioned exists.** Mezzina, R. (2014). Community mental health care in Trieste and beyond: An "open door–no restraint" system of care for recovery and citizenship. *J Nerv Ment Dis, 202 (6)*, 440–45.

p. 297, **The interior of the building is well lit.** Portacolone, E., et al. (2015). A tale of two cities: The exploration of the Trieste Public Psychiatry Model in San Francisco. *Cult Med Psychiatry, 39 (4)*, 680–97.

p. 298, **In Trieste, the cafes at the opera house.** Portacolone, E., et al. (2015). A tale of two cities: The exploration of the Trieste Public Psychiatry Model in San Francisco. *Cult Med Psychiatry, 39 (4)*, 680–97.

p. 298, **The remaining funds finance.** Portacolone, E., et al. (2015). A tale of two cities: The exploration of the Trieste Public Psychiatry Model in San Francisco. *Cult Med Psychiatry, 39 (4)*, 680–97.

p. 298, **In 2012, Trieste had more than four thousand users.** Portacolone, E., et al. (2015). A tale of two cities: The exploration of the Trieste Public Psychiatry Model in San Francisco. *Cult Med Psychiatry, 39 (4)*, 680–97.

p. 301, **In 1948, 30 years before Law 180 was passed.** https://clubhouse-intl.org/.

p. 301, **A directory of Clubhouses.** https://clubhouse-intl.org/what-we-do /international-directory/.

p. 301, **The story of Soteria is entwined with that of its creator.** Mosher, L. R., and Hendrix, V. (2004). *Soteria: Through Madness to Deliverance.* Bloomington, IN: Xlibris.

p. 303, **Six-month and one-year outcome data revealed.** Mosher, L. R., et al. (1975). Soteria: Evaluation of a home-based treatment for schizophrenia. *American Journal of Orthopsychiatry, 45 (3)*, 455–67.

p. 303, **These studies found that two years after the experiment Soteria patients.** Bola, J. R., and Mosher, L. R. (2003). Treatment of acute psychosis without neuroleptics: Two-year outcomes from the Soteria project. *Journal of Nervous and Mental Disease, 191 (4)*, 219–29.

p. 304, **A systematic review of these studies and similar research in Switzerland.** Calton, T., et al. (2008). A systematic review of the Soteria paradigm for the treatment of people diagnosed with schizophrenia. *Schizophrenia Bulletin, 34 (1)*, 181–92.

p. 304, **Mosher says, "I neither prescribed nor avoided neuroleptics."** Mosher, L. R., and Hendrix, V. (2004). *Soteria: Through Madness to Deliverance.* Bloomington, IN: Xlibris (quote on 303).

p. 304, **Antipsychotic medications were ordinarily not used.** Bola, J. R., and Mosher, L. R. (2003). Treatment of acute psychosis without neuroleptics: Two-year outcomes from the Soteria project. *Journal of Nervous and Mental Disease, 191 (4)*, 219–29.

p. 305, **"Thus, for seriously disturbed people, I occasionally recommend."** Mosher, L. R., and Hendrix, V. (2004). *Soteria: Through Madness to Deliverance.* Bloomington, IN: Xlibris (quote on 303).

INDEX